Experimental Stroke

Edited by

Kunlin Jin, M.D., Ph.D.
Associate Research Professor
San Francisco, California, USA

&

Guo-Yuan Yang, M.D., Ph.D.
Professor
San Francisco, California, USA

DEDICATION

To our families

CONTENTS

FOREWORD

Stroke is a global health problem affecting approximately 15 million people annually throughout the world and about 700,000 people in the USA. It is the third leading cause of death and the most common cause of disability in most developed countries. Although extensive research in basic and preclinical studies has been done and significant progress is being made toward an understanding of the pathophysiology and injury mechanisms and treatment of stroke, there is no comprehensive reference or book that compiles the forefront issues in stroke research.

This is the first experimental reference book of its kind, in which a panel of leading experts specifically addresses current knowledge of both basic science and clinical perspectives in the field of ischemic stroke. Evidently, the book is timely. In the following fifteen chapters, various authors give a comprehensive review of experimental stroke, covering the latest advances such as programmed cell death pathways following cerebral ischemia, application of exogenous and endogenous neural stem cells in experimental stroke models, neurogenesis factors, Ca^{2+}-permeable cation channels in glutamate-dependent and independent Ca^{2+} toxicity after stroke, protective effect of postconditioning after global and focal ischemia, neovascularization after stroke, blood-brain barrier and matrix metalloproteinases after cerebral ischemia, and finally, the application of new MRI methodologies and useful global statistical test techniques for clinical trials.

This book is an excellent reference work for a wide range of neuroscientists, physicians and neurologists, as well as for research scientists investigating the underlying neuropathophy-siology after ischemic stroke.

Pak H. Chan
Stanford University

PREFACE

Stroke remains the third leading cause of death in the United States. Even among survivors, disability due to hemiparesis, gait disorders, aphasia and other deficits is common and about 20% of stroke survivors require institutional care at 6 months post-stroke. This long-term disability contributes to the average lifetime cost for stroke care of ~$140,000 and an annual national cost of ~$54 billion. The most recent major advance in clinical ischemic stroke treatment, the use of thrombolytic agents to dissolve clots in the acute aftermath of stroke, appears to be effective only within the first 3 hours after onset of symptoms; therefore, widely effective treatment for stroke remains elusive, and remains one of the biggest medical challenges in the 21st century.

This book compiles the efforts of 13 well-established experts in the stroke field in reviewing the latest advances in the field, with strong emphasis on neurogenesis, angiogenesis and neuroprotection after ischemic stroke. Vosler and Chen begin with a comprehensive review of common cell death pathways, emphasizing how calpain can modify both intrinsic and extrinsic cell death pathways as well as caspase-independent pathways after experimental stroke. Excessive Ca^{2+} accumulation in neurons is essential for neuronal injury after cerebral ischemia. However, the exact mechanisms underlying the toxic Ca^{2+} loading remain elusive. The chapter by Lusardi *et al.* describes the role of several major Ca^{2+}-permeable cation channels in glutamate-dependent and independent Ca^{2+} toxicity associated with cerebral ischemia. Familiarity with the mechanisms of programmed neuronal death pathways is critical for shaping our understanding of neuronal death caused by cerebral ischemia. Studies have demonstrated pre-conditioning's protection against brain ischemia. Zhao introduces the current findings on the protective effect of post-conditioning in global and focal ischemia in both *in vivo* and *in vitro* models. In addition, the potential protective mechanisms of post-conditioning are also reviewed. The chapter by Gabriel and Yang is an excellent summary of neovascularization, including factors involved, after stroke. Neurovascular matrix breakdown and blood-brain barrier (BBB) disruption play critical roles in the risk of hemorrhage and edema formation. Rosell *et al.* summarize the pathophysiologic actions of Matrix Metalloproteinases following cerebral ischemia, and Cramer and Sun examine the interplay between the BBB and the endothelin system in cerebral ischemia. Ding and Clark review recent research progress in hypothermia in the animal model. Neural stem cells may potentially help repair the damaged brain after cerebral ischemia. Keogh *et al.* cover recent advancements in neurogenesis and exogenous stem cell transplantation, and Yan *et al.* summarize the role of growth factors and cytokines in the regulation of neurogenesis following cerebral ischemia. Stroke is a major cause of death and disability in the elderly; therefore, a better understanding of how age affects the response to therapeutic interventions after stroke is crucial for the rational development of effective treatment. Jin integrates what is known about the responses of endogenous neural stem cells residing in the neurogenic regions of aged brain to experimental ischemic stroke. Zhang and Chopp provide the current data on the effect of erythropoietin (EPO) and carbamylated EPO on neurogenesis and angiogenesis in ischemic brain. Jiang introduces the application of new MRI methodologies to critical issues related to the treatment of stroke, including their potential in predicting and detecting hemorrhagic transformation as well as staging ischemic tissue. Huang *et al.* introduce a new useful global statistical test technique and the corresponding global treatment for assessing treatment's global preference when multiple outcomes are evaluated together.

This book may fall short of covering all major areas of the latest research in the experimental stroke field. However, we have endeavored to include examples of some of the most heavily studied areas, which are of interest to a broad range of investigators and researchers studying stroke.

We would like to thank Bentham Science Publishers, particularly Director Mahmood Alam and Manager Bushra Siddiqui for their support and efforts. We also greatly appreciate all authors and co-authors for their hard work and dedication that have made this volume possible. It is our hope that this book provides valuable information for all interested neuroscientists, pharmaceutical scientists, neuroradiologists, and clinicians as well as medical students.

Kunlin Jin, *M.D., Ph.D.*
Associate Research Professor
San Francisco, California, USA

Guo-Yuan Yang, *M.D., Ph.D.*
Professor
San Francisco, California, USA

CONTRIBUTORS

Jun Chen, M.D., Ph.D.
Professor, Department of Neurology, Department of Pharmacology, and Center for Neuroscience
University of Pittsburgh School of Medicine, Pittsburgh, Pennsylvania, USA
Professor, Geriatric Research, Educational and Clinical Center, Veterans Affairs Pittsburgh
Health Care System, Pittsburgh, Pennsylvania, USA

Michael Chopp, Ph.D.
Professor, Departments of Neurology, Henry Ford Health Sciences Center, Detroit, Michigan
48202, USA
Professor, Department of Physics, Oakland University, Rochester, Michigan 48309, USA

Xiangping Chu, M.D.,Ph.D.
Assistant Professor, Robert S. Dow Neurobiology Laboratories, Legacy Research, Portland, OR
97232, USA

Justin Charles Clark, M.D.
Neurosurgery resident, Department of Neurosurgery, the Barrow Neurological Institute, Phoenix,
AZ, USA

Samuel W. Cramer, M.D., Ph.D. candidate
Depts. of Neurosurgery, University of Wisconsin School of Medicine and Public Health,
Madison, WI 53792, USA

Robert J. Dempsey, M.D.
Professor and Chairman, Department of Neurological Surgery, and Cardiovascular Research
Center, University of Wisconsin-Madison, WI 53792, USA

Yuchuan Ding, M.D., Ph.D.
Associate Professor , Director of Research, Neurosurgical Sciences, Department of
Neurosurgery, Division of Plastic and Reconstructive Surgery, the University of Texas Health
Science Center at San Antonio, San Antonio, TX 78229-3900, USA

Rodney Allanigue Gabriel, M.D. candidate
Center for Cerebrovascular Research, Department of Anesthesia and Perioperative Care,
University of California, San Francisco, CA, USA

Ann-Charlotte Granholm, DDS, Ph.D.
Professor, Department of Neurosciences and the Center on Aging, Medical University of South
Carolina, Charleston, SC 29425, USA

Peng Huang, Ph.D.
Associate Professor
Department of Biostatistics, Bioinformatics and Epidemiology

Medical University of South Carolina, Charleston, SC 29425, USA

Quan Jiang, Ph.D.
Henry Ford Hospital, NMR Laboratory, Neurology Department, Detroit, MI 48202, USA

Kunlin Jin, M.D., Ph.D.
Associate Research Professor, Buck Institute for Age Research, California, CA 94945, USA

Christine L Keogh, Ph.D. candidate
Department of Pathology and Laboratory Medicine, Medical University of South Carolina, Charleston, SC 29464, USA

Eng H. Lo, Ph.D.
Professor, Neuroprotection Research Laboratory, Departments of Radiology and Neurology, Massachusetts General Hospital, and Program in Neuroscience, Harvard Medical School. Boston, MA 01810

Theresa A. Lusardi, Ph.D.
Research Associate, Robert S. Dow Neurobiology Laboratories, Legacy Research, Portland, OR 97232, USA

Anna Rosell, Ph.D.
Postdoctoral fellow, Neuroprotection Research Laboratory, Departments of Radiology and Neurology, Massachusetts General Hospital, and Program in Neuroscience, Harvard Medical School. Boston, MA 01810

Dandan Sun, M.D., Ph.D.
Professor, Department of Neurosurgery and Physiology, Neuroscience Training Program, University of Wisconsin School of Medicine and Public Health, Madison, WI 53792, USA

Raghu Vemuganti, Ph.D.
Assistant Professor, Department of Neurological Surgery, Neuroscience Training Program and Cardiovascular Research Center, University of Wisconsin-Madison, WI 53792, USA

P. S. Vosler, M.D., Ph.D. candidate
Department of Neurology, and Center for Neuroscience, University of Pittsburgh School of Medicine, Pittsburgh, Pennsylvania, USA

Xiaoying Wang, M.D., Ph.D.
Assistant Professor
Neuroprotection Research Laboratory, Departments of Radiology and Neurology, Massachusetts General Hospital, and Program in Neuroscience, Harvard Medical School. Boston, MA 01810

Ling Wei, M.D., Ph.D.
Professor, Department of Pathology and Laboratory Medicine, Medical University of South Carolina, Charleston, SC 29464, USA

Department of Anesthesiology, Emory University School of Medicine, Atlanta, GA 30322, USA

Robert F. Woolson, Ph.D.
Professor, Director of Collaborative Unit, Department of Biostatistics, Bioinformatics and Epidemiology, Medical University of South Carolina, Charleston, SC 29425, USA

Zhi-Gang Xiong, M.D., Ph.D.
Senior Scientist, Robert S. Dow Neurobiology Laboratories, Legacy Research, Portland, OR 97232, USA

Guo-Yuan Yang, M.D., Ph.D.
Professor, Center for Cerebrovascular Research, Department of Anesthesia and Perioperative Care, University of California, San Francisco, CA, USA

Yi-Ping Yan, Ph.D.
Assistant Professor, Department of Neurological Surgery, University of Wisconsin-Madison, WI 53792

Shan Ping Yu, M.D.,Ph.D.
Professor, Department of Pathology and Laboratory Medicine, Medical University of South Carolina, Charleston, SC 29464, USA;
Professor, Department of Anesthesiology, Emory University School of Medicine, Atlanta, GA 30322, USA

Zheng Gang Zhang, Ph.D.
Senior Staff, Departments of Neurology, Henry Ford Health Sciences Center, Detroit, Michigan 48202, USA

Heng Zhao, M.D., Ph.D.
Assistant Professor, Department of Neurosurgery, Stanford University School of Medicine, Stanford, CA 94305-5327, USA

Experimental Stroke, 2008, 1, 1-8

Calpain Modulation of Programmed Cell Death Pathways Following Cerebral Ischemia

P.S. Vosler[1] and J. Chen[1,2,*]

[1]*Department of Neurology, University of Pittsburgh School of Medicine, Pittsburgh, Pennsylvania, USA*

[2]*Geriatric Research, Educational and Clinical Center, Veterans Affairs Pittsburgh Health Care System, Pittsburgh, Pennsylvania, USA*

Correspondence: Dr. Jun Chen, Department of Neurology, S-507, Biomedical Science Tower, University of Pittsburgh School of Medicine, Pittsburgh, PA 15213, USA; E-mail:chenj2@upmc.edu

Abstract: Cerebral ischemia causes a massive insult resulting in the eventual death of ischemia-affected neurons. Historically, research efforts have focused on the canonical cell death signaling pathways examining the activation of both caspase-dependent and –independent mechanisms to execute neuronal death due to ischemia. Recently, however, there is evidence that the calcium-activated protease calpain is able to mediate both neuronal death pathways. This chapter briefly outlines the intrinsic and extrinsic caspase-dependent pathways and the caspase-independent pathways. This is followed by a discussion of the role of calpain in abrogating the caspase-dependent pathway and instigating the caspase-independent pathway. Greater understanding of how neurons actuate delayed neuronal death will potentially lead to the development of viable therapeutics to diminish the negative neurological sequelae caused by cerebral ischemia.

INTRODUCTION

The ability of cells to undergo controlled death is essential for normal growth, development and homeostatic maintenance of all multicellular organisms. This highly evolutionarily conserved mechanism allows for the removal of superfluous or malignant cells during development and during maintenance of the organism [1, 2]. Aberrances in this process are implicated in developmental abnormalities, cancer and neurodegenerative diseases. Impaired programmed cell death occurs in developmental abnormalities and cancer; in contrast, excessive neuronal death occurs in neurodegenerative diseases. Excessive death in these diseases is particularly problematic because neurons are terminally differentiated and have very limited regenerative capacity. Even if neurons are regenerated, it is unlikely that new neurons could recoup the myriad alterations in utility gained by older neurons over decades of life. Familiarity with the activation and mechanism of programmed neuronal death pathways is therefore vital for shaping our understanding of the pathology underlying neurodegenerative diseases and specifically for understanding neuronal death caused by ischemia.

Cerebral ischemia and Excitotoxicity

One of the most studied neurodegenerative processes is the acute insult of ischemic stroke. Ischemia in neurons results when blood flow, and thus energy-producing oxygen and glucose, is obstructed by plaques, thrombi or hemorrhage in cerebral blood vessels. The ensuing lack of energy leads to an uncontrolled and massive depolarization of neurons, resulting in widespread release of neurotoxic levels of glutamate [3]. Excessive release of glutamate, or excitotoxicity, activates glutamate receptors such as *N*-methyl-D-aspartate (NMDA), AMPA and kainate receptors, affecting an influx in calcium to the neurons [4].

Subsequent to this event, neurons that are directly supplied by the occluded vessel immediately die via necrosis. This area is termed the core of the infarct. Necrotic cell death results in permeation of the neuronal membrane, which in turn releases cellular contents into the extracellular milieu, and invokes an immune response and further neuronal damage due to release of proinflammatory cytokines [1, 5].

Neurons surrounding the core, called the penumbra, undergo cell death by a different process. These neurons progressively die from hours to days following the insult via programmed cell death. This is actuated by tightly regulated and intricate protein cascades induced by intracellular and extracellular stimuli, appropriately termed the intrinsic and extrinsic pathways, respectively. Due to the delayed manner of death of neurons in the penumbra, it is thought that abrogating delayed neuronal death will provide therapeutic benefit [6].

Calpain

The roles of the canonical intrinsic and extrinsic cell death pathways in cerebral ischemia have been studied extensively. Recent evidence demonstrates, however, that these pathways are both paralleled and complemented by alternative mechanisms to induce cell death. One of the molecules shown to influence both the intrinsic and extrinsic cell death cascades is the protease calpain [7, 8].

Calpains are highly conserved cytoplasmic cysteine proteases with 15 either tissue-specific or ubiquitous isoforms that are activated by calcium. The two prototypical calpains, μ- and m-calpain (or calpain I and II, respectively), require micromolar and millimolar concentrations of calcium for activation, respectively [9]. They possess a common regulatory subunit of 30kDa and a catalytic subunit of 89kDa. Upon activation by calcium, calpain autocatalytically cleaves the regulatory and catalytic subunits to form 18-kDa and 76-kDa fragments, respectively. Calpain then cleaves a number of cellular proteins, possibly by recognizing secondary and tertiary structures of the substrate; as yet, no consensus amino acid sequence has been defined [8]. The hallmark of calpain activation in cells is the cleavage of the cytoskeletal protein α-spectrin into size-specific cleavage products. Cleavage of α-spectrin is often used as a gauge for calpain activation, and it has even been used as a biomarker determining disease severity [10].

Like the programmed death cascades, calpain is required for normal physiologic function during development and in the maintenance of cells [8]. This is has been shown in studies where genetic deletion of m-calpain or the calpain regulatory subunit resulted in embryonic lethality [11, 12]. While calpain is important for normal growth and development, persistent activation could be seen as a pathologic phenomenon detrimental to neurons.

As will be discussed further in this chapter, calpain cleaves a multitude of proteins regulating the intrinsic and extrinsic neuronal death pathways following an ischemic or excitotoxic injury. A brief overview of both pathways, along with a review of alternative neuronal death pathways, is provided. This is followed by a discussion of the consequences of calpain proteolysis of specific neuronal death effectors.

INTRINSIC PATHWAY

In response to a stress stimulus such as ischemia, neurons initiate the intrinsic or mitochondrial death pathway. This pathway consists of pro- and anti-apoptotic Bcl-2 (B-cell lymphoma-2) family proteins, release of cytochrome *c* and other proteins from the mitochondria, apoptosome formation, caspase activation, cleavage of specific proteins leading to DNA damage and, ultimately, neuronal death (Fig. **1**). Each component of the pathway is briefly discussed below.

Bcl-2 Family

The Bcl-2 (B-cell lymphoma gene 2) family proteins are critical contributors to mitochondria-induced cell death by means of their role in release of cytochrome *c*. The Bcl-2 family consists of three subfamilies of proteins, all of which contain at least one Bcl-2 homology (BH) domain. The anti-apoptotic proteins Bcl-2 and Bcl-X$_L$ have BH domains 1-4 and a hydrophobic C-terminus allowing the proteins to interact with the mitochondrial membrane. In fact, Bcl-2 is located exclusively in intracellular membranes, including the outer mitochondrial membrane. Bcl-X$_L$, in contrast, is found in both the mitochondrial membrane and the cytosol. These proteins are thought to bind and inactivate the multi-domain pro-apoptotic proteins [13, 14].

The pro-apoptotic proteins are comprised of two subfamilies—the multi-domain proteins Bax (Bcl-2 associated protein X) and Bak, and the BH3 domain-only proteins Bid, Bad and Bim. The multi-domain Bax is located in the cytosol, whereas Bak is exclusively located in the outer mitochondrial membrane. Subsequent to an apoptotic stimulus, Bax undergoes changes to its tertiary and quaternary structure, translocates to the mitochondria, and inserts into the outer mitochondrial membrane as large oligomers. Bak also undergoes conformational change in its tertiary and quaternary structure and oligomerizes within the outer mitochondrial membrane. The oligomer inserts of Bax and Bak are thought to create a pore in the outer mitochondrial membrane allowing for the release of cytochrome *c* and the initiation of the apoptotic caspase cascade. Interestingly, the mitochondria remain functional despite the presence of the pore, maintaining their electrochemical gradient and ATP functioning. This is particularly important as apoptosis is an energy-dependent process; cells deficient in energy are thought to switch to necrotic cell death [14, 15].

The BH3 domain-only proteins also contribute to the release of cytochrome *c* via indirect means. Bid, following truncation (discussed further in the extrinsic pathway section), binds to Bax and Bak, facilitating their activation. Bad, in its unphosphorylated state, binds both Bcl-2 and Bcl-X$_L$ and deactivates their anti-apoptotic activity. Bim releases into the cytosol and also binds the anti-apoptotic proteins, precluding their binding to Bax and Bak [14, 15].

Apoptosome Formation

Cytochrome *c* released from the mitochondria into the cytosol then combines with Apaf-1 (apoptotic protease-activating factor-1). Apaf-1 resides in the cytoplasm existing as an inactive monomer and possesses an N-terminal caspase recruitment domain (CARD), a nucleotide-binding and oligomerization region and a series of WD-40 repeats necessary for

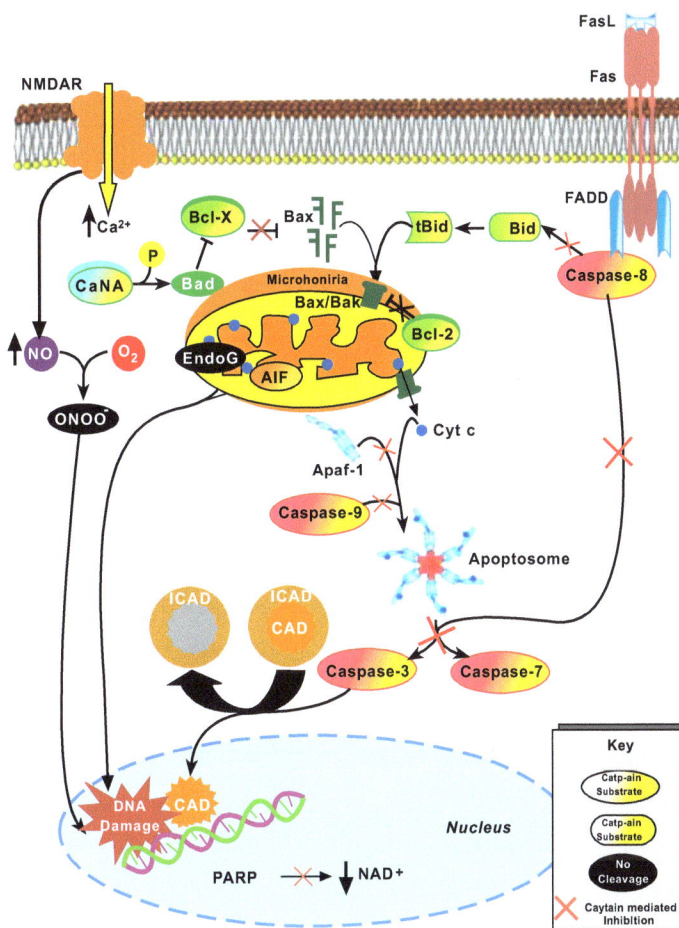

Fig. (1). Ischemia-induced calpain modification of intrinsic and extrinsic pathways. Traditionally, ischemia was thought to activate both the intrinsic and extrinsic pathways. Activation of the pro-apoptotic Bcl-2 family proteins Bax and Bak lead to mitochondrial membrane depolarization and release of cytochrome *c*. Cytochrome *c* release into the cytosol combines with Apaf-1 and dATP, forming the apoptosome. This complex recruits and activates caspase-9, which results in cleavage and activation of effector caspases-3 and -7. Active effector caspases cleave ICAD, releasing CAD to cleave DNA. Inflammation caused by ischemia results in release of pro-inflammatory cytokines such as FasL into the extracellular milieu. The cytokines bind to their respective receptors, causing recruitment of FADD and dimerization of caspase-8. Active capsase-8 cleaves Bid causing further mitochondrial membrane disruption. Additionally, caspase-8 directly cleaves effector caspases. Excitotoxicity due to ischemia, however, causes overactivation of NMDA receptors, leading to increased intracellular calcium and NO activation. Increased intracellular calcium directly activates cytosolic calpain, hijacking both the intrinsic and extrinsic pathways to enact its own neuronal death cascade. Calpain directly cleaves the anti-apoptotic Bcl-2 proteins Bcl-X_L and Bcl-2, and the pro-apoptotic Bcl-2 proteins Bax and Bid. Indirectly, calpain cleaves CaN A, causing dephosphorylation of Bad and sequestration of Bcl-X_L. Combined, these events result in calpain-mediated mitochondrial membrane permeabilization, mitochondrial Ca^{2+} dysregulation, and activation of mitochondrial calpain with cleavage of AIF. Once cleaved, AIF translocates to the nucleus along with EndoG and results in DNA damage. Calpain also cleaves Apaf-1 and apical caspases-8 and -9 to inhibit activation of effector caspases. Finally, rapid induction of NO to form peroxynitrite results in PARP overactivation caused by DNA damage. Overactivated PARP is cleaved by calpain to abrogate detrimental decreases in NAD^+ levels to ensure that programmed neuronal death continues. Abbreviations: AIF, apoptosis-inducing factor; Apaf-1, apoptosis-activating factor 1; CAD, caspase-activated DNase; CaN A, calcineurin A; Cyt *c*, cytochrome *c*; EndoG, endonuclease G; FADD, Fas-associated death domain protein; FasL, Fas ligand; ICAD, inhibitor of caspase-activated DNase; NAD, nicotinamide adenine dinucleotide; NMDAR, *N*-methyl-D-aspartate receptor; NO, nitric oxide; $ONOO^-$, peroxynitrite; PARP, poly (ADP-ribose) polymerase.

cytochrome *c* binding. Upon cytochrome *c* binding, Apaf-1 increases its affinity for dATP. It then undergoes a conformational change resulting in the assembly of seven Apaf-1 molecules into a wheel-shaped configuration—the apoptosome. Apoptosome formation reveals the CARD domains on Apaf-1 and provides a scaffold for caspase-9 dimerization and activation [16].

Caspase Cascade

Caspases, or cysteine-dependent aspartic acid-specific proteases, are categorized as apical (or initiator) caspases, and executioner (or effector) caspases. As their name implies, they all contain a conserved cysteine in their catalytic site and have specificity for cleaving after aspartic acid residues on substrate proteins. They are constitutively expressed as zymogens in the cytosol. The apical caspases, caspases-9 and -8 (discussed in the extrinsic pathway section), exist as inactive monomers, and are activated by dimerization [17]. Following apoptosome formation, caspase-9 dimerizes, becomes activated, and cleaves the executioner caspases-3, -6 and -7. Executioner caspases are present in the cytosol as inactive dimers, and they are activated by cleavage of each monomer into a large and small subunit. This leads to irreversible activation of the executioner caspases known to cleave approximately 400 substrates [18].

Repercussion of Caspase Activation

Executioner caspases cleave a number of proteins that result in the phenotypic appearance of apoptotic cells. During apoptosis, neurons, like other cells of the body, undergo cell rounding, retraction of processes coinciding with detachment from other neurons, nuclear condensation, and nuclear and DNA fragmentation [19]. Cell rounding and retraction of processes are thought to be caused by caspase cleavage of cytoskeletal proteins such as actin, myosin, α-spectrin, tubulin and tau. Nuclear fragmentation can be explained, in part, by caspase cleavage of the nuclear lamins A, B and C. Cleavage of actin filaments also contributes to nuclear fragmentation due to the exten-sive interaction of actin and the nuclear envelope [5].

One of the features pathognomonic of programmed cell death is DNA degradation by endonucleases into a distinctive DNA ladder. Detection of DNA fragmentation by staining the nucleus and examining for chromatin condensation and nuclear fragmentation is a common method to quantify apoptotic cell death. DNA fragmentation occurs due to cleavage of inhibitor of caspase-activated DNase (ICAD) by caspases. This releases caspase-activated DNase (CAD) and results in chromatin destruction. Poly (ADP-ribose) polymerase (PARP), a DNA repair enzyme, is also a substrate of caspases. Cerebral ischemia causes single- and double-strand DNA breaks [20, 21], activating PARP [22]. PARP activation requires considerable amounts of NAD and ATP, and it results in severe energy depletion, causing the damaged neuron to undergo necrosis [23, 24]. Cleavage of PARP inhibits its DNA repair activity, abrogating the PARP-mediated energy sink and conserving energy for programmed cell death [25].

Programmed cell death is not due to the cleavage of any single substrate—it is the orchestrated cleavage of a spectrum of substrates with subsequent alteration of function that directs neurons to ultimate death. As will be discussed further, factors other than caspases contribute to all of the aforementioned processes and can also influence cell death.

EXTRINSIC PATHWAY

As the name implies, the extrinsic pathway of programmed cell death is initiated by extracellular stimuli. Ligands, including Fas ligand (FasL), tumor necrosis factor α (TNFα) and tumor necrosis factor-related apoptosis inducing ligand (TRAIL), bind to transmembrane death receptors (of similar name; i.e. FasL binds Fas receptor). Binding of these ligands induces oligomerization of the receptors and recruitment of Fas-associated death domain protein (FADD), an adaptor protein that attracts and binds aggregates of caspase-8. As stated above, apical caspases are activated by dimerization. The aggregation of caspase-8 on death receptor adaptor proteins activates the caspase to cleave and activate procaspases-3 and -7 [5, 13]. Activation of executioner caspases by the extrinsic pathway generates the same effect as activation by the intrinsic pathway.

There is also cross-talk between the extrinsic and intrinsic pathways through caspase-8 mediated truncation of the Bcl-2 BH3-only protein Bid. Truncated Bid can bind to Bax and Bak causing mitochondrial membrane destabilization with subsequent cytochrome *c* release and further caspase activation [14]. Therefore, while the intrinsic and extrinsic cell death pathways are activated by dissimilar stimuli, they ultimately converge upon the same machinery to effect neuronal death.

CASPASE-INDEPENDENT CELL DEATH PATHWAYS

In addition to the canonical caspase-mediated death pathways discussed above, cells have evolved alternative mechanisms originating from the mitochondria that govern programmed cell death. Collectively dubbed "caspase-independent," these pathways provoke cell death via release of the proteins apoptosis-inducing factor (AIF) and endonuclease G from the mitochondria.

Apoptosis-Inducing Factor

AIF is a flavoprotein that functions as an oxidoreduc-tase within the mitochondrial intermembrane under physiologic conditions. Under periods of excitotoxic stress, however, there is an increase in nitric oxide (NO)-dependent oxygen free radicals, leading to DNA damage [3]. Increased DNA damage activates PARP, resulting in NAD depletion, PAR polymer formation, and release of AIF from the mitochondria [26]. The Bcl-2 proteins Bax and Bid are also necessary for AIF release [27, 28]. Liberated AIF translocates to the nucleus, a necessary event for AIF-induced cell death [29]. Despite the fact that AIF has no inherent endonuclease activity, it causes distinctly high molecular weight (~50kb) fragmentation of DNA [30]. This is in contrast to the finer oligonucleosomal DNA degradation seen following caspase activation. Mechanistically, it is known that AIF possesses DNA binding capability, which is necessary for AIF-induced cell death [31]. Binding of AIF to DNA causes chromatin condensation, a factor that possibly increases DNA susceptibility to endonucleases.

The importance of AIF in neuronal cell death is exemplified by examining the ischemia-resistant phenotype of Harlequin mice. These mice possess a proviral insert within the AIF gene rendering an 80% reduction in total AIF compared to wild-type controls [32]. Despite retinal and cerebellar degeneration likely due to reduced tolerance to oxidative stress, these mice have an approximate 40% reduction in infarct volume following a focal ischemic insult [28].

Endonuclease G

Perturbation of the mitochondrial membrane leads to the release of another factor involved with the apoptotic processing of DNA—endonuclease G. Like AIF, endonuclease G resides in the mitochondrial intermembrane space under physiologic conditions. Genetic deletion of the endonuclease G gene results in embryonic lethality within three days of conception, demonstrating its essential role in normal development [33]. Other than its role in apoptosis, a function of endonuclease G in healthy cells is not yet determined. Currently, it is thought that the mitochondrion houses endonuclease G until appropriate stimuli release it to effect cell death [34].

Similar to AIF, release of endonuclease G from the mitochondria is due to proapoptotic Bcl-2 protein activity and results in its translocation to the nucleus [35]. Again, the release of endonuclease G is caspase independent, as application of caspase inhibitors fails to block its release. However, unlike AIF, endonuclease G directly fragments DNA in concert with DNase I-like enzymes and exonucleases to actuate apoptotic DNA processing [34].

Thus, caspase-independent pathways have also been shown to be imperative for programmed neuronal death. It is suspected that, while these pathways are distinct, there are elements of cross-talk between pathways. For example, AIF in the cytosol can induce the release of cytochrome *c*, activating the intrinsic caspase cascade [30]. Therefore, there are positive feedback loops that activate multiple pathways to ensure neuronal death.

CALPAIN MODULATION OF APOP-TOTIC PATHWAYS

This section will discuss how calpain can modify both the canonical intrinsic and extrinsic pathways as well as the caspase-independent pathways. Further-more, it will be shown that calpain-mediated proteo-lysis of many of calpain's substrates results in a posi-tive feedback loop facilitating further calpain activation.

Calpain and the Bcl-2 Family

Commencing with the apex of the intrinsic apoptotic cascade, following an *in vitro* model of ischemia via oxygen-glucose deprivation (OGD), calpain activation results in cleavage of anti-apoptotic Bcl-X$_L$ within its loop domain into a 25kDa fragment [36]. The cleavage site of calpain is in close proximity to the caspase cleavage site that confers a pro- rather than an anti-apoptotic function to the protein [37, 38]. Thus, the calpain-mediated cleavage product of Bcl-X$_L$ is presumed to promote cell death rather than its normal function of inhibiting pro-apoptotic Bcl-2 family proteins. This may also be the case with Bcl-2, as this anti-apoptotic protein is also cleaved by calpain along with Bcl-X$_L$ following cardiac arrest [39].

Excitotoxic insult also induces calpain-mediated control over the extrinsic apoptotic pathway through cleavage of Bid. Truncation of Bid occurs following excitotoxicity more readily in calpastatin null knockout mice compared to wild-type controls, directly implicating calpain. Again, truncated Bid binds to Bax and Bak, facilitating mitochondrial membrane permeabilization and release of factors such as cytochrome *c*, AIF and endonuclease G. Indeed, truncation of Bid precedes AIF and endonuclease G release, suggesting a causal role in their release [40].

Synergistically, calpain also cleaves cytosolic Bax into a p18 fragment [41]. Overexpression of the p18 fragment of Bax robustly increases cytotoxicity [42], an effect that is blocked by overexpression of anti-apoptotic Bcl-2 [43]. As discussed above, activation of Bax results in mitochondrial membrane permeabili-zation. This diminishes mitochondrial calcium regulation, causing unmitigated rises in intracellular calcium that propagate further calpain activation.

Calpain can also affect the pro-apoptotic Bcl-2 family protein Bad via an indirect mechanism. Calpain cleavage of the protein phosphatase calcineurin (CaN) A removes subunit A, the autoinhibitory domain [44, 45]. The now constitutively active phosphatase dephosphorylates and activates Bad [46], resulting in the sequestration of Bcl-2 and Bcl-X$_L$. Furthermore, CaN A overactivation results in dephosphorylation and translocation of the transcription factors nuclear factor of activated T-cells (NFAT) and forkhead in rhabdomyosarcoma (FKHR) to the nucleus. This results in increased transcription of proapoptotic Bim and FasL [47, 48]. Thus, calpain can modulate neuronal death at multiple levels directly by manipulating Bcl-2 family proteins and indirectly via various signaling mechanisms.

Calpain, Apaf-1 and Caspases

Compromise of the mitochondrial membrane with subsequent cytochrome *c* release suggests activation of the intrinsic apoptotic pathway via activation of

Apaf-1. However, calpain is also known to cleave Apaf-1. Proteolytic cleavage of Apaf-1 by calpain prevents apoptosome formation and subsequent effector caspase activation [49]. Activated calpain has further jurisdiction over caspase activation via cleavage of caspase-9 [50]. Activation of NMDA receptors subsequent to NO administration results in calpain activation, cytochrome *c* and AIF release, and also caspase-9 cleavage. As stated above, activation of apical caspases requires dimerization rather than cleavage; accordingly, caspase-3 is not activated. Similarly, NMDA toxicity in rat hippocampal neurons results in caspase-9 proteolysis and a failure to activate caspase-3 [51]. Calpain also can cleave caspase-8, resulting in inactivation of the extrinsic apoptotic pathway inhibiting caspase-3 and -7 activation [52].

Calpain is also known to cleave effector caspases-3 and -7. The cleavage of these proteins, however, does not result in their activation [52-54]. Calpain proteolysis of caspase-3 and -7 occurs at sites distinct from those caused by apical caspase activation. Following caspase cascade activation, caspase-3 and -7 are cleaved into fragments of 20 and 17kDa, and 20 and 10kDa, respectively. Calpain-mediated cleavage resulted in inactive ~30kDa fragments for caspase-3 and -7 [52, 53]. While these fragments are inactive, there is evidence that they may retain the capacity for activation if later there is cleavage of the entire pro-domain [54]. Alternatively, calpain cleavage of the effector caspases could prevent activator recognition, further precluding their activity-dependent processing. In essence, calpain overrides effector caspase activation via inhibition of both the intrinsic and extrinsic apoptotic pathways at the level of the apical caspases. This allows for calpain-dependent signaling to occur without external interference.

Calpain and PARP

Inactivation of effector caspases is not without its consequences. As discussed above, effector caspases possess numerous substrates necessary not only to achieve neuronal death, but also to maintain energy levels required to complete the process. This is epitomized by caspase cleavage of PARP, which halts the energy-depleting action of the DNA repair enzyme. Excitotoxic insults increase Ca^{2+} influx through NMDA receptors and activate calpain. Activation of NMDA receptors also results in increased NO production, yielding DNA-damaging oxygen free radicals and subsequent PARP activation. In order to ensure that the neuron does not undergo uncontrolled necrosis, calpain also cleaves PARP [53, 55] into a configuration similar to cleavage by caspase-3 that is unlikely to retain DNA repair activity [56]. Moreover, DNA-damaging agents are known to activate PARP-1 upstream of calpain activation. Calpain, in turn, cleaves Bax and leads to AIF release [57]. Thus, calpain acts in a negative feedback manner

in this instance to protect from vast neuronal energy depletion.

Calpain and Caspase-Independent Cell Death

Calpain activation is directly linked to programmed neuronal death following excitotoxicity in a caspase-independent manner [27, 58]. Since calpain prevents caspase activation, calpain must induce an alternate pathway. Until recently, AIF release was linked to PARP activation [26, 57, 59] and to Bax and Bid translocation to the mitochondria [27, 28]; however, a direct mechanism tying these disparate mechanisms together was lacking. Calpain activation is a common phenomenon to these signaling mechanisms.

First tested in isolated mitochondria from brain and liver, calpain mediates truncation of AIF and release from mitochondria in response to truncated Bid [60]. In both *in vitro* and *in vivo* models of ischemia, it was determined that μ-calpain located in the intermitochondrial space is activated and mediates cleavage of AIF, which is responsible for its translocation to the nucleus [61]. While Bid and Bax are not required for AIF truncation, Bid enhances calpain-mediated AIF release.

The identification of a mitochondrial calpain, calpain 10, substantiates the above findings. Although it is an atypical calpain lacking domain IV (calcium binding domain), it is present in the mitochondrial outer membrane, intermembrane space, inner membrane and matrix [62]. Furthermore, mitochondrial calpain has similar calcium activating requirements, as μ-calpain and antibodies directed against μ-calpain recognize the mitochondrial form [63].

A direct link between calpain activation and endonuclease G release and activation has not been identified. Indirectly, calpain could release endonuclease G. Endonuclease G is located in the mitochondrial intermembrane space, and calpain-mediated activation of Bid and Bax with subsequent permeabilization of the outer mitochondrial membrane could permit exodus of the nuclease from the mitochondria. It is also likely that endonuclease G works parallel to AIF in causing DNA damage and facilitating neuronal death.

CONCLUSION

The previous discussion indicates that calpain plays an integral role in enacting programmed neuronal death due to ischemia. Not only does calpain directly mediate neuronal death via AIF truncation and release from the mitochondria, it manipulates the intrinsic and extrinsic programmed death signaling pathways to guarantee its unfettered utility. Calpain is not restricted solely to these pathways, however, as calpain possesses a number of substrates that are implicated in ischemia-induced neuronal death [7]. Further work is necessary to elucidate the entirety of calpain-induced neuronal death mechanisms, and to facilitate the creation of viable therapeutics for alleviating the negative sequelae of cerebral ischemia.

ACKNOWLEDGEMENTS

This work was supported by NIH/NINDS grants (NS43802, NS45048, NS44178, NS 56118 and NS36736) and VA Merit Review to J.C. Additional support was provided by the American Heart Association to P.V. (0715254U). We thank Carol Culver for editorial assistance and Pat Strickler for secretarial support.

REFERENCES

[1]   Kerr JF, Wyllie AH, Currie AR. Apoptosis: a basic biological phenomenon with wide-ranging implications in tissue kinetics. Br J Cancer 1972; 26(4): 239-57.

[2]   Wyllie AH, Kerr JF, Currie AR. Cell death: the significance of apoptosis. Int Rev Cytol 1980; 68: 251-306.

[3]   Hara MR, Snyder SH. Cell signaling and neuronal death. Annu Rev Pharmacol Toxicol 2007; 47: 117-41.

[4]   Olney JW. Brain lesions, obesity, and other disturbances in mice treated with monosodium glutamate. Science 1969; 164(880): 719-21.

[5]   Taylor RC, Cullen SP, Martin SJ. Apoptosis: controlled demolition at the cellular level. Nat Rev Mol Cell Biol 2008; 9(3): 231-41.

[6]   Lo EH. A new penumbra: transitioning from injury into repair after stroke. Nat Med 2008; 14(5): 497-500.

[7]   Bevers MB, Neumar RW. Mechanistic role of calpains in postischemic neurodegeneration. J Cereb Blood Flow Metab 2008; 28(4): 655-73.

[8]   Goll DE, Thompson VF, Li H, Wei W, Cong J. The calpain system. Physiol Rev 2003; 83(3): 731-801.

[9]   Chan SL, Mattson MP. Caspase and calpain substrates: roles in synaptic plasticity and cell death. J Neurosci Res 1999; 58(1): 167-90.

[10] Czogalla A, Sikorski AF. Spectrin and calpain: a 'target' and a 'sniper' in the pathology of neuronal cells. Cell Mol Life Sci 2005; 62(17): 1913-24.

[11] Arthur JS, Elce JS, Hegadorn C, Williams K, Greer PA. Disruption of the murine calpain small subunit gene, Capn4: calpain is essential for embryonic development but not for cell growth and division. Mol Cell Biol 2000; 20(12): 4474-81.

[12] Dutt P, Croall DE, Arthur JS, et al. m-Calpain is required for preimplantation embryonic development in mice. BMC Dev Biol 2006; 6: 3.

[13] Antonsson B. Mitochondria and the Bcl-2 family proteins in apoptosis signaling pathways. Mol Cell Biochem 2004; 256-257(1-2): 141-55.

[14] Youle RJ, Strasser A. The BCL-2 protein family: opposing activities that mediate cell death. Nat Rev Mol Cell Biol 2008; 9(1): 47-59.

[15] Antonsson B. Bax and other pro-apoptotic Bcl-2 family "killer-proteins" and their victim the mitochondrion. Cell Tissue Res 2001; 306(3): 347-61.

[16] Riedl SJ, Salvesen GS. The apoptosome: signalling platform of cell death. Nat Rev Mol Cell Biol 2007; 8(5): 405-13.

[17] Shi Y. Caspase activation: revisiting the induced proximity model. Cell 2004; 117(7): 855-8.

[18] Luthi AU, Martin SJ. The CASBAH: a searchable database of caspase substrates. Cell Death Differ 2007; 14(4): 641-50.

[19] Graham SH, Chen J. Programmed cell death in cerebral ischemia. J Cereb Blood Flow Metab 2001; 21(2): 99-109.

[20] Chen J, Jin K, Chen M, et al. Early detection of DNA strand breaks in the brain after transient focal ischemia: implications for the role of DNA damage in apoptosis and neuronal cell death. J Neurochem 1997; 69(1): 232-45.

[21] Liu PK, Hsu CY, Dizdaroglu M, et al. Damage, repair, and mutagenesis in nuclear genes after mouse forebrain ischemia-reperfusion. J Neurosci 1996; 16(21): 6795-806.

[22] de Murcia G, Menissier de Murcia J. Poly(ADP-ribose) polymerase: a molecular nick-sensor. Trends Biochem Sci 1994; 19(4): 172-6.

[23] Szabo C, Dawson VL. Role of poly(ADP-ribose) synthetase in inflammation and ischaemia-reperfusion. Trends Pharmacol Sci 1998; 19(7): 287-98.

[24] Yu SW, Wang H, Poitras MF, et al. Mediation of poly(ADP-ribose) polymerase-1-dependent cell death by apoptosis-inducing factor. Science 2002; 297(5579): 259-63.

[25] Ha HC, Snyder SH. Poly(ADP-ribose) polymerase-1 in the nervous system. Neurobiol Dis 2000; 7(4): 225-39.

[26] Yu SW, Andrabi SA, Wang H, et al. Apoptosis-inducing factor mediates poly(ADP-ribose) (PAR) polymer-induced cell death. Proc Natl Acad Sci USA 2006; 103(48): 18314-9.

[27] Cregan SP, Fortin A, MacLaurin JG, et al. Apoptosis-inducing factor is involved in the regulation of caspase-independent neuronal cell death. J Cell Biol 2002; 158(3): 507-17.

[28] Culmsee C, Zhu C, Landshamer S, et al. Apoptosis-inducing factor triggered by poly(ADP-ribose) polymerase and Bid mediates neuronal cell death after oxygen-glucose deprivation and focal cerebral ischemia. J Neurosci 2005; 25(44): 10262-72.

[29] Cheung EC, Joza N, Steenaart NA, et al. Dissociating the dual roles of apoptosis-inducing factor in maintaining mitochondrial structure and apoptosis. EMBO J 2006; 25(17): 4061-73.

[30] Susin SA, Lorenzo HK, Zamzami N et al. Molecular characterization of mitochondrial apoptosis-inducing factor. Nature 1999; 397(6718): 441-6.

[31] Ye H, Cande C, Stephanou NC, et al. DNA binding is required for the apoptogenic action of apoptosis inducing factor. Nat Struct Biol 2002; 9(9): 680-4.

[32] Klein JA, Longo-Guess CM, Rossmann MP, et al. The harlequin mouse mutation downregulates apoptosis-inducing factor. Nature 2002; 419(6905): 367-74.

[33] Zhang J, Dong M, Li L, et al. Endonuclease G is required for early embryogenesis and normal apoptosis in mice. Proc Natl Acad Sci U S A 2003; 100(26): 15782-7.

[34] Widlak P, Garrard WT. Discovery, regulation, and action of the major apoptotic nucleases DFF40/CAD and endonuclease G. J Cell Biochem 2005; 94(6): 1078-87.

[35] Li LY, Luo X, Wang X. Endonuclease G is an apoptotic DNase when released from mitochondria. Nature 2001; 412(6842): 95-9.

[36] Nakagawa T, Yuan J. Cross-talk between two cysteine protease families. Activation of caspase-12 by calpain in apoptosis. J Cell Biol 2000; 150(4): 887-94.

[37] Clem RJ, Cheng EH, Karp CL, et al. Modulation of cell death by Bcl-XL through caspase interaction. Proc Natl Acad Sci USA 1998; 95(2): 554-9.

[38] Fujita N, Nagahashi A, Nagashima K, Rokudai S, Tsuruo T. Acceleration of apoptotic cell death after the cleavage of Bcl-XL protein by caspase-3-like proteases. Oncogene 1998; 17(10): 1295-304.

[39] Krajewska M, Rosenthal RE, Mikolajczyk J, et al. Early processing of Bid and caspase-6, -8, -10, -14 in the canine brain during cardiac arrest and resuscitation. Exp Neurol 2004; 189(2): 261-79.

[40] Takano J, Tomioka M, Tsubuki S, et al. Calpain mediates excitotoxic DNA fragmentation via mitochondrial

pathways in adult brains: evidence from calpastatin mutant mice. J Biol Chem 2005; 280(16): 16175-84.

[41]   Wood DE, Thomas A, Devi LA, *et al.* Bax cleavage is mediated by calpain during drug-induced apoptosis. Oncogene 1998; 17(9): 1069-78.

[42]   Wood DE, Newcomb EW. Cleavage of Bax enhances its cell death function. Exp Cell Res 2000; 256(2): 375-82.

[43]   Choi WS, Lee EH, Chung CW, *et al.* Cleavage of Bax is mediated by caspase-dependent or -independent calpain activation in dopaminergic neuronal cells: protective role of Bcl-2. J Neurochem 2001; 77(6): 1531-41.

[44]   Lakshmikuttyamma A, Selvakumar P, Sharma AR, Anderson DH, Sharma RK. *In vitro* proteolytic degradation of bovine brain calcineurin by m-calpain. Neurochem Res 2004; 29(10): 1913-21.

[45]   Wang KK, Roufogalis BD, Villalobo A. Characterization of the fragmented forms of calcineurin produced by calpain I. Biochem Cell Biol 1989; 67(10): 703-11.

[46]   Uchino H, Minamikawa-Tachino R, *et al.* Differential neuroprotection by cyclosporin A and FK506 following ischemia corresponds with differing abilities to inhibit calcineurin and the mitochondrial permeability transition. Neurobiol Dis 2002; 10(3): 219-33.

[47]   Shioda N, Han F, Moriguchi S, Fukunaga K. Constitutively active calcineurin mediates delayed neuronal death through Fas-ligand expression via activation of NFAT and FKHR transcriptional activities in mouse brain ischemia. J Neurochem 2007; 102(5): 1506-17.

[48]   Shioda N, Moriguchi S, Shirasaki Y, Fukunaga K. Generation of constitutively active calcineurin by calpain contributes to delayed neuronal death following mouse brain ischemia. J Neurochem 2006; 98(1): 310-20.

[49]   Reimertz C, Kogel D, Lankiewicz S, Poppe M, Prehn JH. Ca(2+)-induced inhibition of apoptosis in human SH-SY5Y neuroblastoma cells: degradation of apoptotic protease activating factor-1 (APAF-1). J Neurochem 2001; 78(6): 1256-66.

[50]   Volbracht C, Chua BT, Ng CP, Bahr BA, Hong W, Li P. The critical role of calpain versus caspase activation in excitotoxic injury induced by nitric oxide. J Neurochem 2005; 93(5): 1280-92.

[51]   Lankiewicz S, Marc Luetjens C, *et al.* Activation of calpain I converts excitotoxic neuron death into a caspase-independent cell death. J Biol Chem 2000; 275(22): 17064-71.

[52]   Chua BT, Guo K, Li P. Direct cleavage by the calcium-activated protease calpain can lead to inactivation of caspases. J Biol Chem 2000; 275(7): 5131-5.

[53]   McGinnis KM, Gnegy ME, Park YH, Mukerjee N, Wang KK. Procaspase-3 and poly(ADP)ribose polymerase (PARP) are calpain substrates. Biochem Biophys Res Commun 1999; 263(1): 94-9.

[54]   Wolf BB, Goldstein JC, Stennicke HR, *et al.* Calpain functions in a caspase-independent manner to promote apoptosis-like events during platelet activation. Blood 1999; 94(5): 1683-92.

[55]   Boland B, Campbell V. beta-Amyloid (1-40)-induced apoptosis of cultured cortical neurones involves calpain-mediated cleavage of poly-ADP-ribose polymerase. Neurobiol Aging 2003; 24(1): 179-86.

[56]   Pieper AA, Verma A, Zhang J, Snyder SH. Poly (ADP-ribose) polymerase, nitric oxide and cell death. Trends Pharmacol Sci 1999; 20(4): 171-81.

[57]   Moubarak RS, Yuste VJ, Artus C, *et al.* Sequential activation of poly(ADP-ribose) polymerase 1, calpains, and Bax is essential in apoptosis-inducing factor-mediated programmed necrosis. Mol Cell Biol 2007; 27(13): 4844-62.

[58]   Ray SK. Currently evaluated calpain and caspase inhibitors for neuroprotection in experimental brain ischemia. Curr Med Chem 2006; 13(28): 3425-40.

[59]   Du L, Zhang X, Han YY, *et al.* Intra-mitochondrial poly(ADP-ribosylation) contributes to NAD+ depletion and cell death induced by oxidative stress. J Biol Chem 2003; 278(20): 18426-33.

[60]   Polster BM, Basanez G, Etxebarria A, Hardwick JM, Nicholls DG. Calpain I induces cleavage and release of apoptosis-inducing factor from isolated mitochondria. J Biol Chem 2005; 280(8): 6447-54.

[61]   Cao G, Xing J, Xiao X, *et al.* Critical role of calpain I in mitochondrial release of apoptosis-inducing factor in ischemic neuronal injury. J Neurosci 2007; 27(35): 9278-93.

[62]   Arrington DD, Van Vleet TR, Schnellmann RG. Calpain 10: a mitochondrial calpain and its role in calcium-induced mitochondrial dysfunction. Am J Physiol Cell Physiol 2006; 291(6): C1159-71.

[63]   Ozaki T, Tomita H, Tamai M, Ishiguro S. Characteristics of mitochondrial calpains. J Biochem 2007; 142(3): 365-76.

Calcium-permeable Ion Channels and Ischemic Brain Injury

Theresa A. Lusardi, Xiangping Chu and Zhi-Gang Xiong*

Robert S. Dow Neurobiology Laboratories, Legacy Research, Portland, OR 97232, USA;
E-mail: zxiong@Downeurobioogy.org

Abstract: Stroke, or brain ischemia, is a leading cause of morbidity and mortality worldwide. It is also a leading cause for long-term disabilities. Although enormous progresses have been made in recent years towards defining the responses of brain to ischemia, thrombolysis remains the only effective treatment for stroke patients. Unfortunately, thrombolitics have limited success and a serious side effect of intracerebral hemorrhage. It has been well recognized for many years that excessive Ca^{2+} accumulation in neurons is essential for neuronal injury associated with brain ischemia. However, the exact mechanism(s) and pathway(s) underlying the toxic Ca^{2+} loading remain elusive. The objective of this chapter is to discuss the role of several major Ca^{2+}-permeable cation channels, including NMDA-receptor-gated channels, TRPM7 channels, and acid sensing channels, in glutamate-dependent and independent Ca^{2+} toxicity associated with brain ischemia.

INTRODUCTION

Ischemic stroke, or cerebral ischemia, is the second most common cause of death and long-term disabilities worldwide. Because of the aging population, the burden will increase greatly during the next 20 years, especially in developing countries. Although major advances have occurred in the prevention of stroke during the past decades, no effective treatment is currently available other than the use of thrombolytics (e.g. tPA), which has limited success and a major side effect of intracranial hemorrhage [1,2]. Therefore, searching for new cell injury mechanisms and effective therapeutic strategies constitutes a major challenge for stroke research.

Although multiple factors may contribute to ischemic brain injury, it was recognized many years ago that excessive Ca^{2+} entry and resultant cytosolic Ca^{2+} overload plays an essential role in neuronal injury associated with brain ischemia [3]. In the resting condition, free intracellular Ca^{2+} concentration ($[Ca^{2+}]_i$) is maintained at nanomolar levels. Following ischemia, $[Ca^{2+}]_i$ can reach several micromoles or higher. Excessive $[Ca^{2+}]_i$ loading can activate enzyme systems such as proteases, phospholipases, and endonucleases. Over-activation of these enzymes in turn causes breakdown of proteins, lipids and nucleic acids, which leads to final destruction of neurons [4-6]. In addition, overloading Ca^{2+} in mitochondria can cause opening of mitochondria permeability transition pore (PTP), a large conductance channel residing in both the inner and outer mitochondrial membrane [7,8]. Activation of PTP promotes apoptosis through release of cytochrome c and subsequent activation of caspases [9-11].

There are multiple pathways through which $[Ca^{2+}]_i$ may be increased in neurons. For example, Ca^{2+} can enter neurons through various Ca^{2+}-permeable ion channels including voltage-gated (e.g. L-type, N-type, and P/Q type Ca^{2+} channels), ligand-gated (e.g. glutamate-gated channels, ATP gated channels, and acid-sensing ion channels), or through some ion exchange system (e.g. reverse Na^+/Ca^{2+} exchanger). $[Ca^{2+}]_i$ can also be increased through release from the intracellular stores (e.g. endoplasmic reticulum, ER). The exact source (or sources) of Ca^{2+} loading responsible for ischemic neuronal injury, however, remains unclear.

GLUTAMATE RECEPTOR MEDIATED Ca^{2+}-DEPENDENT NEURONAL INJURY - EXCITOTOXICITY

Over the past two decades, the N-methyl-D-aspartate (NMDA) subtype of glutamate receptors was considered as the main entry pathway responsible for toxic Ca^{2+} loading in ischemia [4,12-15]. This was supported by a large number of studies demonstrating neuroprotection by NMDA receptor antagonists [12,15-18].

Glutamate is the major excitatory neurotransmitter in the central nervous system (CNS) [19-21]. Glutamate receptors are widely expressed at the soma, postsynaptic density, and dendrites of CNS neurons. In the normal conditions, activation of glutamate receptors is involved in a variety of physiological functions of neurons including synaptic transmission/plasticity, learning/memory, neuronal development and differentiation, movement and sensation, etc [19,22]. Glutamate receptors can be classified into two major categories: ionotropic receptors, which are ligand-gated cation channels; and metabotropic receptors, which are coupled through G proteins to second messenger systems [23]. One subtype of ionotropic glutamate receptor, the N-methyl-D-aspartate (or NMDA) receptor, is highly permeable to Ca^{2+} ions. The increase in intracellular Ca^{2+} through NMDA receptor-gated channels is critical both for physiological function and for "excitotoxicity" [3,15,24-26].

The term "excitotoxicity" was originally described by Olney and his colleagues as a concept whereby neurons are over-stimulated, or excited, to the point of death through an overabundance of excitatory neurotransmission [27,28]. During ischemia, neurons and glial cells are depolarized due to deprivation of oxygen/glucose and loss of ATP. Membrane depolarization leads to synaptic release of glutamate from neurons and electrogenic transport of glutamate from astrocytes [14,29,30]. Accumulation of glutamate in the extracellular space causes uncontrolled activation of post-synaptic glutamate receptors, particularly the NMDA receptor-gated channels, leading to overload of intracellular Ca^{2+} beyond what neurons can handle. Studies in neuronal cultures have shown two distinct phases involved in excitotoxicity [31,32]. The first phase of glutamate toxicity, which develops within minutes after exposure to glutamate, is neuronal swelling, likely caused by excessive entry of Na^+ ions and water into the neurons. The 2nd phase of toxicity develops slowly and depends on the presence of extracellular Ca^{2+} [33-35]. It is known that the 2nd phase is triggered by excessive Ca^{2+} influx directly through the glutamate receptor channels or, to some extent, indirectly through voltage-dependent Ca^{2+} channels following the depolarization of neurons [36,37]. A recent study indicated that cleavage of Na^+/Ca^{2+} exchanger by Ca^{2+}-dependent protease plays an important role in delayed calcium deregulation and injury caused by glutamate receptor activation [38].

In contrast to overwhelming success in cell culture and animal studies which demonstrated clear neuroprotection by glutamate antagonists, none of the human trials using the glutamate antagonists showed a satisfactory protection. The reasons for the failure of multiple clinical trials have been extensively discussed [4,39-42]. It is believed that multiple factors, including difficulty in early initiation of treatment and intolerance of severe side effects, may have contributed to the failures. It is worth mentioning that, even with well-controlled animal studies, NMDA antagonists only have a short effective time-window of less than 1 hour post-ischemia [39,43-45]. This factor may have already predicted the failure of human trials but was somehow overlooked.

Despite intensive research on glutamate-induced Ca^{2+} toxicity, the precise link between NMDA receptor-mediated Ca^{2+} loading and the subsequent neurotoxicity was unclear. Particularly interesting is the factor that an equal amount of Ca^{2+} loading from voltage-gated Ca^{2+} channels is not as toxic as the Ca^{2+} entry through glutamate receptor-gated channels, suggesting that Ca^{2+} influx through NMDA channels is functionally coupled to neurotoxic signaling pathways [15]. Based on the finding that NMDA receptors closely interact with postsynaptic density proteins [46,47], Sattler and colleagues hypothesized that interaction of postsynaptic density protein 95

(PSD-95) with NMDA receptors and nitric oxide synthase (NOS) may play a role in glutamate toxicity. Using a combination of anti-sense approach, electrophysiology technique, fluorescent calcium imaging, and *in vitro* cell toxicity assays, they demonstrated that disruption of PSD-95 dramatically reduced NMDA receptor-mediated neurotoxicity [48]. Since targeting PSD-95 disrupts only the toxic event of the Ca^{2+} loading, but leaves normal physiological functions of NMDA receptors undisturbed, this approach may point to a new direction for neuroprotection. It is known that one of the factors contributing to the failure of human stroke trials using the glutamate antagonists is the presence of severe side effects such as psychosis, largely due to the blockade of physiological functions of this important receptor [4,41]. Further investigation demonstrated that disrupting the interaction between PSD-95 and NMDA receptors, by using a short peptide that competes for the binding site of PSD-95 to NMDA receptors, is also neuroprotective if delivered either before or 1h after an ischemic insult [49]. Thus, targeting PSD-95, which blocks the toxic effect of NMDA receptor activation but leaves the normal channel function un-touched, may therefore have significant implications in the search for precisely targeted therapeutic agents for a range of neurological disorders where activation of NMDA receptors plays an important role.

TRPM CHANNELS AND ISCHEMIC NEURONAL INJURY

Brain ischemia initiates a complex cascade of metabolic events, several of which involve the generation of nitrogen and oxygen free radicals. These free radicals and related reactive chemical species may mediate much of the damage that occurs after brain ischemia. Ischemia causes a surge in nitric oxide synthase (NOS) activity in neurons and possibly glia [50,51]. In the context of brain ischemia, the activity of NOS is broadly deleterious, and its inhibition or inactivation is neuroprotective [51,52]. Production of nitric oxide (NO), triggered by the action of NOS, for example, is highly enhanced during ischemia. In addition to causing the synthesis of NO, brain ischemia leads to the generation of superoxide, through the action of NOS, xanthine oxidase, leakage from the mitochondrial electron transport chain, and other mechanisms [51,53]. NO and superoxide are themselves highly reactive but can also combine to form a highly toxic anion, peroxynitrite [54]. The toxicity of the free radicals results largely from their direct modification of macromolecules, especially DNA. However, recent studies also demonstrated that oxidative stress may promote Ca^{2+} toxicity through the activation of several Ca^{2+}-permeable cation channels [55,56].

Transient receptor potential (TRP) channels are an exciting new family of cation channels that are highly expressed in various tissues including the brain

[57,58]. Several members can be activated by oxidative stress and oxygen free radicals, both of which play important roles in neurodegeneration. Recent work has indicated that members of the melastatin subfamily (TRPM) of TRP proteins, particularly TRPM7, may play a key role in neuronal death associated with brain ischemia [56,59-61].

The TRP superfamily is a diverse group of voltage-independent calcium-permeable cation channels expressed in mammalian cells [57,58]. These channels have been divided into six subfamilies, and two of them, TRPC and TRPM, have members that are widely expressed and activated by oxidative stress. TRPC3 and TRPC4 are activated by oxidants, which induce Na^+ and Ca^{2+} entry into cells through phospholipase C-dependent mechanisms. TRPM2 is activated by oxidative stress or TNFalpha, and the mechanism involves production of ADP-ribose, which binds to an ADP-ribose binding cleft in the TRPM2 C-terminus. Treatment of neurons or HEK 293T cells expressing TRPM2 with H_2O_2 resulted in Ca^{2+} influx and increased susceptibility to cell death [59]. Inhibition of endogenous TRPM2 function, in contrast, protected cell viability [55,59]. Nevertheless, the exact role of TRPM2 in Ca^{2+} toxicity associated with ischemic brain injury remains to be explored.

The potential role of TRPM7 channels in ischemic neuronal death has been described recently [56]. The failure of stroke trials using the glutamate receptor antagonists (anti-excitatory therapy) suggests the presence of glutamate-independent cell injury pathways. To explore these potential pathways, Aarts and colleagues re-examined the mechanism by which neurons die in ischemic conditions. Cultured mouse cortical neurons were exposed to oxygen-glucose deprivation (OGD), an insult reported to mediate neuronal death through NMDA receptor activation [62,63]. Blocking the glutamate excitotoxicity in these cultures unmasked a potent, previously unappreciated mechanism of non-excitotoxic death, which became increasingly responsible for neurodegeneration as the duration of OGD was prolonged [56]. Further studies demonstrated that the mechanism of cell death involves activation of a non-selective cation current with Ca^{2+} permeability. The current showed outward rectifying properties, was sensitive to reactive oxygen/nitrogen species (ROS) potentiation, and was blocked by Gd^{3+}. These electrophysiological characteristics and pharmacological properties suggest that the currents are likely carried by TRPM7, a widely expressed Ca^{2+}-permeable non-selective cation conductance [64] belonging to the TRP (transient receptor potential) cation channel super-family. Further molecular biological approaches (e.g. siRNA) confirmed the involvement of TRPM7 channels in anoxic neuronal injury [56]. These studies indicated that, in ischemic conditions, TRPM7 is activated by ROS produced by the nitric oxide signaling pathway. A lethal positive feedback loop is established when Ca^{2+} influx through TRPM7 stimulates further ROS production, causing further TRPM7 activation. Blocking TRPM7 channels or suppressing its expression by RNA interference is sufficient to prevent the death of neurons in OGD.

ACID-SENSING ION CHANNELS AND ISCHEMIC BRAIN INJURY

Various biochemical reactions and cellular metabolisms depend on a stable acid-base balance [65]. Therefore, maintaining a stable pH value is critical for normal brain functions. In physiological conditions, extracellular pH (pH_o) and intracellular pH (pH_i) in the brain are maintained at ~7.3 and ~7.0 through H^+ transporting mechanisms including Na^+/H^+ exchange, Na^+-driven $Cl^-/HCO3^-$ exchange, Na^+-HCO_3^- co-transport, and passive Cl^-/HCO_3^- exchange [66]. In acute neurological conditions such as brain ischemia, neurotrauma, and epileptic seizure, however, marked reductions of tissue pH, or acidosis takes place [67-72]. In brain ischemia, for example, the shortage of oxygen supply promotes anaerobic glycolysis, leading to lactic acid accumulation [73,74]. Lactic acid accumulation, along with H^+ released from ATP hydrolysis, results in decreased tissue pH. At the same time, cessation of local circulation results in carbon dioxide accumulation and carbonic acid build up, which also contributes to the decrease of tissue pH [70]. During ischemia, brain pH typically falls to ~6.5. It can also fall to 6.0 or below during severe ischemia or under hyperglycemic conditions [68,71,72,75,76].

Acidosis has long been known to play an important role in ischemic brain injury [70,73,74,77-79], and a direct correlation of brain acidosis with infarct size has been described [70,80]. However, the exact mechanism underlying acidosis-mediated neuronal injury remained vague and ill defined. Severe acidosis may cause non-selective denaturation of proteins and nucleic acids [81]; trigger cell swelling via stimulation of Na^+/H^+ and Cl^-/HCO_3^- exchangers, which leads to cellular edema and osmolysis [82]; hinder postischemic metabolic recovery by inhibiting mitochondrial energy metabolism and impairing postischemic blood flow via vascular edema [83]. The stimulation of pathologic free radical formation by acidosis has also been described [84]. At the neurotransmitter level, profound acidosis inhibits astrocytic glutamate uptake, which may contribute to excitatory neuronal injury [85]. Marked acidosis, with tissue pH <5.5, may influence neuronal vulnerability indirectly by damaging glial cells [74,79,86].

Interestingly, mild acidosis has actually been shown to be beneficial in protecting neurons from excitotoxic injury [87-89]. An explanation for this effect is that low pH_o inhibits NMDA channel activity [90,91]. This finding may suggest that, during brain ischemia where acidosis takes place, Ca^{2+} entry through NMDA channels does not play a major role in neuronal injury since the activity of NMDA channels is inhibited by the ischemic acidosis.

In contrast to its modulating effect on other ion channels, studies in recent years demonstrated that external protons can activate a distinct family of ligand-gated channels, the acid-sensing ion channels (ASICs), highly expressed in neurons of peripheral sensory and central nervous systems [92-103]. ASICs belong to the amiloride-sensitive epithelial Na^+-channel/degenerin (ENaC/Deg) superfamily [92,104], which contains two transmembrane spanning regions (TM1 and TM2) flanked by a large cysteine-rich extracellular loop and short intracellular N and C termini [92,93,105-110]. To date, four genes encoding six ASIC subunits have been cloned and their electrophysiological and pharmacological properties characterized. ASIC1a subunits (also named ASIC or BNaC2) are widely expressed in peripheral sensory neurons and in CNS neurons [93,97,111]. These channels can be activated by moderate decreases of pH_o to ~7.0, with a pH for half maximal activation ($pH_{0.5}$) at ~6.2 [93,112]. In addition to Na^+, homomeric ASIC1a channels are also permeable to Ca^{2+} ions [93,113,114]. ASIC1b (or ASIC1β) is a splice variant of ASIC1a, which is expressed only in sensory neurons [115,116]. Similar to ASIC1a, homomeric ASIC1b channels have high sensitivity to H^+ with a $pH_{0.5}$ at ~5.9 [116]. Unlike ASIC1a, however, ASIC1b has no detectable Ca^{2+} permeability [115,116]. ASIC2a subunits (also named MDEG, or BNaC1) have widespread distribution in both peripheral sensory and central neurons [95,111,117]. However, homomeric ASIC2a channels have very low sensitivity to H^+ with a $pH_{0.5}$ of 4.4 [95,117,118]. It is unlikely that homomeric ASIC2a channels can be activated in any physiological or pathological conditions in the brain. ASIC2b subunits (or MDEG2) are expressed in peripheral sensory and in central neurons [118]. They do not form functional homomeric channels, but may associate with other ASIC subunits (e.g. ASIC3) to form heteromultimeric channels with distinct properties [118]. ASIC3 subunits (also named DRASIC) are predominantly expressed in neurons of dorsal root ganglia [119,120]. Homomeric ASIC3 channels respond to pH drops biphasically, with a fast desensitizing current followed by a sustained component [119-121]. ASIC4 subunits are highly expressed in the pituitary gland [122,123]. Similar to ASIC2b, they do not seem to form functional homomeric channels [123]. ASICs were initially believed to assemble as a tetramer with either identical (homomeric) or different (heteromeric) ASIC subunits [93,109]. However, recent analysis of crystal structure suggested that ASICs exist only as trimers [124].

The main function of ASICs in peripheral sensory neurons include nociception, mechanosensation, and taste transduction [125-137]. The presence of ASICs in the brain, which lacks nociceptors, suggests that these channels have functions beyond nociception. Indeed, recent studies have indicated that ASIC1a is

involved in synaptic plasticity, learning and memory [96,138], while ASIC2a may be required for the maintenance of retinal integrity [139] and survival of neurons following global ischemia [140]. In pathological conditions, activation of Ca^{2+}-permeable ASIC1a is also responsible for glutamate-independent, acidosis mediated, ischemic brain injury [103,113,141] and axon degeneration [142].

The presence of ASIC1a in the brain, its activation by pH drop to a level commonly seen in ischemia, and its permeability to Ca^{2+} all make it likely that activation of ASIC1a is involved in acidosis-mediated ischemic brain injury. A series of recent studies, performed both in neuronal cell culture (cortical and hippocampal) and in whole animal models, have provided strong evidence supporting this hypothesis [103,113,141]. In cultured mouse cortical neurons, for example, brief acid incubation at pH 6.0 induced significant neuronal injury, as indicated by increased LDH release and fluorescent live/dead cell staining. This acid-induced neuronal injury was glutamate-independent, but was inhibited by amiloride, a non-specific ASIC blocker, or PcTX1, a specific ASIC1a inhibitor, indicating the involvement of ASIC1a activation. In contrast to the neurons from $ASIC1^{+/+}$ mice, neurons cultured from the $ASIC1^{-/-}$ mice did not show increased cell death following brief acid incubation. Reducing the concentration of extracellular Ca^{2+}, which lowers the driving force for Ca^{2+} entry, also decreased acid-induced injury of CNS neurons [103,113].

Further evidence supporting a role of ASIC1a activation in ischemic brain injury was provided by in vivo studies using both rat and mouse models of focal ischemia [103,141]. In rats, intracerebral ventricular injection of either amiloride or PcTX1 significantly reduced the infarct volume by up to 60%. Similarly, in a mouse model of ischemia, ASIC1a knockout provided a similar protection against the ischemic brain injury. Furthermore, ASIC1a blockade and ASIC1 gene knockout provided additional protection in the presence of the glutamate receptor antagonist memantine [103]. The protection by ASIC1a blockade has an time window of efficacy of up to 5 hours, and the protection persists for at least 7 days [143]. Attenuating brain acidosis by intracerebroventricular administration of $NaHCO_3$ is also protective, further suggesting that acidosis is the effector of injury.

Since activation of NMDA receptors and subsequent Ca^{2+} toxicity has been known to play an important role in ischemic brain injury, the outcome of co-application of both blockers has also been investigated. Compared to ASIC1a or NMDA blockade alone, co-application of NMDA and ASIC blockade produces additional neuroprotection, and the presence of ASIC1a blockade prolongs the time window of effectiveness of NMDA blockade [143]. Therefore, the Ca^{2+}-permeable ASIC1a channel represents a novel pharmacological target for ischemic brain injury.

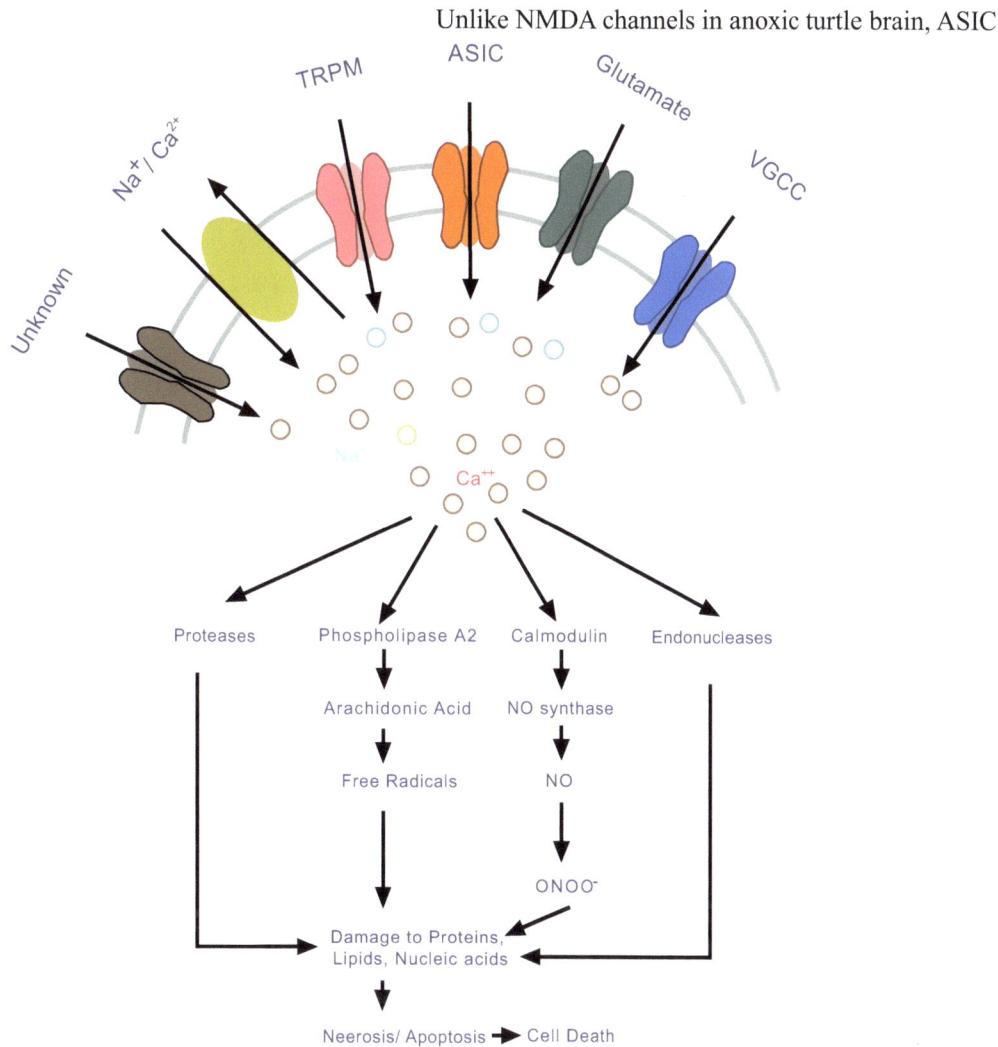

Fig. (1). Potential Ca^{2+} entry pathways in neurons and the mechanisms of Ca^{2+}-mediated cell toxicity. VGCC - voltage-gated calcium channel; Na^+/Ca^{2+} - sodium/calcium exchanger.

HYPOXIA/ISCHEMIA MODULATES THE PROPERTIES OF ION CHANNELS

Activation of various ion channels and/or membrane receptors (e.g. NMDA channels) is known to be involved in the pathology of brain ischemia. On the other hand, ischemia itself may induce dramatic changes to the properties of certain ion channels. For example, following anoxia, NMDA channel activity decreases dramatically (by ~80%) in turtle brain, a phenomena termed "channel arrest" [144,145]. Similarly, in rat brain and cultured neurons, K^+ channel gene expression and channel activity decrease substantially following a sub-lethal ischemia, a process partially responsible for ischemic tolerance [146]. These findings suggest that the properties of various ion channels may be subjected to modulation by ischemic signals. To better understand the role of ASICs in brain ischemia, ASIC currents were also recorded in neurons following oxygen-glucose deprivation (OGD), an *in vitro* model of ischemia.

activity in cultured mouse cortical neurons was enhanced by OGD treatment [103]. Brief OGD not only increased the peak amplitude of the ASIC currents but also reduced the current desensitization. These changes of ASICs are expected to dramatically increase the amount of Ca^{2+} entry through these channels. Accordingly, OGD treatment enhanced acidosis-mediated injury of cultured mouse cortical neurons [103]. The exact cellular and molecular mechanisms underlying ischemia-induced increase of ASIC activity remain unclear. One explanation is that OGD treatment induces increased affinity of ASICs for the proton. This is demonstrated by a shift in the H^+-dose response relationship towards less acidic pH following sublethal OGD treatement [147]. A recent study by Allen and Attwell demonstrated that arachidonic acid, a lipid metabolite released in ischemia, can increase the amplitude of the ASIC current in rat cerebellar Purkinje neurons [148]. Gao and colleagues demonstrated that an increased CaMKII phosphorylation of the ASIC1a subunits by NMDAR activation may be involved in ischemia-induced enhancement of the ASIC responses [141]. These findings, together with the reports that chelation of the extracellular Ca^{2+} by lactate enhances the activation of ASIC3 [149,150], further suggest that ASICs are actively involved in the pathology of brain ischemia.

PERSPECTIVES

Stroke/brain ischemia is a leading health problem worldwide. Although in recent years enormous progresses have been made in the prevention of stroke, unfortunately, there is still no effective treatment for stroke patients. Searching for new cell injury mechanisms and effective therapeutic strategies is therefore a major challenge in the field. Brain ishcmia initiates various biochemical changes such as glutamate release, production of oxygen free radicals, and acidosis. These changes may facilitate the opening of several Ca^{2+}-permeable ion channels such as glutamate-receptor-gated channels, TRPM7 channels, acid-sensing ion channels, etc. Activation of these channels induces entry of Ca^{2+} and accumulation of intracellular Ca^{2+}. Un-controlled accumulation or overload of neurons with Ca^{2+} activates a panel of enzymes including proteases, phospholipases and endonucleases, leading to destruction of neurons either through necrotic or apoptotic processes (Fig. **1**). Targeting these channels may lead to effective neuroprotective interventions for stroke patients. The recent failure of clinical trials using the antagonists of glutamate receptors indicated a need for new approaches, e.g. by targeting some of the harmful down-stream signaling pathways, instead of blocking the function of the entire receptor. It may also suggest that future effort should focus on glutamate-independent Ca^{2+} toxicity in ischemia, e.g. through activation of TRPM7 channels or ASICs.

REFERENCES

[1]   Weintraub MI. Thrombolysis (tissue plasminogen activator) in stroke: a medicolegal quagmire. Stroke 2006; 37(7): 1917-1922.

[2]   Wang X, Tsuji K, Lee SR, *et al*. Mechanisms of hemorrhagic transformation after tissue plasminogen activator reperfusion therapy for ischemic stroke. Stroke 2004; 35(11 Suppl 1): 2726-2730.

[3]   Choi DW. Calcium-mediated neurotoxicity: relationship to specific channel types and role in ischemic damage. Trends Neurosci 1988; 11(10): 465-469.

[4]   Lee JM, Zipfel GJ, Choi DW. The changing landscape of ischaemic brain injury mechanisms. Nature 1999; 399(6738 Suppl): A7-14.

[5]   Simonian NA, Coyle JT. Oxidative stress in neurodegenerative diseases. Annu Rev Pharmacol Toxicol 1996; 36: 83-106.

[6]   Coyle JT, Puttfarcken P. Oxidative stress, glutamate, and neurodegenerative disorders. Science 1993; 262(5134): 689-695.

[7]   Zoratti M, Szabo I. The mitochondrial permeability transition. Biochim Biophys Acta 1995; 1241(2): 139-176.

[8]   Bernardi P, Colonna R, Costantini P, *et al*. The mitochondrial permeability transition. Biofactors 1998; 8(3-4): 273-281.

[9]   Liu X, Kim CN, Yang J, Jemmerson R, Wang X. Induction of apoptotic program in cell-free extracts: requirement for dATP and cytochrome c. Cell 1996; 86(1): 147-157.

[10]   Hengartner MO. The biochemistry of apoptosis. Nature 2000; 407(6805): 770-776.

[11]   Polster BM, Fiskum G. Mitochondrial mechanisms of neural cell apoptosis. J Neurochem 2004; 90(6): 1281-1289.

[12]   Simon RP, Swan JH, Griffiths T, Meldrum BS. Blockade of N-methyl-D-aspartate receptors may protect against ischemic damage in the brain. Science 1984; 226(4676): 850-852.

[13]   Choi DW, Rothman SM. The role of glutamate neurotoxicity in hypoxic-ischemic neuronal death. Annu Rev Neurosci 1990; 13: 171-182.

[14]   Siesjo BK. Pathophysiology and treatment of focal cerebral ischemia. Part II: Mechanisms of damage and treatment. J Neurosurg 1992; 77(3): 337-354.

[15]   Tymianski M, Charlton MP, Carlen PL, Tator CH. Source specificity of early calcium neurotoxicity in cultured embryonic spinal neurons. J Neurosci 1993; 13(5): 2085-2104.

[16]   Choi DW, Koh JY, Peters S. Pharmacology of glutamate neurotoxicity in cortical cell culture: attenuation by NMDA antagonists. J Neurosci 1988; 8(1): 185-196.

[17]   Albers GW, Goldberg MP, Choi DW. N-methyl-D-aspartate antagonists: ready for clinical trial in brain ischemia? Ann Neurol 1989; 25(4): 398-403.

[18]   Wieloch T. Hypoglycemia-induced neuronal damage prevented by an N-methyl-D- aspartate antagonist. Science 1985; 230(4726): 681-683.

[19]   Nakanishi S. Molecular diversity of glutamate receptors and implications for brain function. Science 1992; 258: 597-603.

[20]   Curtis DR, Watkins JC. Acidic amino acids with strong excitatory actions on mammalian neurones. J Physiol 1960; 166: 1-14.

[21]   Krnjevic K. Glutamate and gamma-aminobutyric acid in brain. Nature 1970; 228(267): 119-124.

[22]   Gasic GP, Hollmann M. Molecular neurobiology of glutamate receptors. Annu Rev Physiol 1992; 54: 507-536.

[23]   Hollmann M, Heinemann S. Cloned glutamate receptors. Annu Rev Neurosci 1994; 17: 31-108.

[24]   Mori H, Mishina M. Structure and function of the NMDA receptor channel. Neuropharmacology 1995; 34(10): 1219-1237.

[25]   Sucher NJ, Awobuluyi M, Choi YB, Lipton SA. NMDA receptors: from genes to channels. Trends Pharmacol Sci 1996; 17(10): 348-355.

[26]   Rothman SM, Olney JW. Excitotoxicity and the NMDA receptor--Still lethal after eight years. Trends Neurosci 1995; 18: 57-58.

[27]   Olney JW, Ho OL, Rhee V. Cytotoxic effects of acidic and sulphur containing amino acids on the infant mouse central nervous system. Exp Brain Res 1971; 14(1): 61-76.

[28]   Olney J, Price M, Salles KS, Labruyere J, Frierdich G. MK-801 powerfully protects against N-methyl aspartate neurotoxicity. Eur J Pharmacol 1987; 141(3): 357-361.

[29]   Nicholls D, Attwell D. The release and uptake of excitatory amino acids. Trends Pharmacol Sci 1990; 11: 462-467.

[30]   Benveniste H, Drejer J, Schousboe A, Diemer NH. Elevation of the extracellular concentrations of glutamate and aspartate in rat hippocampus during transient cerebral ischemia monitored by intracerebral microdialysis. J Neurochem 1984; 43(5): 1369-1374.

[31]   Choi DW. Excitotoxic cell death. J Neurobiol 1992; 23(9): 1261-1276.

[32]   Shaw PJ, Ince PG. Glutamate, excitotoxicity and amyotrophic lateral sclerosis. J Neurol 1997; 244 (Suppl 2): S3-14.

[33]   Choi DW. Calcium: still center-stage in hypoxic-ischemic neuronal death. Trends Neurosci 1995; 18(2): 58-60.

[34]   Randall RD, Thayer SA. Glutamate-induced calcium transient triggers delayed calcium overload and

neurotoxicity in rat hippocampal neurons. J Neurosci 1992; 12(5): 1882-1895.

[35] Tymianski M, Charlton MP, Carlen PL, Tator CH. Secondary Ca2+ overload indicates early neuronal injury which precedes staining with viability indicators. Brain Res 1993; 607(1-2): 319-323.

[36] Sucher NJ, Lipton SA, Dreyer EB. Molecular basis of glutamate toxicity in retinal ganglion cells. Vis Res 1997; 37(24): 3483-3493.

[37] Murphy EJ, Horrocks LA. Mechanisms of hypoxic and ischemic injury. Use of cell culture models. Mol Chem Neuropathol 1993; 19(1-2): 95-106.

[38] Bano D, Young KW, Guerin CJ, Lefeuvre R, Rothwell NJ, Naldini L et al. Cleavage of the plasma membrane Na+/Ca2+ exchanger in excitotoxicity. Cell 2005; 120(2): 275-285.

[39] Gladstone DJ, Black SE, Hakim AM. Toward wisdom from failure: lessons from neuroprotective stroke trials and new therapeutic directions. Stroke 2002; 33(8): 2123-2136.

[40] Ikonomidou C, Turski L. Why did NMDA receptor antagonists fail clinical trials for stroke and traumatic brain injury? Lancet Neurol 2002; 1(6): 383-386.

[41] Hoyte L, Barber PA, Buchan AM, Hill MD. The rise and fall of NMDA antagonists for ischemic stroke. Curr Mol Med 2004; 4(2): 131-136.

[42] Wahlgren NG, Ahmed N. Neuroprotection in cerebral ischaemia: facts and fancies--the need for new approaches. Cerebrovasc Dis 2004; 17 Suppl 1: 153-166.

[43] Rod MR, Auer RN. Pre- and post-ischemic administration of dizocilpine (MK-801) reduces cerebral necrosis in the rat. Can J Neurol Sci 1989; 16(3): 340-344.

[44] Chen M, Bullock R, Graham DI, Frey P, Lowe D, McCulloch J. Evaluation of a competitive NMDA antagonist (D-CPPene) in feline focal cerebral ischemia. Ann Neurol 1991; 30: 62-70.

[45] Biegon A, Fry PA, Paden CM, Alexandrovich A, Tsenter J, Shohami E. Dynamic changes in N-methyl-D-aspartate receptors after closed head injury in mice: Implications for treatment of neurological and cognitive deficits. Proc Natl Acad Sci USA 2004; 101(14): 5117-5122.

[46] Kornau HC, Schenker LT, Kennedy MB, Seeburg PH. Domain interaction between NMDA receptor subunits and the postsynaptic density protein PSD-95. Science 1995; 269(5231): 1737-1740.

[47] Hunt CA, Schenker LJ, Kennedy MB. PSD-95 is associated with the postsynaptic density and not with the presynaptic membrane at forebrain synapses. J Neurosci 1996; 16(4): 1380-1388.

[48] Sattler R, Xiong Z, Lu WY, Hafner M, MacDonald JF, Tymianski M. Specific coupling of NMDA receptor activation to nitric oxide neurotoxicity by PSD-95 protein. Science 1999; 284(5421): 1845-1848.

[49] Aarts M, Liu Y, Liu L, et al. Treatment of ischemic brain damage by perturbing NMDA receptor- PSD-95 protein interactions. Science 2002; 298(5594): 846-850.

[50] Samdani AF, Dawson TM, Dawson VL. Nitric oxide synthase in models of focal ischemia. Stroke 1997; 28(6): 1283-1288.

[51] Love S. Oxidative stress in brain ischemia. Brain Pathol 1999; 9(1): 119-131.

[52] Wei G, Dawson VL, Zweier JL. Role of neuronal and endothelial nitric oxide synthase in nitric oxide generation in the brain following cerebral ischemia. Biochim Biophys Acta 1999; 1455(1): 23-34.

[53] Traystman RJ, Kirsch JR, Koehler RC. Oxygen radical mechanisms of brain injury following ischemia and reperfusion. J Appl Physiol 1991; 71(4): 1185-1195.

[54] Beckman JS, Beckman TW, Chen J, Marshall PA, Freeman BA. Apparent hydroxyl radical production by peroxynitrite: implications for endothelial injury from nitric oxide and superoxide. Proc Natl Acad Sci USA 1990; 87(4): 1620-1624.

[55] Miller BA. The role of TRP channels in oxidative stress-induced cell death. J Membr Biol 2006; 209(1): 31-41.

[56] Aarts M, Iihara K, Wei WL, et al. A key role for TRPM7 channels in anoxic neuronal death. Cell 2003; 115(7): 863-877.

[57] Nilius B, Voets T. TRP channels: a TR(I)P through a world of multifunctional cation channels. Pflugers Arch 2005; 451(1): 1-10.

[58] Venkatachalam K, Montell C. TRP channels. Annu Rev Biochem 2007; 76: 387-417.

[59] Kaneko S, Kawakami S, Hara Y, Wakamori M, Itoh E, Minami T et al. A critical role of TRPM2 in neuronal cell death by hydrogen peroxide. J Pharmacol Sci 2006; 101(1): 66-76.

[60] Aarts MM, Tymianski M. TRPM7 and ischemic CNS injury. Neuroscientist 2005; 11(2): 116-123.

[61] Nicotera P, Bano D. The enemy at the gates. Ca2+ entry through TRPM7 channels and anoxic neuronal death. Cell 2003; 115(7): 768-770.

[62] Kiedrowski L, Costa E, Wroblewski JT. Glutamate receptor agonists stimulate nitric oxide synthase in primary cultures of cerebellar granule cells. J Neurochem 1992; 58: 335-341.

[63] Grassi F, Giovannelli A, Fucile S, Eusebi F. Activation of the nicotinic acetylcholine receptor mobilizes calcium from caffeine-insensitive stores in C2C12 mouse myotubes. Pflugers Arch 1993; 422: 591-598.

[64] Nadler MJ, Hermosura MC, Inabe K, Perraud AL, Zhu Q, Stokes AJ et al. LTRPC7 is a Mg.ATP-regulated divalent cation channel required for cell viability. Nature 2001; 411(6837): 590-595.

[65] Chesler M. The regulation and modulation of pH in the nervous system. Prog Neurobiol 1990; 34(5): 401-427.

[66] Chesler M. Regulation and modulation of pH in the brain. Physiol Rev 2003; 83(4): 1183-1221.

[67] Crowell JW, Kaufmann BN. Changes in tissue pH after circulatory arrest. Am J Physiol 1961; 200: 743-745.

[68] Ljunggren B, Norberg K, Siesjo BK. Influence of tissue acidosis upon restitution of brain energy metabolism following total ischemia. Brain Res 1974; 77(2): 173-186.

[69] Thorn W, Heitmann R. Hydrogen ion concentration of cerebral cortex of rabbit in situ during peracute total ischemia, pure anoxia and during recuperation. Pflugers Arch 1954; 258(6): 501-510.

[70] Siesjo BK. Acidosis and ischemic brain damage. Neurochem Pathol 1988; 9: 31-88.

[71] Rehncrona S. Brain acidosis. Ann Emerg Med 1985; 14(8): 770-776.

[72] Nedergaard M, Kraig RP, Tanabe J, Pulsinelli WA. Dynamics of interstitial and intracellular pH in evolving brain infarct. Am J Physiol 1991; 260(3 Pt 2): R581-R588.

[73] Siesjo BK, Katsura K, Kristian T. Acidosis-related damage. Adv Neurol 1996; 71: 209-233.

[74] Tombaugh GC, Sapolsky RM. Evolving concepts about the role of acidosis in ischemic neuropathology. J Neurochem 1993; 61(3): 793-803.

[75] Kraig RP, Pulsinelli WA, Plum F. Hydrogen ion buffering during complete brain ischemia. Brain Res 1985; 342(2): 281-290.

[76] Siemkowicz E, Hansen AJ. Brain extracellular ion composition and EEG activity following 10 minutes ischemia in normo- and hyperglycemic rats. Stroke 1981; 12(2): 236-240.

[77] Kraig RP, Petito CK, Plum F, Pulsinelli WA. Hydrogen ions kill brain at concentrations reached in ischemia. J Cereb Blood Flow Metab 1987; 7(4): 379-386.

[78] Kristian T, Katsura K, Gido G, Siesjo BK. The influence of pH on cellular calcium influx during ischemia. Brain Res 1994; 641(2): 295-302.

[79] Goldman SA, Pulsinelli WA, Clarke WY, Kraig RP, Plum F. The effects of extracellular acidosis on neurons and glia in vitro. J Cereb Blood Flow Metab 1989; 9(4): 471-477.

[80] Back T, Hoehn M, Mies G, et al. Penumbral tissue alkalosis in focal cerebral ischemia: relationship to energy metabolism, blood flow, and steady potential. Ann Neurol 2000; 47(4): 485-492.

[81]   Kalimo H, Rehncrona S, Soderfeldt B, Olsson Y, Siesjo BK. Brain lactic acidosis and ischemic cell damage: 2. Histopathology. J Cereb Blood Flow Metab 1981; 1(3): 313-327.

[82]   Kimelberg HK, Barron KD, Bourke RS, Nelson LR, Cragoe EJ. Brain anti-cytoxic edema agents. Prog Clin Biol Res 1990; 361: 363-385.

[83]   Hillered L, Smith ML, Siesjo BK. Lactic acidosis and recovery of mitochondrial function following forebrain ischemia in the rat. J Cereb Blood Flow Metab 1985; 5(2): 259-266.

[84]   Rehncrona S, Hauge HN, Siesjo BK. Enhancement of iron-catalyzed free radical formation by acidosis in brain homogenates: differences in effect by lactic acid and CO2. J Cereb Blood Flow Metab 1989; 9(1): 65-70.

[85]   Swanson RA, Farrell K, Simon RP. Acidosis causes failure of astrocyte glutamate uptake during hypoxia. J Cereb Blood Flow Metab 1995; 15(3): 417-424.

[86]   Giffard RG, Monyer H, Choi DW. Selective vulnerability of cultured cortical glia to injury by extracellular acidosis. Brain Res 1990; 530(1): 138-141.

[87]   Giffard RG, Monyer H, Christine CW, Choi DW. Acidosis reduces NMDA receptor activation, glutamate neurotoxicity, and oxygen-glucose deprivation neuronal injury in cortical cultures. Brain Res 1990; 506(2): 339-342.

[88]   Kaku DA, Giffard RG, Choi DW. Neuroprotective effects of glutamate antagonists and extracellular acidity. Science 1993; 260: 1516-1518.

[89]   Sapolsky RM, Trafton J, Tombaugh GC. Excitotoxic neuron death, acidotic endangerment, and the paradox of acidotic protection. Adv Neurol 1996; 71: 237-244.

[90]   Tang CM, Dichter M, Morad M. Modulation of the N-methyl-D-aspartate channel by extracellular H+. Proc Natl Acad Sci USA 1990; 87(16): 6445-6449.

[91]   Traynelis SF, Cull-Candy SG. Proton inhibition of N-methyl-D-aspartate receptors in cerebellar neurons. Nature 1990; 345(6273): 347-350.

[92]   Waldmann R, Lazdunski M. H(+)-gated cation channels: neuronal acid sensors in the ENaC/DEG family of ion channels. Curr Opin Neurobiol 1998; 8(3): 418-424.

[93]   Waldmann R, Champigny G, Bassilana F, Heurteaux C, Lazdunski M. A proton-gated cation channel involved in acid-sensing. Nature 1997; 386(6621): 173-177.

[94]   Baron A, Waldmann R, Lazdunski M. ASIC-like, proton-activated currents in rat hippocampal neurons. J Physiol 2002; 539(Pt 2): 485-494.

[95]   Price MP, Snyder PM, Welsh MJ. Cloning and expression of a novel human brain Na+ channel. J Biol Chem 1996; 271(14): 7879-7882.

[96]   Wemmie JA, Chen J, Askwith CC, Hruska-Hageman AM, Price MP, Nolan BC et al. The acid-activated ion channel ASIC contributes to synaptic plasticity, learning, and memory. Neuron 2002; 34(3): 463-477.

[97]   De La Rosa DA, Krueger SR, Kolar A, Shao D, Fitzsimonds RM, Canessa CM. Distribution, subcellular localization and ontogeny of ASIC1 in the mammalian central nervous system. J Physiol 2003; 546(Pt 1): 77-87.

[98]   Krishtal OA, Pidoplichko VI. A receptor for protons in the nerve cell membrane. Neuroscience 1980; 5(12): 2325-2327.

[99]   Kovalchuk Y, Krishtal OA, Nowycky MC. The proton-activated inward current of rat sensory neurons includes a calcium component. Neurosci Lett 1990; 115(2-3): 237-242.

[100]   Grantyn R, Perouansky M, Rodriguez-Tebar A, Lux HD. Expression of depolarizing voltage- and transmitter-activated currents in neuronal precursor cells from the rat brain is preceded by a proton- activated sodium current. Brain Res Dev Brain Res 1989; 49(1): 150-155.

[101]   Ueno S, Nakaye T, Akaike N. Proton-induced sodium current in freshly dissociated hypothalamic neurones of the rat. J Physiol (Lond) 1992; 447: 309-327.

[102]   Varming T. Proton-gated ion channels in cultured mouse cortical neurons. Neuropharmacology 1999; 38(12): 1875-1881.

[103]   Xiong ZG, Zhu XM, Chu XP et al. Neuroprotection in ischemia: blocking calcium-permeable Acid-sensing ion channels. Cell 2004; 118(6): 687-698.

[104]   Kellenberger S, Schild L. Epithelial sodium channel/degenerin family of ion channels: a variety of functions for a shared structure. Physiol Rev 2002; 82(3): 735-767.

[105]   Benos DJ, Stanton BA. Functional domains within the degenerin/epithelial sodium channel (Deg/ENaC) superfamily of ion channels. J Physiol 1999; 520: 631-644.

[106]   Bianchi L, Driscoll M. Protons at the gate: DEG/ENaC ion channels help us feel and remember. Neuron 2002; 34(3): 337-340.

[107]   Corey DP, Garcia-Anoveros J. Mechanosensation and the DEG/ENaC ion channels. Science 1996; 273(5273): 323-324.

[108]   Alvarez dlR, Canessa CM, Fyfe GK, Zhang P. Structure and regulation of amiloride-sensitive sodium channels. Annu Rev Physiol 2000; 62: 573-594.

[109]   Krishtal O. The ASICs: signaling molecules? Modulators? Trends Neurosci 2003; 26(9): 477-483.

[110]   Saugstad JA, Roberts JA, Dong J, Zeitouni S, Evans RJ. Analysis of the membrane topology of the acid-sensing ion channel 2a. J Biol Chem 2004; 279(53): 55514-55519.

[111]   Garcia-Anoveros J, Derfler B, Neville-Golden J, Hyman BT, Corey DP. BNaC1 and BNaC2 constitute a new family of human neuronal sodium channels related to degenerins and epithelial sodium channels. Proc Natl Acad Sci USA 1997; 94(4): 1459-1464.

[112]   Chu XP, Wemmie JA, Wang WZ, et al. Subunit-dependent high-affinity zinc inhibition of acid-sensing ion channels. J Neurosci 2004; 24(40): 8678-8689.

[113]   Yermolaieva O, Leonard AS, Schnizler MK, Abboud FM, Welsh MJ. Extracellular acidosis increases neuronal cell calcium by activating acid-sensing ion channel 1a. Proc Natl Acad Sci USA 2004; 101(17): 6752-6757.

[114]   Chu XP, Miesch J, Johnson M, Root L, Zhu XM, Chen D et al. Proton-Gated Channels in PC12 Cells. J Neurophysiol 2002; 87(5): 2555-2561.

[115]   Bassler EL, Ngo-Anh TJ, Geisler HS, Ruppersberg JP, Grunder S. Molecular and functional characterization of acid-sensing ion channel (ASIC) 1b. J Biol Chem 2001; 276(36): 33782-33787.

[116]   Chen CC, England S, Akopian AN, Wood JN. A sensory neuron-specific, proton-gated ion channel. Proc Natl Acad Sci USA 1998; 95(17): 10240-10245.

[117]   Waldmann R, Champigny G, Voilley N, Lauritzen I, Lazdunski M. The mammalian degenerin MDEG, an amiloride-sensitive cation channel activated by mutations causing neurodegeneration in Caenorhabditis elegans. J Biol Chem 1996; 271(18): 10433-10436.

[118]   Lingueglia E, De Weille JR, Bassilana F, et al. A modulatory subunit of acid sensing ion channels in brain and dorsal root ganglion cells. J Biol Chem 1997; 272(47): 29778-29783.

[119]   Waldmann R, Bassilana F, de Weille J, Champigny G, Heurteaux C, Lazdunski M. Molecular cloning of a non-inactivating proton-gated Na+ channel specific for sensory neurons. J Biol Chem 1997; 272(34): 20975-20978.

[120]   Sutherland SP, Benson CJ, Adelman JP, McCleskey EW. Acid-sensing ion channel 3 matches the acid-gated current in cardiac ischemia-sensing neurons. Proc Natl Acad Sci USA 2001; 98(2): 711-716.

[121]   De Weille J, Bassilana F, Lazdunski M, Waldmann R. Identification, functional expression and chromosomal localisation of a sustained human proton-gated cation channel. FEBS Lett 1998; 433(3): 257-260.

[122]   Akopian AN, Chen CC, Ding Y, Cesare P, Wood JN. A new member of the acid-sensing ion channel family. Neuroreport 2000; 11(10): 2217-2222.

[123]   Grunder S, Geissler HS, Bassler EL, Ruppersberg JP. A new member of acid-sensing ion channels from pituitary gland. Neuroreport 2000; 11(8): 1607-1611.

[124]   Jasti J, Furukawa H, Gonzales EB, Gouaux E. Structure of acid-sensing ion channel 1 at 1.9 A resolution and low pH. Nature 2007; 449(7160): 316-323.

[125]   Benson CJ, Eckert SP, McCleskey EW. Acid-evoked currents in cardiac sensory neurons: A possible mediator of myocardial ischemic sensation. Circ Res 1999; 84(8): 921-928.

[126]   Bevan S, Yeats J. Protons activate a cation conductance in a sub-population of rat dorsal root ganglion neurones. J Physiol (Lond) 1991; 433: 145-161.

[127]   Krishtal OA, Pidoplichko VI. A receptor for protons in the membrane of sensory neurons may participate in nociception. Neuroscience 1981; 6(12): 2599-2601.

[128]   Ugawa S, Ueda T, Ishida Y, Nishigaki M, Shibata Y, Shimada S. Amiloride-blockable acid-sensing ion channels are leading acid sensors expressed in human nociceptors. J Clin Invest 2002; 110(8): 1185-1190.

[129]   Sluka KA, Price MP, Breese NM, Stucky CL, Wemmie JA, Welsh MJ. Chronic hyperalgesia induced by repeated acid injections in muscle is abolished by the loss of ASIC3, but not ASIC1. Pain 2003; 106(3): 229-239.

[130]   Chen CC, Zimmer A, Sun WH, Hall J, Brownstein MJ, Zimmer A. A role for ASIC3 in the modulation of high-intensity pain stimuli. Proc Natl Acad Sci USA 2002; 99(13): 8992-8997.

[131]   Wu LJ, Duan B, Mei YD, et al. Characterization of acid-sensing ion channels in dorsal horn neurons of rat spinal cord. J Biol Chem 2004; 279(42): 43716-43724.

[132]   Price MP, Lewin GR, McIlwrath SL, et al. The mammalian sodium channel BNC1 is required for normal touch sensation. Nature 2000; 407(6807): 1007-1011.

[133]   Price MP, McIlwrath SL, Xie J, et al. The DRASIC cation channel contributes to the detection of cutaneous touch and acid stimuli in mice. Neuron 2001; 32(6): 1071-1083.

[134]   Page AJ, Brierley SM, Martin CM, et al. Different contributions of ASIC channels 1a, 2, and 3 in gastrointestinal mechanosensory function. Gut 2005; 54(10): 1408-1415.

[135]   Ugawa S, Yamamoto T, Ueda T, et al. Amiloride-insensitive currents of the acid-sensing ion channel-2a (ASIC2a)/ASIC2b heteromeric sour-taste receptor channel. J Neurosci 2003; 23(9): 3616-3622.

[136]   Ugawa S. Identification of sour-taste receptor genes. Anat Sci Int 2003; 78(4): 205-210.

[137]   Lin W, Ogura T, Kinnamon SC. Acid-activated cation currents in rat vallate taste receptor cells. J Neurophysiol 2002; 88(1): 133-141.

[138]   Wemmie JA, Askwith CC, Lamani E, Cassell MD, Freeman JH, Jr., Welsh MJ. Acid-sensing ion channel 1 is localized in brain regions with high synaptic density and contributes to fear conditioning. J Neurosci 2003; 23(13): 5496-5502.

[139]   Ettaiche M, Guy N, Hofman P, Lazdunski M, Waldmann R. Acid-sensing ion channel 2 is important for retinal function and protects against light-induced retinal degeneration. J Neurosci 2004; 24(5): 1005-1012.

[140]   Johnson MB, Jin K, Minami M, Chen D, Simon RP. Global ischemia induces expression of acid-sensing ion channel 2a in rat brain. J Cereb Blood Flow Metab 2001; 21(6): 734-740.

[141]   Gao J, Duan B, Wang D, et al. Coupling between NMDA receptor and acid-sensing ion channel contributes to ischemic neuronal death. Neuron 2005; 48(4): 635-646.

[142]   Friese MA, Craner MJ, Etzensperger R, et al. Acid-sensing ion channel-1 contributes to axonal degeneration in autoimmune inflammation of the central nervous system. Nat Med 2007; 13(12): 1483-1489.

[143]   Pignataro G, Simon RP, Xiong ZG. Prolonged activation of ASIC1a and the time window for neuroprotection in cerebral ischaemia. Brain 2007; 130(Pt 1): 151-158.

[144]   Lutz PL. Mechanisms for anoxic survival in the vertebrate brain. Annu Rev Physiol 1992; 54: 601-618.

[145]   Buck LT, Bickler PE. Adenosine and anoxia reduce N-methyl-D-aspartate receptor open probability in turtle cerebrocortex. J Exp Biol 1998; 201(Pt 2): 289-297.

[146]   Stenzel-Poore MP, Stevens SL, Xiong Z, et al. Effect of ischaemic preconditioning on genomic response to cerebral ischaemia: similarity to neuroprotective strategies in hibernation and hypoxia-tolerant states. Lancet 2003; 362(9389): 1028-1037.

[147]   Chu XP, Zhu XM, Chen D, Simon RP, Xiong ZG. Metabolic inhibition enhances the activities of acid-sensing ion channels. Soc Neurosci Abstr 2002; 95.10.

[148]   Allen NJ, Attwell D. Modulation of ASIC channels in rat cerebellar Purkinje neurons by ischemia-related signals. J Physiol (Lond) 2002; 543(2): 521-529.

[149]   Immke DC, McCleskey EW. Lactate enhances the acid-sensing Na+ channel on ischemia-sensing neurons. Nat Neurosci 2001; 4(9): 869-870.

[150]   Immke DC, McCleskey EW. Protons open acid-sensing ion channels by catalyzing relief of Ca2+ blockade. Neuron 2003; 37(1): 75-84.

The Protective Effect of Ischemic Postconditioning Against Ischemic Brain Injury

Heng Zhao

Department of Neurosurgery, Stanford University School of Medicine, Stanford, CA 94305-5327, USA;
E-mail: hzhao@stanford.edu

Abstract: Ischemic postconditioning is an emerging concept for stroke treatment. It refers to a series of mechanical interruptions of reperfusion after ischemia, preventing ischemia/reperfusion injury in both myocardial and cerebral infarction. This review article reveals that the earliest study about ischemic postconditioning was performed more than 50 years ago in the research field of myocardial ischemia, and only thrilled in recent 5 years, and it was shifted from myocardial ischemia to cerebral ischemia only 2 to 3 years ago. The protective effect of postconditioning has been studied in focal and global ischemia *in vivo*, and in slice or primary neuronal cultures *in vitro*. In addition, protective parameters of postconditioning in various ischemic models are discussed. Thereafter, this article provides insights on postconditioning's protective mechanisms associated with reperfusion injury, the Akt, MAPK and PKC cell signaling pathways, suggesting that postconditioning attenuates free radical generation, that the Akt pathway contribute to its protection, and that the MAPK and PKC pathways are closely associated with its protection.

INTRODUCTION

Stroke is the third leading cause of mortality in the United States. A vast majority of stroke survivors live with physical disabilities, and many suffer from post-stroke depression. Although many neuroprotectants have been shown to reduce infarction and improve neurological functions in animal models of stroke in the laboratory, almost no neuroprotectant can offer protective effects in translational studies from the basic research to clinical applications [1]. This situation necessitates the exploration of novel therapeutic strategies; ischemic postconditioning being one that has recently emerged.

The term 'ischemic postconditioning' was coined to contrast with ischemic preconditioning [2, 3]. While preconditioning is performed before ischemic onset, postconditioning is conducted after reperfusion. Ischemic preconditioning refers to a brief, sublethal ischemia that prevents ischemic injury caused by a subsequent prolonged, lethal ischemia [4, 5]. Preconditioning has served as a powerful tool for understanding the endogenous mechanisms by which the ischemic organs are protected [4]. Although preconditioning has been considered a golden standard for ischemic protection both in the heart and in the brain, its clinical application has been disappointing. This is because the predictability of ischemia occurrence is required for clinical applications of preconditioning, which significantly limits its clinical translation. Nevertheless, ischemic postconditioning is performed after ischemia/reperfusion. Thus, its clinical application does not count on the predictability of stroke occurrence.

Postconditioning is first clearly defined in the research field of myocardial ischemia as a series of mechanical interruptions performed during initial reperfusion [2, 3]. Earliest studies about postconditioning were conducted more than five decades ago, when it was well-established that a sudden restoration of the arterial flow after heart ischemia results in ventricular fibrillation [6]. Sewell and colleagues [6], however, found that intermittent reperfusion over several minutes block ventricular fibrillations in dogs, leading to a normal rhythm. This phenomenon was repeated by Na and colleagues in 1996 [3], who first coined the term of 'postconditioning', and found that postconditioning was as effective as preconditioning in preventing ventricular fibrillations in cats. However, postconditioning studies did not thrive until 2003, when Z.Q Zhao and colleagues published their first study on postconditioning [2]. In this study, the protective effect of postconditioning and that of preconditioning were compared in dogs [2]. Lethal heart ischemia of 60 minutes was induced by occluding the left anterior descending artery (LAD). Preconditioning of 5 minutes LAD occlusion was conducted 10 minutes before the onset of the lethal ischemia, whereas postconditioning was conducted by three cycles of 30-second reperfusion and 30-second occlusion at the start of reperfusion [2]. Postconditioning reduced infarct size by ~44 %, which was comparable with the protective effects of preconditioning [2]. Thereafter, many groups have confirmed that the protective effects of postconditioning in myocardial ischemia [7], and the intensive research on the postconditioning in the heart has led to clinical trials. Statt *et al.* reported that postconditioning, which was performed by 4 cycles of 1 minute reperfusion/ 1 minute occlusion via an angioplasty balloon, reduced acute myocardial injury in patients who had ongoing myocardial infarction [8].

The question is if ischemic postconditioning can also apply to stroke brains. The rationale of extrapolating postconditioning from treating heart ischemia to brain ischemia largely depends on whether the principle for stroke treatment is similar to that for heart ischemia therapy. Past studies have revealed that the mechanisms of ischemic brain injury have many similar aspects compared with those of myocardial ischemic injury [9]. For instance, both apoptosis and necrosis occur in the ischemic brain or heart [10-12], and free radical products after reperfusion play critical roles in inducing ischemia/reperfusion injury in both the brain and the heart. In addition, similar cell signaling pathways contribute to cell death or regulate cell survival in both the brain and the heart. These pathways include calpain mediated necrotic pathways [13], cytochrome c/caspase mediated apoptotic pathways [14], MAPK pathways [15], the PKC pathway [16, 17], and the Akt/PKB survival pathways [18]. Finally, as previously discussed, preconditioning robustly reduces ischemic damage in both the brain and the heart [4, 5]. Based on these similarities, it is a logical and intriguing idea to test whether postconditioning also protects against cerebral ischemia.

In the past 2 to 3 years, a few groups have demonstrated postconditioning's protection against brain ischemia [9, 19-22], which has opened a novel avenue for research of stroke treatment. Here we review the protective effect of postconditioning in global and focal ischemia *in vivo*, and in an OGD model *in vitro*, which mimics *in vivo* stroke. In addition, the protective effect of postconditioning on ischemia-induced neurobehavioral alterations, and the potential protective mechanisms of postconditioning are also reviewed.

ISCHEMIC POSTCONDITIONING MODELS AND PROTECTIVE PARA-METERS OF POSTCONDITIONING AGAINST CERE-BRAL ISCHEMIA

1. Focal ischemia

Our laboratories have demonstrated that postconditioning reduces infarct size in focal ischemia in rats [21, 23]. In our first study, we compared the protective effects of postconditioning in a focal ischemia model with various severities. Stroke was induced by transiently occluding the bilateral common carotid artery (bCCA) for 15, 30 or 60 min combined with permanent occlusion of the distal middle cerebral artery (dMCA) [21]. Ischemic postconditioning, which consists of three cycles of 30 second bCCA release and 10 seconds of bCCA occlusion, was conducted after 15, 30 or 60 min's bCCA occlusion [21]. As a result, postconditioning reduced infarct size by ~80, ~51,~17%, respectively, in 15, 30 or 60 min CCA occlusion combined with permanent dMCA occlusion. Thus, postconditioning reduces infarct size

as a function of ischemic severity – that is, it is less effective with longer periods of ischemia.

The reasons for us to focus on this focal cerebral ischemia model to study postconditioning are multiple. First, we have previously found that partial reperfusion generates about 10% smaller infarction than the total reperfusion in this model [24]. In that study, total reperfusion was achieved by three vessel releases (bilateral CCA plus dMCA); partial reperfusion was generated by two vessel releases (bilateral CCA) while the MCA remained occluded. Since incomplete reperfusion reduces infarction, we assumed that postconditioning, which disrupts reperfusion, would also protect against ischemic injury in this unique model. Second, this model generates well-defined, reproducible cortical infarcts [18, 25]. We believe that a highly reproducible model is necessary to characterize the protective effects of postconditioning. Third, the bilateral CCAs are accessible; reperfusion can simply be manipulated by occluding or releasing the bilateral CCA, which allows us to conduct postconditioning.

We then examined the temporal factors of postconditioning using the ischemic model of 30 min bCCA occlusion combined with permanent dMCA occlusion [26], since it generates a prominent cortical infarction, against which postconditioning offers a reliable and reproducible protection. We compared the impact of cycle numbers and duration of reperfusion/occlusion on the protective effect of postconditioning. The results showed that postconditioning with 3 cycles, but not with 10 cycles, of 30 sec release and 10 sec occlusion (30s/10s) of the bilateral CCA reduced infarction measured at 2 days after stroke. In contrast, postconditioning with 3 cycles of 10s/10s offered no protection, while postconditioning with 10 cycles generated the strongest protection. In these experiments, postconditioning was conducted immediately after reperfusion. However, postconditioning did not reduce infarction when it was initiated at 3 min after reperfusion. Therefore, postconditioning's protection depends on the number of cycles and duration of each cycle of reperfusion and occlusion, and the onset time of postconditioning.

Nevertheless, some neuroprotectants, such as post-ischemic hypothermia [27], and rapid ischemic preconditioning [4], have been shown to provide protection for only a few days after ischemia. In addition, reducing injured brain tissue may not translate into the preservation of neurological function [28]. Therefore, it is essential to test whether postconditioning has chronic protection and preserves brain function. We further found that postconditioning reduced lesion size ~40% in rats subjected to ischemia when measured 30 days after ischemia, suggesting a long-term protection of postconditioning. In the same study, neurological functions were assayed by the vibrissae test, a well-established method of detecting asymmetric usage of the forelimb caused by stroke.

We found that the percentage of contralateral forelimb placements dropped from 100% before ischemia to ~25 - ~60% after ischemia, indicating an asymmetrical deficit in forelimb use, of which the overall deficit was attenuated by postconditioning from 2 through 30 days after ischemia, suggesting postconditioning also improves neurological function [29].

In our experiments, robust protection of postconditioning is observed only in moderate or mild brain ischemia in which the bilateral CCA occlusion time was 15 or 30 min [21], while the protection is mild in more severe ischemia (60 min of CCA occlusion). Xing and colleagues have recently confirmed our findings, showing that postconditioning reduced infarction by about only 16% [30]. In their study, focal ischemia was induced by MCA suture occlusion for 60 min; postconditioning was performed by 6 cycles of 30 sec reperfusion/30 sec occlusion initiated immediately after reperfusion [30]. Therefore, it seems that postconditioning does not generate the same level of protection in the ischemic brain as in the ischemic heart. However, we have not tested if the optimized parameter has better protection in a longer period of ischemia, and Xing and colleagues did not compare the protective effect of postconditioning with different parameters. Therefore, we can not exclude the possibility that the relatively weak protection is due to the usage of sub-optimal parameters of postconditioning.

In contrast with our finding, Pignataro and colleagues have demonstrated a very strong protection of postconditioning in a severe focal ischemic model [22, 31], in which the MCA was occluded for 100 minutes. Postconditioning's protection with three conditions were compared: 5 cycles of 2 min MCA release and 2 min occlusion (2min/2min); 3 cycles of 5 min release and 5 min occlusion; one time of 10 min occlusion performed at 10 min reperfusion. They found that postconditioning with 5 cycles of 2min/2min offered no protection, while with 3 cycles of 5min/5min it reduced infarction by 38% and 1 cycle of 10 minutes reperfusion/occlusion reduced infarct size by ~70 % compared with rats subjected to control ischemia. However, postconditioning with 10 min of occlusion and 30 min reperfusion had no protection. Again, this study suggests that onset time of postconditioning is critical for its neuroprotective effect.

2. Global ischemia

A few groups have studied the protective effects of postconditioning on transient global cerebral ischemia. Wang *et al.* showed postconditioning's protection in a 10 min transient global ischemia model in rats [20]. In their study, postconditioning was applied immediately after reperfusion. Postconditioning consists of 3 cycles of reperfusion/occlusion with periods of 15 sec/15 sec, 30sec/30sec, 60 sec/15sec; in another group, postconditioning with 3 cycles of 15sec/15sec was

applied at 45 sec reperfusion [20]. The results showed that at 7 days of reperfusion, 85.8% of CA1 hippocampal neurons and 64.1% of parietal cortical neurons were either lost or dead. Postconditioning with 15 sec/15 sec, 30sec/30sec applied immediately after reperfusion, and with 5sec/15sec applied at 45 sec reperfusion attenuated neuronal death to about 10-20% in the hippocampus, and to about 0-6% in the parietal cortex; however, postconditioning with 60sec/15sec applied immediately after reperfusion offered no protection [20]. Among these tested protective conditions, postconditioning with 15/15 applied at 45 sec after reperfusion showed the strongest protection in the hippocampus, but no difference was reported in the cortex. Consistent with its protective effects on neuronal survival, postconditioning improves subject performance on spatial learning and memory in a water maze test three weeks after reperfusion [20], suggesting that postconditioning executes long-term protection in global ischemia. Rehni and Singh have also shown that postconditioning with 3 cycles of 10 s/10s attenuated behavioral deficits after global ischemia in mice [19]. However, they did not report how postconditioning affects neuronal loss.

In all of the studies discussed above, postconditioning was conducted during early reperfusion after stroke. Postconditioning applied at later time points may also execute protection. Burda *et al.* showed that postconditioning can be conducted at 2 days after reperfusion in rat global ischemia [32]. In their studies, global ischemia was induced by 4-vessel occlusion in rats, and postconditioning was conducted by 4 techniques: short ischemia, injection of 3-nitropropionic acid (3-NP), norepinephrine and bradykinin [32, 33]. Ischemia for 8 min caused 60% CA1 neuronal loss measured at 7d after reperfusion [34]. Postconditioning with 5 min ischemia applied at 2d, or with intraperitoneal injection of norepinephrine or 3NP at 2d, recovered neuronal survival to about 100%. In addition, 10 min ischemia caused about 70 % of CA 1 neuronal loss, but postconditioning with 6 min ischemia applied at 2 d nearly completely prevented neuronal loss while with 3-NP injection at 2d, neuronal survival was returned to about 80% [34]. In a separate study by the same group [35], 8 min of ischemia caused 52% neuronal loss in the CA 1 at 3 days after reperfusion while postconditioning with a bradykinin injection at 2 days saved more than 97% of CA 1 neurons.

3. *In vitro* ischemia

Pignataro *et al.* also established an *in vitro* ischemic model in which postconditioning reduced neuronal death [22]. Cortical culture was used in their study. *In vitro* ischemia was induced by 120 min-OGD, which caused more than 50% cell death. Postconditioning with 30 min of OGD conducted at 10min, 30 min or 60 min after reperfusion did not reduce cell death; however, with 10 min OGD initiated at 10 min of reperfusion, postconditioning robustly blocked cell death [22]. This study suggests that onset time of postconditioning and period of postconditioning is critical for generating neuroprotection.

Combination of postconditioning with pre-conditioning offers no synergistic protection

There are at least two reasons to study whether the combination of postconditioning with preconditioning has a synergistic effect. First, the combination study may provide some clues to understand the protective mechanisms of both preconditioning and postconditioning. The protective mechanisms of preconditioning and postconditioning have received extensive studies in the heart. The results suggest that they have some mechanisms in common. For example, both pre- and postconditioning protect the ischemic organ by enhancing adenosine activity, reducing the products of reactive oxygen species and lipid peroxidation [2, 36], inhibiting JNK/P38 activities [37] but promoting ERK1/2 activity [38]. Most of the recent studies in the brain have also suggested that both preconditioning and postconditioning act through some common pathways, such as the Akt pathways [22, 29]. Therefore, one may speculate if they do share mechanisms in common thus their combination would have a stronger protection. Second, because both preconditioning and postconditioning may be feasible in certain clinical settings in which stroke occurrence is predictable, a combination study may help clinicians to decide if a combination of both preconditioning and postconditioning is an option for clinical applications.

We have recently compared the protective effect of rapid and delayed preconditioning with that of postconditioning, and studied the protective effect of postconditioning combined with either rapid or delayed preconditioning [26]. Rapid preconditioning was induced by transiently occluding the left dMCA for 15 min, and the prolonged ischemia of 30 min CCA occlusion, combined with permanent dMCA occlusion was induced 60 min later [26]. Delayed preconditioning was induced by occluding the left dMCA for 5 or 15 min at 3 d before the prolonged ischemia. Postconditioning of 10 cycles of 10s/10s was conducted immediately after reperfusion. We found that the protective effect of postconditioning is comparable with that of rapid preconditioning, but it is less effective than delayed preconditioning. We further addressed whether postconditioning plus preconditioning can generate a synergistic effect [26]. We found that postconditioning combined with either rapid or delayed preconditioning provides additional reductions in infarction. Our results are consistent with a previous study [22]: Pignataro and colleagues reported that postconditioning's protection is comparable with that of delayed preconditioning in a suture MCA occlusion model in rats, while a

combination of postconditioning with preconditioning provided no greater protection.

PROTECTIVE MECHANISMS OF POST-CONDITIONING AGAINST STROKE

1. Postconditioning primarily targets early reperfusion, reduces free radical generation and inflammation, and blocks apoptosis

A primary therapeutic strategy for ischemic stroke is to recannalize the occluded blood vessels to allow early reperfusion, which is made possible by administrating the thrombolytic agent, t-PA [39], or by inserting mechanical devices to remove the occluding clot [40]. However, reperfusion is a double edged sword, which generates an overproduction of reactive oxygen species (ROS) or free radicals, leading to reperfusion injury in the ischemic brain [41]. Reperfusion injury has been repeatedly confirmed in many studies. For example, 6 hours of MCA occlusion generated a smaller infarct size than 3 hours of MCA occlusion plus 3 hours of reperfusion [42]. In addition, 72% of infarction was reduced by permanent unilateral CCA/MCA occlusion compared with transient occlusion for 2 to 5 hours in rats when infarction was measured 24h after ischemia onset [43]. These studies suggest that reperfusion exacerbates ischemic injury. In addition, as we have discussed, partial reperfusion leads to a reduction in infarct size. Moreover, our most recent study further showed that controlled reperfusion, in which CBF was allowed to recover gradually, also attenuates brain injury after stroke. Similarly, an *in vitro* study has demonstrated that gradual re-oxygenation after *in vitro* ischemia (OGD) produces less neuronal death in cell culture. In contrast to the protective effect of partial reperfusion, hyperemic response has been suspected to be detrimental to ischemic brain. In addition, hyperemic response is often followed by hypotension or no-reflow phenomenon, which further damages the ischemic brain.

Since postconditioning is primarily instituted to disrupt reperfusion, it is important to confirm if postconditioning attenuates the hyperemic response, and if it mitigates hypotension thereafter. As a result, we initially measured cerebral blood flow (CBF) in the penumbra in rats subjected to 15 or 30 min of bilateral CCA occlusion combined with permanent MCA occlusion [21, 26]. A clear hyperemic response was detected after reperfusion in rats subjected to 15 min, and CBF was recovered to pre-ischemic levels in rats with 30 min of CCA occlusion [21, 26]. We showed that postconditioning interrupts reperfusion in these two models. Most importantly, postconditioning improves CBF at 30 min after reperfusion [26], which is confirmed by another study using a global ischemia model [20]. Taken together, postconditioning reduces cerebral ischemic injury by disrupting the early reperfusion and improving reperfusion thereafter.

It is well-known that the sudden, abrupt reperfusion leads to overproduction of ROS, which leads to apoptosis [41]. In addition, inflammatory response also exacerbates ischemic injury [44]. Therefore, it is reasonable to examine whether postconditioning attenuates ROS production and apoptosis, and if it inhibits inflammatory response. Indeed, we found that postconditioning profoundly attenuated the amount of superoxide at 30 minutes after reperfusion in the model of 30 minutes CCA occlusion plus permanent MCA occlusion [21]. Consistent with our findings, postconditioning has been shown to attenuate lipid peroxidate levels in a focal ischemia model [30]. Moreover, other reports demonstrated that postconditioning performed 2 days after global ischemia increased activities of antioxidant enzymes, including superoxide dismutase and catalase [33]

Furthermore, we have shown that postconditioning blocked terminal deoxynucleotidyl transferase-mediated uridine 5'-triphosphate-biotin nick end labeling (TUNEL) positive staining, a marker of apoptosis, in the penumbra 2 days after stroke [21]. In more recent findings, Wang and colleagues further showed that postconditioning reduced cytochrome c release from the mitochondria to the cytosol, a critical cascade for apoptosis induction [20]. Taken together, postconditioning may reduce ischemic injury by blocking apoptosis.

Postconditioning may also inhibit inflammation after stroke. During inflammatory response, leukocytes extravagate into the brain tissue, releasing ROS, thus attacking lipid membrane, DNA and proteins [41]. Inflammation is mediated by cytokines, such as IL-1beta and TNF-alpha, and adhesion molecules, such as ICAM-1 [45]. A recent study showed that postconditioning inhibits myeloperoxidase (MPO) activity, an indicator of leukocytes accumulation, in the cortex at 24h after stroke [30]. In addition, postconditioning attenuates the expression of IL-1beta and TNF-alpha mRNA, and ICAM-1 protein expression in the ischemic cortex at 24h after ischemia [30]. These results suggest that postconditioning may produce an anti-inflammation effect.

2. Akt pathway contributes to the protective effect of postconditioning

Many cell signaling pathways are involved in ischemic injury after stroke, and neuronal death and survival is determined by a balance between cell death and survival in signaling pathways. We and others have recently demonstrated that the occurrence of apoptosis is probably due to a dysfunction of the Akt pathway, a critical signaling pathway for neuronal survival (Zhao *et al.* 2006, review). In the Akt pathway, Akt is activated by the phosphorylation of

Ser-473 and Thr-308 [46, 47], which is regulated by phosphoinositide 3-kinase (PI3K) and phosphoinositide-dependent protein kinase-1 (PDK1) phosphorylation. In contrast, Akt is inactivated by *phosphatase and tensin homologue deleted on chromosome 10* (PTEN) [46]. Activated Akt translocates from the membrane to the cytosol, mitochondria or the nuclei to block apoptosis by phosphorylating its substrates, such as Bcl-2 associated death protein (Bad) and glycogen synthase kinase 3β (GSK3β) [46, 48]. In the absence of Akt kinase activity, nonphosphorylated Bad translocates into the mitochondria and triggers cytochrome c release, caspase-3 activation and apoptosis [49]. Dephosphorylation of GSK3β leads to its activation and phosphorylation of β-catenin, thus resulting in β-catenin degradation.

Past studies have demonstrated that the Akt pathway contributes to neuronal survival after stroke. As we have recently reviewed (Zhao *et al.* 2006), the level of Akt phosphorylation at Ser 473 (P-Akt) transiently increases after cerebral ischemia, while the levels of phosphorylation of PTEN, PDK1, FKHR and GSK 3 β decrease. Compounds such as growth factors, estrogen, and free radical scavengers upregulate P-Akt, which may contribute to their effects in reducing ischemic damage.

It has recently been demonstrated that postconditioning increases Akt phosphorylation (as measured by Western blot) [22, 29], and has further shown that postconditioning increases Akt activity (assayed by an *in vitro* kinase assay) (Gao *et al.* 2008). Furthermore, Akt inhibition partially blocks the protective effect of postconditioning [22, 29]. However, postconditioning does not affect PTEN or PDK1 phosphorylation but it does inhibit an increase in GSK3β phosphorylation. Finally, we found that postconditioning blocks β-catenin phosphorylation subsequent to GSK3β, but have no effect on total or non-phosphorylated, active β-catenin protein levels [29]. We concluded that the Akt pathway plays a critical role in postconditioning's protection.

3. MAPK pathways are involved in postconditioning's protection

The MAPK pathways, including extracellular signal regulated kinase 1/2 (ERK1/2), P38. and c-Jun N-terminal kinases (JNK) pathways, are also closely related with ischemic injury and neuronal survival, though whether their roles are protective or detrimental remain controversial [50].

In the MAPK pathways, extracellular signal regulated kinase 1/2 (ERK1/2), p38 and c-Jun N-terminal kinases (JNK) are the three best characterized modules [50]. The ERK1/2 is activated through the three-tiered Raf/MEK/ERK cascade by growth factors and various stressors such as cytokines [51, 52]. Activated Raf phosphorylates the dual specificity kinases MEK1 and MEK2, which in turn phosphorylate ERK1/2. ERK activation can typically be inhibited by the MEK inhibitor, U0126 [50]. As with ERK, JNK or P38 is activated through their respective three-tiered cascades by a variety of stressors, including DNA damage, growth factor deprivation, cytokines, and UV irradiation [50].

Both ERK1/2 and JNK are well-known to be involved in cerebral ischemia [50]. JNK and p38 appear to be clearly detrimental after stroke, and their inhibition blocks apoptosis in many neuronal death paradigms [50]. However, ERK1/2's activity is involved in both neuroprotection and injury exacerbation. We have recently reviewed this dual role of ERK1/2 [50]. In general, ERK1/2 phosphorylation is increased after cerebral ischemia/reperfusion. This increase is apparently involved in the beneficial effects of growth factors, estrogen, preconditioning, and hypothermia on the ischemic brain, but it also promotes inflammation and oxidative stress, and its inhibition reduces ischemic damage [50]. We suggest that the dual potential of ERK1/2 actions in the ischemic brain is likely related to its responses to a diverse array of agonists and cell surface receptors. For instance, the ERK1/2 activity generated by cytokines and free radicals or other inflammatory factors after stroke may worsen ischemic damage, while the ERK1/2 activity produced by exogenous growth factors, estrogen, and preconditioning favors neuroprotection. Therefore, to achieve neuroprotection, the protective effect of ERK1/2 should be optimized while its detrimental actions should be blocked [50]. To study the changes in ERK1/2 in the protective effect of postconditioning may facilitate our understanding in its roles.

Our study confirmed that ERK1/2 phosphorylation (P-ERK1/2) was increased from 1 to 24 hours after stroke, and found that postconditioning reduced its level in the penumbra [29]. Our results implicate a detrimental role of P-ERK1/2 after ischemia, so its inhibition may contribute to the protection of postconditioning, which conflicts with the findings from Pignataro *et al.* that postconditioning enhanced ERK1/2 phosphorylation [22]. However, in their study, increases in P-ERK1/2 may be unrelated with the protective effect of postconditioning, since U0126, the antagonist of ERK1/2, did not block postconditioning's protection. The discrepancy between our result and that of Pignataro *et al.* is probably due to differing ischemic models and postconditioning parameters employed in these two studies [22, 29].

Therefore, the puzzle regarding the role of ERK1/2 in rapid postconditioning has not been resolved. Previous studies, including our own, have some limitations. First, the activity of ERK1/2 was evaluated by its phosphorylation alone [29, 50]. As we saw in the case of Akt, the *in vitro* Akt kinase assay suggested that Akt phosphorylation alone does not represent Akt activity [18]. We deem that the same experiment about kinase activity assay for ERK should be performed. Second, the subcellular localization of ERK1/2 after stroke was not studied. However, ERK1/2 subcellular translocation may play a critical role in its actual neuroprotective and detrimental effects [50]. Third, its spatial distribution in different cell types has not been analyzed. Fourth, in our own study, ERK1/2 antagonists have not been tested in postconditioning [29]. Therefore, it warrants to further study the role of ERK1/2 in ischemic postconditioning.

4. Postconditioning inhibits δPKC cleavage and improves εPKC phosphorylation

Stroke induced apoptosis is also mediated by PKC pathways. There are at least 11 isozymes of the PKC family, including δPKC and εPKC [53]. PKC isozymes differ as to their intracellular location and function, and their activities are regulated by their subcellular location, cleavage form and phosphorylation. While δPKC activity usually leads to cell death [17], εPKC promotes neuronal survival [16]. δPKC has been implicated in mediating ischemic and reperfusion brain injury. For instance, δPKC mRNA increases after ischemia in both global [54] and focal ischemia [55]. Furthermore, a single injection of the δPKC-specific inhibitor, δV1-1, up to 6 h after reperfusion reduces infarct size following transient cerebral ischemia [56]. We have recently shown that mild hypothermia protects the ischemic brain by inhibiting δPKC's particulate (membrane), mitochondrial and nuclear subcellular translocation [17]. In contrast with the worsening effect of δPKC, δPKC activities promote neuronal survival. For instance, we have shown that mild to moderate hypothermia protects the brain by preserving δPKC activity [16].

We recently studied the protective effect of postconditioning on the PKC pathways [29]. Changes in total and cleaved δPKC, phosphorylated δPKC (thr 505) (P- δPKC), and phosphorylated εPKC (P-εPKC) were examined. We found that postconditioning had no effect on the protein levels of total δPKC, but blocks the increase in levels of the cleaved form of δPKC, indicative of δPKC activity at 1 h after stroke in the penumbra [29]. Although postconditioning had no effect on P-δPKC levels, which were decreased by 24 h after stroke onset, it strongly inhibited decreases in p-εPKC after stroke. Our results suggest that postconditioning may reduce ischemic damage by inhibiting the worsening effect of δPKC while promoting a beneficial effect of εPKC activity [29].

CONCLUSION

The protective effects of postconditioning against cerebral ischemia have been established and confirmed by several independent groups, from focal ischemia to global ischemia, and from *in vivo* to *in vitro* models:

Postconditioning not only reduces infarction in acute stages but it also provides long-term protection, and improves animal's neurobehavioral functions. Postconditioning primarily disrupts the early reperfusion, attenuates hyperemic response after reperfusion, but improves CBF after 30 min of reperfusion. In addition, postconditioning seems to reduce ischemic injury by blocking the overproduction of ROS and lipid peroxidation, and inhibit apoptosis. Furthermore, the underlying cellular and molecular mechanisms of postconditioning are being revealed: the Akt survival signaling pathway contributes to postconditioning's protection; the MAPK pathways may also be involved in its protection; and changes in δPKC and εPKC activities are associated with postconditioning.

REFERENCES

[1]   Hoyte L, Kaur J, Buchan, AM. Lost in translation: taking neuroprotection from animal models to clinical trials. Exp Neurol 2004; 188(2): 200-4.

[2]   Zhao ZQ, Corvera JS, Halkos ME, *et al.* Inhibition of myocardial injury by ischemic postconditioning during reperfusion: comparison with ischemic preconditioning. Am J Physiol Heart Circ Physiol 2003; 285(2): H579-88.

[3]   Na, HS, Kim YI, Yoon YW, Han HC, Nahm SH, Hong SK. Ventricular premature beat-driven intermittent restoration of coronary blood flow reduces the incidence of reperfusion-induced ventricular fibrillation in a cat model of regional ischemia. Am Heart J 1996; 132(1 Pt 1): 78-83.

[4]   Perez-Pinzon MA. Neuroprotective effects of ischemic preconditioning in brain mitochondria following cerebral ischemia. J Bioenerg Biomembr 2004; 36(4): 323-7.

[5]   Murry CE, Jennings RB, Reimer KA. Preconditioning with ischemia: a delay of lethal cell injury in ischemic myocardium. Circulation 1986; 74(5): 1124-36.

[6]   Sewell WH, Koth DR, Huggins CE. Ventricular fibrillation in dogs after sudden return of flow to the coronary artery. Surgery 1955; 38(6): 1050-3.

[7]   Zhao ZQ, Vinten-Johansen J. Postconditioning: reduction of reperfusion-induced injury. Cardiovasc Res 2006; 70(2): 200-11.

[8]   Staat P, Rioufol G, Piot C, *et al.* Postconditioning the human heart. Circulation 2005; 112(14): 2143-8.

[9]   Zhao H. The protective effect of ischemic postconditioning against ischemic injury: from the heart to the brain. J Neuroimmune Pharmacol 2007; 2(4): 313-8.

[10]   Zhao H, Wang JQ, Sun G, Schaal DW, Sapolsky RM, Steinberg GK. Conditions of protection by hypothermia and effects on apoptotic pathways in a model of permanent middle cerebral artery occlusion. J Cereb Blood Flow Metab 2005; 25: S474 .

[11]   Zhao H, Yenari M, Cheng D, Sapolsky RM, Steinberg GK. Biphasic cytochrome c release after transient global ischemia and its inhibition by hypothermia. J Cereb Blood Flow Metab 2005; 25: 1119-1129.

[12]   Merkle S, Frantz S, Schon MP, *et al.* A role for caspase-1 in heart failure. Circ Res 2007; 100(5): 645-53.

[13]   Yamashima T, Implication of cysteine proteases calpain, cathepsin and caspase in ischemic neuronal death of primates. Prog Neurobiol 2000; 62(3): 273-95.

[14]   Chen, J, Nagayama T, Jin K, Stetler RA, Zhu RL, Graham SH, *et al.* Induction of caspase-3-like protease may mediate delayed neuronal death in the hippocampus after transient cerebral ischemia. J Neurosci 1998; 18(13): 4914-28.

[15]   Noshita N, Sugawara T, Hayashi T, Lewen A, Omar G, Chan PH. Copper/zinc superoxide dismutase attenuates neuronal cell death by preventing extracellular signal-

[16]   regulated kinase activation after transient focal cerebral ischemia in mice. J Neurosci 2002; 22(18): 7923-30.

[16]   Shimohata T, Zhao H, Steinberg GK. Epsilon PKC may contribute to the protective effect of hypothermia in a rat focal cerebral ischemia model. Stroke 2007; 38(2): 375-80.

[17]   Shimohata T, Zhao H, Sung JH, Sun G, Mochly-Rosen D, Steinberg GK. Suppression of deltaPKC activation after focal cerebral ischemia contributes to the protective effect of hypothermia. J Cereb Blood Flow Metab 2007; 27(8): 1463-75.

[18]   Zhao H, Shimohata T, Wang JQ, *et al.* Akt contributes to neuroprotection by hypothermia against cerebral ischemia in rats. J Neurosci 2005; 25(42): 9794-806.

[19]   Rehni AK, Singh N. Role of phosphoinositide 3-kinase in ischemic postconditioning-induced attenuation of cerebral ischemia-evoked behavioral deficits in mice. Pharmacol Rep 2007; 59(2): 192-8.

[20]   Wang JY, Shen J, Gao Q, *et al.* Ischemic postconditioning protects against global cerebral ischemia/reperfusion-induced injury in rats. Stroke 2008; 39(3): 983-90.

[21]   Zhao H, Sapolsky RM, Steinberg GK. Interrupting reperfusion as a stroke therapy: ischemic postconditioning reduces infarct size after focal ischemia in rats. J Cereb Blood Flow Metab 2006; 26(9): 1114-21.

[22]   Pignataro G, Meller R, Inoue K, *et al. In vivo* and *in vitro* characterization of a novel neuroprotective strategy for stroke: ischemic postconditioning. J Cereb Blood Flow Metab 2008; 28(2): 232-41.

[23]   Zhao H. The protective effect of ischemic postconditioning against ischemic injury: from the heart to the brain. J Neuroimmune Pharmacol 2007; 2(4): 313-8.

[24]   Zhao H, Yenari MA, Cheng D, Sapolsky RM, Steinberg GK. Bcl-2 overexpression protects against neuron loss within the ischemic margin following experimental stroke and inhibits cytochrome C translocation and caspase-3 activity. J Neurochem 2003; 85(4): 1026-36.

[25]   Zhao H, Yenari MA, Cheng D, Barreto-Chang OL, Sapolsky RM, Steinberg GK. Bcl-2 transfection via herpes simplex virus blocks apoptosis-inducing factor translocation after focal ischemia in the rat. J Cereb Blood Flow Metab 2004; 24(6): 681-92.

[26]   Gao X, Ren C, Zhao H. Protective effects of ischemic postconditioning compared to gradual reperfusion or preconditioning. J Neurosci Res 2008: p in press.

[27]   Dietrich WD, Busto R, Alonso O, Globus MY, Ginsberg MD. Intraischemic but not postischemic brain hypothermia protects chronically following global forebrain ischemia in rats. J Cereb Blood Flow Metab1993; 13(4): 541-9.

[28]   Dumas TC, Sapolsky RM. Gene therapy against neurological insults: sparing neurons versus sparing function. Trends Neurosci 2001; 24(12): 695-700.

[29]   Gao X, Zhang H, Takahashi T, *et al.* The Akt signaling pathway contributes to postconditioning's protection against stroke; the protection is associated with the MAPK and PKC pathways. J Neurochem 2008: p in press.

[30]   Xing B, Chen H, Zhang M, *et al.* Ischemic post-conditioning protects brain and reduces inflammation in a rat model of focal cerebral ischemia/reperfusion. J Neurochem 2008; 105(5): 1737-45.

[31]   Pignataro G, Xiong Z, Simon RP. Ischemic post-conditioning: a new neuroprotective strateg. Program No 7603 2006 Neuroscience Meeting Planner Atlanta, GA: Society for Neuroscience 2006 (Online).

[32]   Burda J, Danielisova V, Nemethova M, *et al.* Delayed postconditionig initiates additive mechanism necessary for survival of selectively vulnerable neurons after transient ischemia in rat brain. Cell Mol Neurobiol 2006; 26(7-8): 1139-49.

[33]   Danielisova V, Nemethova M, Gottlieb M, Burda J. The changes in endogenous antioxidant enzyme activity after postconditioning. Cell Mol Neurobiol 2006; 26(7-8): 1181-91.

[34]   Burda J, Danielisova V, Nemethova M, *et al.* Delayed postconditionig initiates additive mechanism necessary for

survival of selectively vulnerable neurons after transient ischemia in rat brain. Cell Mol Neurobiol 2006; 26(7-8): 1141-51.

[35]   Danielisova V, Gottlieb M, Nemethova M, Burda J. Effects of bradykinin postconditioning on endogenous antioxidant enzyme activity after transient forebrain ischemia in rat. Neurochem Res 2008; 33(6); 1057-64.

[36]   Halkos ME, Kerendi F, Corvera JS, *et al.* Myocardial protection with postconditioning is not enhanced by ischemic preconditioning. Ann Thorac Surg 2004; 78(3): 961-9; discussion 969.

[37]   Sun HY, Wang NP, Halkos M, *et al.* Postconditioning attenuates cardiomyocyte apoptosis via inhibition of JNK and p38 mitogen-activated protein kinase signaling pathways. Apoptosis 2006; 11(9): 1583-93.

[38]   Yang XM, Proctor JB, Cui L, Krieg T, Downey JM, Cohen MV. Multiple, brief coronary occlusions during early reperfusion protect rabbit hearts by targeting cell signaling pathways. J Am Coll Cardiol 2004; 44(5): 1103-10.

[39]   Fisher M, Brott TG. Emerging therapies for acute ischemic stroke: new therapies on trial. Stroke 2003; 34(2): 359-61.

[40]   Smith WS, Sung G, Starkman S, *et al.* Safety and efficacy of mechanical embolectomy in acute ischemic stroke: results of the MERCI trial. Stroke 2005; 36(7): 1432-8.

[41]   Chan PH. Role of oxidants in ischemic brain damage. Stroke 1996; 27(6): 1124-9.

[42]   Yang GY, Betz AL. Reperfusion-induced injury to the blood-brain barrier after middle cerebral artery occlusion in rats. Stroke 1994; 25(8): 1658-64, discussion 1664-5.

[43]   Aronowski J, Strong R, Grotta JC. Reperfusion injury: demonstration of brain damage produced by reperfusion after transient focal ischemia in rats. J Cereb Blood Flow Metab 1997; 17(10): 1048-56.

[44]   Bowen KK, Naylor M, Vemuganti R. Prevention of inflammation is a mechanism of preconditioning-induced neuroprotection against focal cerebral ischemia. Neurochem Int 2006; 49(2): 127-35.

[45]   Kriz J. Inflammation in ischemic brain injury: timing is important. Crit Rev Neurobiol 2006; 18(1-2): 145-57.

[46]   Franke TF, Hornik CP, Segev L, Shostak GA, Sugimoto C. PI3K/Akt and apoptosis: size matters. Oncogene 2003; 22(56): 8983-98.

[47]   Fresno Vara JA, Casado E, de Castro J, Cejas P, Belda-Iniesta C, Gonzalez-Baron M. PI3K/Akt signalling pathway and cancer. Cancer Treat Rev 2004; 30(2): 193-204.

[48]   Hanada M, Feng J, Hemmings BA. Structure, regulation and function of PKB/AKT--a major therapeutic target. Biochim Biophys Acta 2004; 1697(1-2): 3-16.

[49]   Jiang X, Wang X. Cytochrome C-mediated apoptosis. Annu Rev Biochem 2004; 73: 87-106.

[50]   Sawe N, Steinberg GK, Zhao H. Dual roles of the MAPK/ERK1/2 cell signaling pathway after stroke. J Neurosci Res 2008; 86(8): 1659-69.

[51]   Kamme F, Campbell K, Wieloch T. Biphasic expression of the fos and jun families of transcription factors following transient forebrain ischemia in the rat effect of hypothermia. Eur J Neurosci 1995; 7(10): 2007-16.

[52]   Sutton LN, Clark BJ, Norwood CR, Woodford EJ, Welsh FA. Global cerebral ischemia in piglets under conditions of mild and deep hypothermia. Stroke 1991; 22(12): 1567-73.

[53]   Casabona G. Intracellular signal modulation: a pivotal role for protein kinase C. Prog Neuropsychopharmacol Biol Psychiatry 1997; 21(3): 407-25.

[54]   Koponen S, Goldsteins G, Keinanen R, Koistinaho J. Induction of protein kinase C-delta subspecies in neurons and microglia after transient global brain ischemia. J Cereb Blood Flow Metab 2000; 20(1): 93-102.

[55]   Miettinen S, Roivainen R, Keinanen R, Hokfelt T, Koistinaho J. Specific induction of protein kinase C delta subspecies after transient middle cerebral artery occlusion in the rat brain: inhibition by MK-801. J Neurosci 1996; 16(19): 6236-45.

[56]   Bright R, Raval AP, Dembner JM, Perez-Pinzon MA, Steinberg GK, Yenari MA, Mochly-Rosen D. Protein kinase C delta mediates cerebral reperfusion injury *in vivo*. J Neurosci 2004; 24(31): 6880-8.

26   *Experimental Stroke, 2008, 1, 26-37*

Neovascularization Following Cerebral Ischemia

Rodney Allanigue Gabriel[1] and Guo-Yuan Yang[1,2,*]

[1]*Center for Cerebrovascular Research, Department of Anesthesia and Perioperative Care, University of California San Francisco, San Francisco, CA, USA;* [2]*Med-X Research Institute, Shanghai JiaoTong University, Shanghai, China; E-mail: gyyang@sjtu.edu.cn*

Abstract: Neovascularization is the generation of new blood vessels and is made possible either through vasculogenesis, arteriogenesis, or angiogenesis. This process is far from simple as a plethora of growth factors, cytokines and chemokines, and various cell types are required to interact in a collaborative manner in order to initiate and maintain neovasculature. Because neovascularization process occurs following ischemia or traumatic injury, promoting neovascularization is a potential therapeutic approach to these insults. Exogenous regulation of blood vessel formation is therapeutic when it produces functional and stable capillaries, in which newly proliferating microvessels minimally increase blood-brain-barrier permeability and produce adequate regional cerebral blood flow. To review this issue of cerebral neovascularization, we discuss: 1) important angiogenic growth factors, cytokines, extracellular matrix proteins, and cell types involved in brain angiogenesis; 2) involvement of inflammation in cerebral neovascularization; 3) stem cells play a role in cerebral neovascularization; 4) neovascularization following cerebral ischemia in animal model or in clinical cases; and finally 5) neovascularization as a therapeutic target for cerebral ischemic injury.

INTRODUCTION

Cerebral ischemic stroke is burdened by its high morbidity and mortality. Initially caused by the limitation of blood supply to the brain, cerebral ischemia is a pathological process that may be rescued by physiological mechanisms of neo -vascularization. This concept is widely understood in a sense that various growth factors and pathways have been identified; however, the precise framework at which these entities interact in a synergistic, additive, or antagonistic manner still needs to be clarified. Neovascularization is the generation of new blood vessels and is made possible either through vasculogenesis, arteriogenesis, or angiogenesis. Vasculogenesis is a *de novo* process, in which progenitor stem cells give rise to new vascular networks [1]. Arteriogenesis is a process in which the diameter of an existing arterial vessel increases in order to redirect blood flow to areas of higher demand [2]. Angiogenesis is the development of new capillaries from preexisting microvessels that are involved in the normal development of the vascular system [3, 4] and in pathological processes in the central nervous system (CNS). Due to the wide spectrum of fields related to angiogenesis alone, the scope of this book chapter will not discuss vasculogenesis and arteriogenesis, but instead provide a basic resource for conceptualizing the key players in angiogenesis that follows cerebral ischemia in humans, animal models, and cell culture. We then discuss literature that has elucidated cerebral ischemia-induced angiogenesis in animal models and in the clinical setting, and then conclude with how exogenously-induced neovascularization may be therapeutic for stroke recovery.

MEDIATORS OF NEOVASCULARIZA-TION IN THE BRAIN

Angiogenesis, rather than vasculogenesis, is the main process of organ vascularization during the development of the cerebrovascular system [5]. New vessels sprout from the perineural vascular system and migrate into the developing neuroectoderm [3, 5]. During adulthood, new vessel formation in the brain is virtually absent and present only during pathological and regenerative conditions, as seen in cerebral ischemia, traumatic injury, neoplastic disease, and vascular malformations.

The basis of many neurological diseases is contingent on the disruption of the blood brain barrier (BBB), which is comprised of a single layer of endothelial cells (EC) closely bound together by tight junction proteins [6]. Angiogenic mechanisms that give rise to new microvessels within this complex capillary network involve an array of growth factors, inflammatory mediators, structural proteins, and cell-types interacting with the extracellular matrix (ECM). Several reviews have already described the roles of these growth factors in angiogenesis [3, 4, 7, 8], and therefore, we focus our discussion on the specific roles of these angiogenic mediators in the development and maintenance of the cerebrovasculature and their mitogenic potential specifically to brain micro -vascular ECs.

1. VEGF in brain angiogenesis

VEGF is a soluble glycosylated homodimeric protein with diverse and potent functionality in angiogenesis that can induce EC differentiation, survival, and migration. It promotes vasodilation via upregulation of downstream nitric oxide, thereby permitting microvascular permeability and vessel sprouting [3, 4, 9]. VEGF receptor-1 and -2, termed Flt-1 and Flk-1/KDR, respectively, are tyrosine kinases that are exclusively located on EC membranes. Deficiency of VEGF leading to the impairment of directed growth and invasion of brain capillaries in the embryo suggests that vascularization of the CNS during embryonic development is dependent on this angiogenic mediator [10]. Mice deficient in VEGF-A die *in utero*, while mice lacking VEGF-B, although they survive birth, exhibit impaired protection against cerebral ischemic injury [11]. In the fetal brain, VEGF protein localizes to multiple cell types and its expression levels correlate with angiogenesis [12]. Neuroepithelial cells in the ventricular zone produce VEGF that further attracts blood vessel growth into the brain [10]. During BBB maturation, a latter stage in CNS vasculature development, src-suppressed C-kinase substrate instead reduces VEGF expression, regulates tight junction protein formation, and decreases BBB permeability [13].

By the time the cerebrovasculature system has completed its development, VEGF expression is largely absent in this quiescent state, but is upregulated during some vascular processes in the brain [14-17]. Fibroblast growth factor (FGF), platelet-derived growth factor (PDGF), epidermal growth factor, tumor necrosis factor-α, interleukin-6 (IL-6), and hypoxia-inducible factor-1 alpha (HIF-1α) upregulate VEGF expression in brain diseases [4]. During hypoxic conditions, HIF-1α is stabilized and transactivated to the nucleus where it stimulates target genes, such as VEGF, mounting an angiogenic response to the inciting hypoxia [18-20]. Although appropriate upregulation of VEGF by HIF-1α can lead to pro-angiogenic activity that protects against neurological injury seen following cerebral ischemia, overexpression can be pathological in neoplastic lesions such as gliomas [3, 21].

Phosphorylation of focal adhesion kinase (FAK), Src, Ras, protein kinase B (Akt), and mitogen-activated protein kinase (MAPK) are downstream signaling pathways that follow VEGF-induced activation of Flk-1 and Flt-1 on brain microvascular ECs [22-25]. Cell-to-cell contact and ECM adherence contribute to cell migration and focal adhesion functionality made possible by the activation of these pathways. Downstream signals induce expression of integrins such as αvβ5 and α6β1, but not α6β4, thus subsequently promoting focal cell adhesion and migration of brain ECs [22, 23]. In addition, VEGF promotes brain microvascular EC migration by upregulating intracellular adhesion molecule-1 via phosph-stidylinositol 3 kinase (PI3K) and Akt signaling [24]. Activation of PI3K/Akt by VEGF also upregulates nitric oxide production, a molecule known for its vasodilating and pro-angiogenic ability [26].

Matrix metalloproteinases (MMPs), a class of zinc-dependant endopeptidases, in concert with VEGF, activate vascular remodeling in the brain by promoting ECM breakdown and BBB disruption. VEGF and the angiopoietins are upstream regulators for MMP activity during cerebral angiogenesis [27-30]. Exogenous transduction of VEGF into the brain causes a large increase in MMP-9 expression with an associated increase in cerebral microvessel formation, while inhibition of MMP-9 with doxycycline attenuates this VEGF-induced angiogenesis [30]. Various cells synthesize and release MMPs into the ECM; these include neutrophils, which are a major source of these enzymes during cerebral angiogenesis [31, 32]. MMPs release ECM-bound VEGF in blood vessels by cleaving the matrix-binding domain associated with VEGF [33]. Disruption of the BBB is accomplished by MMP-9 attacking vulnerable tight junction proteins, including occludin and claudin-5, as well as basal lamina proteins, such as type I collagen, fibronectin, laminin, and heparan sulfate [33, 34]. Of particular importance is the tight junction protein zona occludens-1 (ZO-1), which is important for ECM-cell and cell-cell contact, specifically in the maintenance of tight junction formations between brain capillary ECs comprising the BBB. After cerebral ischemia and traumatic brain injury, MMP-9 knockout mice demonstrate decreased degradation of ZO-1 and depressed BBB disruption compared to wild-type mice-- this highlights the direct relationship between MMP-9, tight junction proteins, and BBB integrity [35, 36]. On the other hand, a decrease in ZO-1 and an increase in MMP-9 activity are asso-ciated with exacerbated BBB disruption and vessel remodeling in induced cerebral angiogenesis [37].

2. Angiopoietins in brain angiogenesis

Ang-1 and Ang-2 are the angiopoeitins that serve a dynamic role in brain angiogenesis and exhibit competing functions, made possible by their contrasting interaction with the tyrosine kinase receptor, Tie-2. The former is a natural agonist for the Tie-2 receptor while the latter antagonizes Ang-1-mediated phosphorylation of the receptor. However, Ang-2 may weakly induce Tie-2 autophosphorylation on brain ECs at higher concentrations [3, 38, 39]. The p85 sub-unit of PI3K, Grb2, Shp-2, and Dok-R is bound to the intracellular domain of activated Tie-2 [40]. Phosphorylation of Tie-2 in brain ECs activates PI3K/Akt and MAPK signaling pathway [41]. This downstream signaling following Tie-2 activation, promoted by Ang-1, directs stabilization of endothelial interactions and smooth muscle cells and is therefore coupled to vascular maturation in the cerebrovasculature [3, 39]. Thus, downregulation of Tie-2 phosphorylation, promoted by Ang-2 expression, leads to vascular remodeling as opposed to stabilization.

Angiopoietins are involved in cerebral vascular formation during fetal brain development [13, 42, 43]. For instance, during the development of neural tube vascularization, appropriate Ang-1 expression in motor neurons is a requisite for mediating vessel sprouting from the perineural vascular plexus [42]. Ang-2 is associated with retraction of cerebral blood vessels during embryonic development [43]. During BBB maturation when VEGF expression is decreased, src-suppressed C-kinase substrate functions upstream to the upregulation of Ang-1, which further contributes to the integrity of the BBB [13]. In the adult brain, Ang-1 is constitutively expressed in all cerebral vessels while Ang-2 is largely absent, except within the choroid plexus epithelium and ependymal cells [44].

Although it has no effect on brain EC proliferation *in vitro*, Ang-2 stimulates chemotaxis when these cells are plated on fibronectin plates, and tube-like structure formation when plated on collagen gels [38]. Ang-2 prevents Ang-1 activation of Tie-2; however, higher concentrations of Ang-2 can weakly induce Tie-2 phosphorylation *in vitro* [38, 40]. Autophosphorylation of Tie-2 by high concentrations of Ang-2 leads to activation of downstream mediators including c-Fyn, c-Fes, and PI3K (but not MAPK nor Ras), which together activates tube formation and migration of murine brain capillary ECs [38]. In contrast, Ang-1 dose-dependently induces cell proliferation in brain microvascular ECs *in vitro* by a mechanism that involves activation of PI3K, as well as MAPK [40]. *In vitro* studies for brain microvessel ECs have demonstrated that although both Ang-1 and high con-centrations of Ang-2 phosphorylated Tie-2, the former produced markedly higher phosphorylation [38, 40].

Transplantation of recombinant Ang-2 into the normal rat cortex demonstrates the *in vivo* functionality of Ang-2 in increasing BBB breakdown [45]. Unlike Ang-2, Ang-1 promotes BBB integrity during brain angiogenesis [37, 46]. Moreover, angiopoietins play an important role in pathological angiogenesis, espe-cially in tissue environments following cerebral ische-mia and traumatic brain injury; or during the progre-ssion of cerebrovascular malformations, such as caver-nous malformations and arteriovenous malformations [3, 7, 17, 47].

3. Other Pro-angiogenic factors in brain angiogenesis

PDGF, brain-derived neurotrophic factor (BDNF), FGF, and nitric oxide, to name a few, are other angiogenic factors in cerebral angiogenesis worth mentioning. PDGF is important for cell growth and division, particularly in blood vessel formation [7], and participates in the development and maturation of the CNS [4]. During embryonic development, for example, PDGF-B and its receptor are required for the recruitment of pericytes into brain capillaries [48]. Absence of pericytes covering brain capillaries is phenotypic for PDGF-B-deficient mice and consequently leads to irregularly shaped, unstable blood vessels with increased capillary diameter and transendothelial permeability within the cerebrovasculature system [48, 49].

BDNF is part of a larger group of neurotrophins that promotes EC survival and induces angiogenesis in ischemic tissues [50]. It activates its tyrosine kinase receptor TrkB on brain-derived ECs to induce angiogenic sprouting and cell survival via downstream activation of the PI3K/Akt pathway [51]. Furthermore, brain-derived ECs exhibit increased production of BDNF in hypoxic environments [51].

FGF and its receptor are widely distributed throughout the CNS [4]. Within the BBB environment, FGF-2 is primarily produced by the astrocytes that are at close proximity to the ECs [52]. Activation of phospholipase C, Src, and MAPK by FGF receptor-1 direct brain endothelial proliferation and differentiation [53]. FGF-2 stimulates Src-dependent tube formation in murine brain capillary ECs when cultured on collagen-coated surfaces; however, it promotes cell proliferation and migration without tube formation in these cells grown on fibronectin-coated surfaces [53, 54]. FGF-2 also induces sustained MAPK activation, which is necessary for brain endothelial proliferation *in vitro* [54], and is also important for chemotaxis and focal adhesion interactions in brain capillary ECs [55, 56]. Specifically, it activates Fes, a non-receptor protein tyrosine kinase, which enhances FAK-dependant activation of Src within focal adhesions, thereby promoting disassembly of focal adhesions and cell migration [57]. This growth factor induces maintenance of tight junction proteins ZO-1, occludin, claudin-5, and claudin-3 in an *in vitro* cortical organotypic slice culture, suggesting that this growth factor potentially influences BBB integrity [58, 59].

During the initial phases of angiogenesis, nitric oxide mediates vasodilation prior to vessel sprouting, among other functions important for angiogenesis [4]. Endothelial nitric oxide synthase (eNOS) is an EC enzyme that synthesizes nitric oxide from the terminal L-arginine. During embryonic development of the CNS vasculature, eNOS is widely expressed in the endothelial lining of all types of blood vessels and the choroid plexus in the developing fetal rat brain [60]. During adulthood, eNOS protein is also present in ECs of the vasculature and choroid plexus of the rat brain [60, 61]. Nitric oxide donor promotes capillary tube formation in cultured brain ECs via activation of guanylate cyclase [62, 63]. *In vivo*, it induces Ang-1/Tie2 expression in the brain and stabilizes angiogenic vessels following stroke [63]. Induction of a nitric oxide donor into the mouse brain also enhances SDF-1 and CXCR4 expression, which further promotes bone marrow cell (BMC) migration into the angiogenic focus [64].

INVOLVEMENT OF INFLAMMATION IN CEREBRAL NEOVASCULARIZATION

Inflammatory response is a cardinal element of angiogenesis, especially for leukocyte recruitment and signaling in vascular remodeling. Interleukins are produced by ECs and leukocytes, which is a dynamic group of inflammatory cytokines involved in acute phase reactions, chemotaxis, leukocytic activation, and temperature regulation. Various interleukins, including IL-1, IL-6, and IL-8, also contribute to the regulation of brain microvessel ECs involved in angiogenesis [65-67]. During CNS vascular development, interleukin expression coincides with VEGF mRNA expression and is decreased following birth [68].

In brain vascular endothelial and smooth muscle cells, some interleukins induce angiogenic activity through mechanisms involving VEGF and MMPs [16, 68-70]. Specifically, IL-1β favors plasticity and permeability in the BBB by a mechanism that involves inducing the expression of HIF-1α and its target, VEGF, in astrocytes [69]. IL-6 is a multifunctional cytokine with potent roles in inducing cell proliferation, differentiation, and apoptosis [66]. This interleukin induces vascular smooth muscle cell activation by stimulating smooth muscle cell proliferation, VEGF release, and upregulation of VEGFR and MMP-9 *in vitro* [16]. Furthermore, IL-6 increases proliferation and migration of cerebral ECs *in vitro* by a mechanism that involves successive upregulation of MMP-3 and MMP-9 [68, 71]. Interestingly, transgenic mice that overexpress IL-6 present with a neurological disease manifested with increased angiogenesis in the cerebellum [72]. IL-6 also stimulates proliferation, migration, and tube formation in endothelial progenitor cell (EPC) angiogenesis *in vitro* [66]. IL-8 mediates angiogenesis by enhancing proliferation, survival, and MMP expression in ECs [67, 73]. Induction of IL-8 in brain microvessel ECs by VEGF promotes leukocyte infiltration into active angiogenic sites [25].

STEM CELLS PLAY A ROLE IN CEREBRAL NEOVASCULARIZATION

BMCs have been well defined in their ability to differentiate into multiple cell-types that are essential for new blood vessel formation. Notably, cells originating from bone marrow-derived EPC and myeloid cells contribute to angiogenic activity in the brain. BMCs' differentiation travels along a step-by-step process that ultimately produces committed cells within the myeloid or lymphoid lineage. Less frequently, BMCs may also differentiate into endothelial and smooth muscle cells [74-76]. Macrophages are important cells for angiogenesis in both inflammatory response and tumorigenic processes. It is known that macrophages are a source for various angiogenic factors (including urokinase-type tissue plasminogen activator, angiotropin, MMPs, transforming growth factor-β, fibronectin, and PDGF [77]), and are able to release bFGF [78]. Increased macrophage infiltration induced by granulocyte-macrophage colony-stimulating factor promotes cerebrovascular arteriogenesis and improves functional improvement of brain hemodynamic patterns [79]. Similarly, neutrophil plays an important role in facilitating focal angiogenesis in the brain by providing a major source of VEGF, MMPs, and elastases [31, 80].

Rapid mobilization of BMCs is initiated following acute tissue injury. Subpopulations of BM-derived EPCs exist within specialized regions in the BM that are ready for rapid release into the circulation [74]. Following ischemic damage, HIF-1α expression is enhanced and induces the expression of stromal cell-derived factor-1 (SDF-1, also named CXCL12), a chemokine largely accountable for progenitor cell trafficking [19]. With its high reactivity with the BMC receptor CXCR4, this chemokine has a pivotal role in the recruitment and retention of BMCs to sites requiring revascularization of ischemic tissue [19]. Once homed to the angiogenic focus, BMCs introduce a rich source of growth factors or lay resident as structural cells for new blood vessel development in the brain.

Recruitment and proliferation of various cell-types involved in post-ischemic vessel formation are contingent on the locally increased growth factors, cytokines, and chemokines. An increase in SDF-1 occurs within the ischemic region following stroke and is further associated with homing of BMCs [81, 82]. During cerebral stroke, BMCs are recruited to the site of injury, with most vessel-associated and parenchymal-associated BMCs resembling pericytes or perivascular microglia and activated microglia, respectively [82, 83]. Increased number of macrophages is regionally distributed to the area of increased microvessel density following ischemia [84]. Furthermore, bone marrow-derived EPCs participate in the angiogenesis process taking place at the boundary of the infarct zone following cerebral ischemic onset [75].

CEREBRAL ISCHEMIA INDUCES NEOVASCULARIZATION IN ANIMAL MODELS

In rodents, it is clear that after transient middle cerebral artery occlusion (tMCAO), microvessel density increases especially within the inner margin of the cystic infarct; this hyperdense vasculature is accompanied by increased leakiness [85]. By 30-90 days after ischemic onset, vessel hyperdensity regresses significantly [85]. T2-weighted MRI imaging demonstrates increased angiogenesis 4 weeks after initiation of embolic stroke in mice [86].

HIF-1α expression in hypoxic tissue is upregulated in a time-related manner around the ischemic boundary zone and induces various signaling pathways, one of which involves the upregulation of VEGF [87, 88]. VEGF mRNA expression is evident 1 hour after reperfusion following MCAO in rat and peaks at 3 to 24 hours thereafter [14, 15]. The length of ischemia makes no difference in the degree and temporal profile of VEGF mRNA [14]; however, VEGF immunoreactivity is more pronounced in permanent MCAO (pMCAO) than tMCAO in rats [89]. ECs and glial-like cells within the ischemic core and perifocal area are some cell-types co-stained with VEGF expression [90]. Flt-1 increases in neurons, glial cells, and ECs while Flk-1 is prominent in glial cells and ECs following cerebral ischemia [89].

VEGF mediates eNOS expression of nitric oxide following cerebral ischemia [91]. Interestingly, the phosphorylation state of eNOS is important in regards to vascular reactivity following stroke. Specifically, the phosphorylation state of the serine 1179 position for eNOS protein, which is associated with increased NO expression, correlates with better response to stroke and improvement of regional cerebral blood flow (rCBF) following tMCAO in animals [92].

Two to four hours following induction of embolic MCAO in a rat model, a decrease in Ang-1 mRNA occurs simultaneously with an increase in VEGF within the boundary of the infarct lesion [93]. However, Ang-1 and Tie-2 receptor expression remain unchanged within the infarct region after permanent MCAO in mice [90]. After 2 to 28 days following MCAO, Ang-1 and its receptor are increased instead [93]. Since Ang-1 expression is normally increased in non-angiogenic states, which is characterized by quiescent and stable vasculature, its reduction in expression early after stroke may complement VEGF's role in angiogenesis. As VEGF induces angiogenesis, reduction of Ang-1 partially explains the consequent BBB leakage. In contrast to Ang-1, Ang-2 mRNA expression increases early within the infarct and peri-infarct zone, as shown in a mouse model for pMCAO, which also coincides with an upregulation of VEGF expression [90]. Protein receptors for angiopoietins and Tie-1/Tie-2 have a biphasic pattern of expression post-ischemia and are expressed exclusively on ECs [94]. Early gene expression for VEGF and Ang-2 following stroke is involved with vascular sprouting, while later gene expression for Ang-1 is implicated in vessel maturation and stabilization.

VEGF and Ang-2 also regulate MMP expression during ischemia, which is partly responsible for breakdown of the BBB and subsequent vascular remodeling [27-29]. In addition, extracellular MMP inducer (EMMPRIN) may play a key regulatory role for MMP production following cerebral ischemia. Following pMCAO, EMMPRIN localizes to endothelial and perivascular astrocytes, and its expression is correlated with MMP-9 levels in both a spatial and temporal manner [95]. Clinical data demonstrate that an increase in plasma MMP levels is correlated with outcome in stroke patients [96]. Following MCAO in animals, reperfusion leads to biphasic opening of the BBB with early stages high in MMP-2 activation and later stages (24-48 hours after) with more intense expression of MMP-9 and MMP-3 [27, 34]. Temporal profiling of MMP-9 after pMCAO demonstrates that MMP-9 is upregulated after 12 hours, peaks after 24 hours for 5 days, and returns to basal levels after 15 days; MMP-9 co-localized with ECs, macrophages and neutrophils within the periphery of the infarct [97]. Early expression levels of MMP-9 following stroke promote BBB disruption and hemorrhage by degrading the ECM; however, delayed expression of MMP-9, 7 to 14 days after stroke in animals, is associated with neurovascular modeling and affords beneficial cortical responses [98]. Interestingly, treatment of MMP-9 inhibitor at a later versus earlier period after stroke suppresses neurovascular modeling and increases ischemic brain injury [98].

bFGF is part of the heparin-binding protein family and serves as an EC mitogen, angiogenic factor, and neurotophic factor [99]. After tMCAO in the rodent brain, bFGF mRNA expression increases 2.5-fold within the ischemic cortex after 60 minutes and remains elevated for 2 weeks, whereby localization of bFGF mRNA remains proximal to areas with increased blood vessel density and co-localizes primarily with astrocytes and other cells [99]. Peak expression of bFGF mRNA is noted at 12 to 24 hours after tMCAO [100]. Upregulation of PDGF follows tMCAO in rats and is localized especially in the perifocal area [101]. PDGF-B and its receptor are upregulated in vascular structures, mainly on pericytes, after cerebral ischemia [102, 103].

NEOVASCULARIZATION FOLLOWING CLINICAL CEREBRAL ISCHEMIA INJURY

Most of what we know in regards to post-ischemic pathological angiogenesis has been derived from studies in rodent models. Whether these findings are translatable to the clinical arena remains an unanswered question. Magnetic resonance imaging (MRI) analysis demonstrates that angiogenesis is activated following stroke incidence in humans and that this restorative process coupled with neurogenesis is correlated to better neurological outcome [104]. Although the temporal and spatial profile of various angiogenic growth factors are better understood in animal models, there is some understanding in the similarities of expression profiles in humans versus in the laboratory. Various isotypes of VEGF protein as well as its receptor, KDR, are upregulated in human brain ischemic tissue within the perifocal region, specifically in neurons, ECs, and astrocytes [105]. Compared to age-matched controls, VEGF expression peaked at seven days after stroke onset and remained elevated by day 14. Furthermore, expression of VEGF correlates with infarct volume and clinical outcome [106]. Downstream signaling induced by VEGF, including MAPK tyrosine phosphorylation, may also be activated specifically in the grey matter of the penumbra [107]. Within the infarct core and penumbral region, FGF-2 and PDGF are also upregulated, mainly in neurons, astrocytes, macrophages, and ECs [103, 108]. Additionally, high levels of active TGF-β are found in the ischemic penumbra [109]. Interestingly, circulating EPCs are increased in ischemic stroke patients compared to healthy individuals. In fact, lower levels of these stem cells are predictive of worse stroke outcome in humans, whereas higher levels are associated with good functional outcome and reduced infarct growth [110, 111].

Changes in the ECM are also important in post-ischemic cerebral angiogenesis in humans. Hyaluronan is important in cerebral ECM for the regulation of angiogenesis. Overexpression of hyaluronan regulators, including hyaludinodases and hyaluronan synthases, are apparent days after stroke onset in humans–these regulators are upregulated in microvessels and neurons located in peri-infarcted areas [112]. Furthermore, MMP-9 levels are increased in both the infarct core and peri-infarct tissue within stroke patients, mainly co-localized with neutrophilic infiltrates and activated microglial cells [113]. These ECM components as well as the mentioned growth factors may play similar roles in animal stroke models and human stroke pathophysiology. Perhaps a proper balance of each of these components is necessary for ideal clinical recovery following ischemic injury in the brain. More interesting research can focus on relative levels of angiogenic factors like VEGF, FGF-2, MMP-9, etc., and how their expression levels in both a temporal and spatial entity can predict clinical outcome.

On the other hand, studies have shown the potential usefulness of interleukins as predictors for clinical outcome in stroke patients. Interleukins are important inflammatory mediators involved in the patho-physiology of stroke and are key players in angiogenesis. How they specifically contribute to post-ischemic cerebral angiogenesis is better understood in animal and cell culture models than in the human disease. IL-6, IL-8, and IL-10, and IL-18 are some cytokines released following stroke in humans [114-116]. Plasma levels of these molecules show promise in their ability to predict stroke outcome. IL-18 levels are an independent predictor for outcome after MCAO in humans, whereby higher levels (>780 pg/mL) demonstrate significantly higher incidences of recurrent stroke and accumulative death within 90 days after initial onset [114]. Peak plasma IL-6 levels correlate with CT brain infarction volume [117]. Levels of this interleukin are also an independent risk factor for early clinical worsening [118, 119]. Other inflammatory mediators associated with worsening stroke outcome include ICAM-1, C-reactive protein, and serum amyloid A [119, 120]. Interestingly, leukocyte counts, mainly neutrophils, are independent risk factors for recurrent ischemic events within one week following initial onset in humans [121]. Contrarily, lower concentrations of IL-10, an anti-inflammatory interleukin, are correlated with neurological worsening in stroke patients, specifically in patients with subcortical infarcts or lacunar strokes but not with cortical lesions [115]. Aside from their functions in recruiting leukocytes that may damage prone tissue, the impact of the levels of these inflammatory mediators on stroke outcome may also be partly explained by its contribution to angiogenesis. Any imbalance in angiogenic factors can either lead to reduced collateral growth or overgrowth of leaky edematous vessels, which both can lead to worse clinical outcome. In any case, the value of elucidating the mechanisms at which angiogenesis is regulated in clinical stroke is obvious.

NEOVASCULARIZATION AS A THERAPEUTIC TARGET FOR CEREBRAL ISCHEMIC INJURY

Strategies that inhibit angiogenesis in brain tumors have amassed promising therapeutic results in numerous clinical trials [3]. Although progression of these diseases is dependent on angiogenesis, in others, such as cerebral ischemia or brain injury, pro-angiogenic effects are instead curative. Various methodologies and the mechanisms of activating angiogenesis in animal models have been extensively explored [37, 46, 122-124]. We introduce the term "functional cerebral angiogenesis" (FCA) to describe an overall attempt to induce "healthy" blood vessel formation in the brain that minimally disrupts the BBB and improves rCBF. By inducing single angiogenic factor, multiple angiogenic factors, or pro-angiogenic cell types, it is possible to modulate FCA in the brain.

1. Single angiogenic factor hyperstimulation

Viral delivery or protein transfusion of $VEGF_{165}$ [123-125] and $VEGF_{164}$ [126] induces actively proliferating microvessel formation in the mouse brain, which is observed one to two weeks after transplantation and can be maintained for up to 12 weeks. Neurons, astrocytes, and ECs are co-localized to VEGF during this exogenous stimulating angiogenesis. VEGF is able to improve rCBF after gene transfer in the ischemic brain; however, the formation of leaky, immature, and unstable vessels follows after early administration of VEGF following MCAO, which demonstrates deleterious effects that compromise the BBB and increase brain edema [127-129]. VEGF has an effect on enlarging small vessels and its mechanism in cerebral angiogenesis includes upregulation of MMP-9 and downregulation of ZO-1, which may further contribute to the apparent VEGF-induced edema [37, 46, 130].

Addressing these consequent deleterious effects of VEGF on angiogenic factor-induced cerebral vessel formation is not trivial, highlighted by evidence that prior sequestration of VEGF with the fusion protein mFlt(1-3)-IgG attenuates infarct volume by means of reducing edema and vascular leakiness [131]. Inhibition of VEGF via gene transfer of soluble Flt-1, a natural inhibitor of VEGF, also attenuates cerebral ischemic injury when transduced shortly after artery occlusion [132]. Although the observation that VEGF is deleterious to a disease characterized by insufficient blood flow sounds counterintuitive, it instead corroborates the multidimensional nature of angiogenesis and how a specific balance of growth factors needs to be maintained during an appropriate temporal profile in order develop FCA. To address this issue, one option is to implement methods that induce angiogenesis by introducing other growth factors that can perhaps concomitantly minimize BBB disruption, increase rCBF, and upregulate new vessel formation.

HOXD3, insulin growth factor-1 (IGF-1), HGF, FGF, BDNF, and nitric oxide each are promising and attractive agents. HOXD3 is part of the homeobox family of transcription factors that can upregulate angiogenesis by inducing integrin, urokinase-type plasminogen activator, and type I collagen expression [133, 134]. Retroviral delivery of HOXD3 into the mouse brain greatly induces microvessel formation, increases rCBF, and maintains vascular leakage [122]. IGF-1 participates in vascular remodeling in the adult brain and has been demonstrated *in vitro* to induce growth of brain ECs by a mechanism involving HIF-1α and VEGF upregulation [135]. After systemic injection, IGF-1 localizes to the luminal side of brain vessels and increases brain vessel density [135]. In a stroke model in rodents, long-term cerebral IGF-1 overexpression contributes to increased vascular density and local vascular perfusion in the peri-infarct region, which is related to better functional outcome and reduced

infarct volume [136]. FGF-2 and FGF-18 are able to improve rCBF following MCAO, whereby FGF-18 demonstrates better outcomes relative to FGF-2 [137]. HGF is originally characterized as a potent mitogen for hepatocytes, but currently found to have pro-angiogenic functions in human ECs and haemopoietic progenitor cells [138]. HGF stimulates angiogenesis with limited cerebral edema or BBB destruction in the rodent brain and has been used to improve rCBF and collateral formation after cerebral hypoperfusion [127, 139]. Also, adenovirus-mediated transfer of heparin-binding EGF-like growth factor can enhance angiogenesis in the peri-infarct striatum in a model for cerebral ischemia in mice [140].

Nitric oxide and eNOS also have potential in therapeutic cerebral angiogenesis, which has been shown in stroke and traumatic brain injury animal studies of active angiogenesis [62, 64, 141]. Nitric oxide levels in stroke patients are associated with severity and outcome, with lower levels associated with poorer outcome [142]. Following cerebral ischemia, increased physical activity can upregulate eNOS in the vasculature, which leads to increased newly generated cells in vascular sites, increased density of perfused microvessels, and sustained augmentation of rCBF within the ischemic striatum; these protective effects are abolished with eNOS inhibitor and are lacking in eNOS-deficient mice [143]. Furthermore, MCAO-induced cerebral ischemia in eNOS-deficient mice presents with decreased post-ischemic angiogenesis, demonstrated by decreased EC proliferation and vascular density within the ischemic border [91]. This is associated with a decrease in BDNF expression, but not VEGF and bFGF in the ischemic brain [91]. Other mechanisms whereby nitric oxide may be protective following ischemic attack in the brain include enhanced expression of SDF-1, which further promotes more bone marrow derived cells to the injured tissue, and downregulation of ischemia-induced heat shock proteins [64]. Administration of sildenafil, a phosphodiesterase inhibitor that can potentially enhance NO-induced cGMP production in vascular beds, promotes angiogenesis and improves rCBF following embolic stroke in rats, demonstrated by MRI imaging [86, 144]. Inhibition of Rho kinase, a mediator that downregulates eNOS under hypoxic conditions, similarly increases rCBF and reduces cerebral infarct size in a stroke model [145].

The chemokine CCL2 contributes to angiogenesis by recruiting macrophages to wound injury sites. This chemokine can induce expression of several angiogenic factors in brain ECs, some of which include β3 integrins [146]. The glycoprotein hormone, erythropoietin, is a cytokine for erythryocyte precursors that reduce ischemic injury in a VEGF-dependent manner [147, 148]. Known to be a key signal for blood cell production, EPO may also contribute to angiogenesis in injured tissue. This is confirmed by its ability to induce FCA by promoting endothelial proliferation and improving rCBF [147-149]. Pro-angiogenic genes, Tie-2, Ang-2, and VEGF are upregulated downstream to erythropoietin induction [148]. Furthermore, erythropoietin reduces brain edema formation in experimental traumatic brain injury [150].

Transplantation of growth factors that stimulate BMC mobilization, especially granulocyte colony-stimulating factor (G-CSF) and SDF-1, is an alternative strategy for inducing cerebral angiogenesis. Exogenous introduction of G-CSF is successful in reducing ischemic damage while attenuating edema formation [151-156]. G-CSF enhances the availability of bone marrow-derived hematopoietic stem cells in the damaged brain tissue, increasing vascularization in that focal area [154]. Co-introduction of G-CSF and Stem Cell Factor, a cytokine important for hematopoietic survival and differentiation, contributes to a significant increase in vessel formation and endothelial cell migration in the brain following MCAO [157]. SDF-1 induces vascularization within the perifocal area of a pig myocardial infarct model; however, it failed to improve myocardial perfusion [158]. SDF-1 gene transfer enhances vasculogenesis and angiogenesis via VEGF/eNOS-dependant pathway in the ischemic limb [159]. When introduced intracerebrally into stroke rats, an increase in vascular density along with enhanced functional rCBF occurred [160].

2. Multiple angiogenic factor hyperstimulation

Multiple factor hyper-stimulation of angiogenesis may provide a novel means to synergistically induce FCA in the brain. Because angiogenesis is a complex process, in which multiple factors cooperate to produce functional vessels, exogenous delivery of a single factor may not be sufficient to induce healthy vasculature. Both timing and balance of various factors are crucial for FCA; therefore, single angiogenic factor-induced angiogenesis may disrupt this balance and temporal profile. For example, VEGF is highly potent in inducing microvessel formation in the brain; however it also overly disrupts BBB integrity and consequently produces microvessel leakage [27]. SDF-1 improves angiogenesis in myocardial ischemia, but it does not improve overall perfusion [158]. To address this issue, exogenous delivery of multiple factors may produce more efficient and healthier vessels.

Co-expression of other angiogenic factors that can modulate and maintain BBB integrity with VEGF is a potential strategy for angiogenic therapy. Early administration of VEGF after MCAO demonstrates deleterious effects, which compromises BBB and increases brain edema [129]. Although co-administration of Ang-2 and VEGF protein into the mouse brain increases microvessel proliferation compared to VEGF alone, it further exacerbates vascular leakage by a mechanism that involves downregulation of ZO-1 and upregulation of MMP-9 [37]. This is expected as Ang-2 antagonizes the Tie2/Tek signal pathway and is involved in vascular remodeling and BBB breakdown. On the other hand, co-administration of VEGF protein with Ang-1 induces microvessel formation while reducing BBB leakage compared to VEGF alone, as confirmed by subsequent increased ZO-1 level and decreased MMP-9 activity [27, 46]. Ang-1 induces microvessel sprouting, branching, and further stabilizes and protects the adult vasculature. Its usefulness in reducing infarct volume and edema formation following cerebral ischemia demonstrates potential for combining these mediators [27].

3. Cell-induced angiogenesis in the brain

Stem cells from multiple sources, such as BMC, embryonic, and peripheral blood stem cells, can promote angiogenesis within ischemic tissue [161-164]. Post-ischemic angiogenesis requires participation of bone-marrow derived EPCs [75], peri-vascular microglia [82], and pericytes [165]. BM-derived stromal cells induce capillary-like tube formation in mouse brain ECs *in vitro* and upregulate angiogenesis *in vivo* as well [166-169]. Intravenously administered BMCs reduce ischemic injury and enhance vascular density and angiogenic factor expression in rodents exposed to MCAO [170]. The mechanism by which these stem cells can activate angiogenesis is dependent on downstream upregulation of angiogenic factors VEGF and Flk-1 [171], upregulation of homing factors SDF-1 receptor and CXCR4 [169], increase in β-integrin expression [167], and differentiation into various cells including ECs [167]. Induction of vessel growth by BM-derived stromal cells in cerebral ischemia also exhibits decreased BBB leakage by a mechanism that involves an increase in Ang-1, Tie-2, and occludin expression [172]. The therapeutic effects of BMCs in stroke are evident even after one year following MCAO in rats, in which BM derived cells differentiated to astrocytes, neurons, microglial cells, and ECs, in that order [169]. Interestingly, BMCs transfected with Ang-1 activates angiogenesis and improves rCBF after cerebral ischemia in mice at a greater extent than BMCs alone [173]. A similar finding is shown in Ang-1-modified human mesenchymal cells [174]. Likewise, BDNF gene-modified mesenchymal cells and FGF-2 gene-modified stem cells provided added benefit to stroke outcome versus non-modified stem cells [175, 176].

Circulating EPCs from peripheral blood home into sites of angiogenesis and differentiate into mature ECs [177, 178]. Here, EPCs contribute to *de novo* vascular formation during wound healing, post-myocardial infarction, and limb ischemia [177, 179, 180]. EPCs' ability to aid in endothelial repair after ischemia in cardiac or peripheral circulation has been studied [181]. Higher circulating EPCs are actually correlated to better functional outcome and reduced infarct volume in stroke patients [111]. After 48 hours of cerebral ischemia in rats that were intravenously transplanted with EPCs, attenuation of ischemic brain injury was indicated, demonstrated by reduced infarct volume and improved rCBF [182].

Embryonic stem cells (ESCs) are distinguished by their unlimited capacity for self-renewal and pluripotency. In cell culture, human ESCs can differentiate into ECs and can participate in vasculogenesis by matrigel assay [163, 166]. Although ESCs can successfully induce capillary and venule formation within infarct zones in the mouse heart [183], more studies need to be undertaken that confirm the angiogenic potential of EPCs and ESCs in the brain vasculature, including its contribution to BBB integrity.

SUMMARY

Angiogenesis is a central component of tissue rescue in response to ischemic injury to the brain. This is mainly an embryological process in the CNS in that when occurring in the adult brain, it is associated with pathological processes, especially stroke. Neovascularization in this regard is a complicated aspect of science as various growth factors interplay with many different cell-types, extracellular components, and inflammatory mediators. Understanding the mechanism at which these growth factors, both at the temporal and spatial level, are critical to other components of angiogenesis is currently under rigorous investigation. With this knowledge, new angiogenic therapies can be innovated in a way that enhances regeneration following cerebral ischemia.

REFERENCES

[1]   Schmidt A, Brixius K, Bloch W. Endothelial precursor cell migration during vasculogenesis. Circ Res 2007 Jul 20; 101(2): 125-36.

[2]   Grundmann S, Piek JJ, Pasterkamp G, Hoefer IE. Arteriogenesis: basic mechanisms and therapeutic stimulation. Eur J Clin Invest 2007 Oct; 37(10): 755-66.

[3]   Zadeh G, Guha A. Angiogenesis in nervous system disorders. Neurosurgery 2003 Dec; 53(6): 1362-74; discussion 74-6.

[4]   Harrigan MR. Angiogenic factors in the central nervous system. Neurosurgery 2003 Sep; 53(3): 639-60; discussion 60-1.

[5]   Greenberg DA, Jin K. From angiogenesis to neuropathology. Nature 2005 Dec 15; 438(7070): 954-9.

[6]   Persidsky Y, Ramirez SH, Haorah J, Kanmogne GD. Blood-brain barrier: structural components and function under physiologic and pathologic conditions. J Neuroimmune Pharmacol 2006 Sep; 1(3): 223-36.

[7]   Lim M, Cheshier S, Steinberg GK. New vessel formation in the central nervous system during tumor growth, vascular malformations, and Moyamoya. Curr Neurovasc Res 2006 Aug; 3(3): 237-45.

[8]   Fan Y, Yang GY. Therapeutic angiogenesis for brain ischemia: a brief review. J Neuroimmune Pharmacol 2007 Sep; 2(3): 284-9.

[9]   Ahmad S, Hewett PW, Wang P, et al. Direct evidence for endothelial vascular endothelial growth factor receptor-1 function in nitric oxide-mediated angiogenesis. Circ Res 2006 Sep 29; 99(7): 715-22.

[10]   Raab S, Beck H, Gaumann A, et al. Impaired brain angiogenesis and neuronal apoptosis induced by conditional homozygous inactivation of vascular endothelial growth factor. Thromb Haemost 2004 Mar; 91(3): 595-605.

[11]   Sun Y, Jin K, Childs JT, Xie L, Mao XO, Greenberg DA. Increased severity of cerebral ischemic injury in vascular endothelial growth factor-B-deficient mice. J Cereb Blood Flow Metab 2004 Oct; 24(10): 1146-52.

[12]   Virgintino D, Errede M, Robertson D, Girolamo F, Masciandaro A, Bertossi M. VEGF expression is developmentally regulated during human brain angiogenesis. Histochem Cell Biol 2003 Mar; 119(3): 227-32.

[13]   Lee SW, Kim WJ, Choi YK, et al. SSeCKS regulates angiogenesis and tight junction formation in blood-brain barrier. Nat Med 2003 Jul; 9(7): 900-6.

[14]   Hayashi T, Abe K, Suzuki H, Itoyama Y. Rapid induction of vascular endothelial growth factor gene expression after transient middle cerebral artery occlusion in rats. Stroke 1997 Oct; 28(10): 2039-44.

[15]   Plate KH, Beck H, Danner S, Allegrini PR, Wiessner C. Cell type specific upregulation of vascular endothelial growth factor in an MCA-occlusion model of cerebral infarct. J Neuropathol Exp Neurol 1999 Jun; 58(6): 654-66.

[16]   Yao JS, Zhai W, Fan Y, et al. Interleukin-6 upregulates expression of KDR and stimulates proliferation of human cerebrovascular smooth muscle cells. J Cereb Blood Flow Metab 2007 Mar; 27(3): 510-20.

[17]   Hashimoto T, Wu Y, Lawton MT, Yang GY, Barbaro NM, Young WL. Coexpression of angiogenic factors in brain arteriovenous malformations. Neurosurgery 2005 May; 56(5): 1058-65; discussion -65.

[18]   Post DE, Van Meir EG. Generation of bidirectional hypoxia/HIF-responsive expression vectors to target gene expression to hypoxic cells. Gene Ther 2001 Dec; 8(23): 1801-7.

[19]   Ceradini DJ, Kulkarni AR, Callaghan MJ, et al. Progenitor cell trafficking is regulated by hypoxic gradients through HIF-1 induction of SDF-1. Nat Med 2004 Aug; 10(8): 858-64.

[20]   Gillespie DL, Whang K, Ragel BT, Flynn JR, Kelly DA, Jensen RL. Silencing of hypoxia inducible factor-1alpha by RNA interference attenuates human glioma cell growth in vivo. Clin Cancer Res 2007 Apr 15; 13(8): 2441-8.

[21]   Shen F, Fan Y, Su H, et al. Adeno-associated viral vector-mediated hypoxia-regulated VEGF gene transfer promotes angiogenesis following focal cerebral ischemia in mice. Gene Ther 2008 Jan; 15(1): 30-9.

[22]   Avraham HK, Lee TH, Koh Y, et al. Vascular endothelial growth factor regulates focal adhesion assembly in human brain microvascular endothelial cells through activation of the focal adhesion kinase and related adhesion focal tyrosine kinase. J Biol Chem 2003 Sep 19; 278(38): 36661-8.

[23]   Lee TH, Seng S, Li H, Kennel SJ, Avraham HK, Avraham S. Integrin regulation by vascular endothelial growth factor in human brain microvascular endothelial cells: role of alpha6beta1 integrin in angiogenesis. J Biol Chem 2006 Dec 29; 281(52): 40450-60.

[24]   Radisavljevic Z, Avraham H, Avraham S. Vascular endothelial growth factor up-regulates ICAM-1 expression via the phosphatidylinositol 3 OH-kinase/AKT/Nitric oxide pathway and modulates migration of brain microvascular endothelial cells. J Biol Chem 2000 Jul 7; 275(27): 20770-4.

[25]   Lee TH, Avraham H, Lee SH, Avraham S. Vascular endothelial growth factor modulates neutrophil transendothelial migration via up-regulation of interleukin-8 in human brain microvascular endothelial cells. J Biol Chem 2002 Mar 22; 277(12): 10445-51.

[26]   Vogel C, Bauer A, Wiesnet M, et al. Flt-1, but not Flk-1 mediates hyperpermeability through activation of the PI3-K/Akt pathway. J Cell Physiol 2007 Jul; 212(1): 236-43.

[27]   Valable S, Montaner J, Bellail A, et al. VEGF-induced BBB permeability is associated with an MMP-9 activity increase in cerebral ischemia: both effects decreased by Ang-1. J Cereb Blood Flow Metab 2005 Nov; 25(11): 1491-504.

[28]   Das A, Fanslow W, Cerretti D, Warren E, Talarico N, McGuire P. Angiopoietin/Tek interactions regulate mmp-9 expression and retinal neovascularization. Lab Invest 2003 Nov; 83(11): 1637-45.

[29]   Wang H, Keiser JA. Vascular endothelial growth factor upregulates the expression of matrix metalloproteinases in vascular smooth muscle cells: role of flt-1. Circ Res 1998 Oct 19; 83(8): 832-40.

[30]   Lee CZ, Xu B, Hashimoto T, McCulloch CE, Yang GY, Young WL. Doxycycline suppresses cerebral matrix metalloproteinase-9 and angiogenesis induced by focal hyperstimulation of vascular endothelial growth factor in a mouse model. Stroke 2004 Jul; 35(7): 1715-9.

[31]   Hao Q, Chen Y, Zhu Y, et al. Neutrophil depletion decreases VEGF-induced focal angiogenesis in the mature mouse brain. J Cereb Blood Flow Metab 2007 Nov; 27(11): 1853-60.

[32]   Chakraborti S, Mandal M, Das S, Mandal A, Chakraborti T. Regulation of matrix metalloproteinases: an overview. Mol Cell Biochem 2003 Nov; 253(1-2): 269-85.

[33]   Page-McCaw A, Ewald AJ, Werb Z. Matrix metalloproteinases and the regulation of tissue remodelling. Nat Rev Mol Cell Biol 2007 Mar; 8(3): 221-33.

[34]   Rosenberg GA, Yang Y. Vasogenic edema due to tight junction disruption by matrix metalloproteinases in cerebral ischemia. Neurosurg Focus 2007; 22(5): E4.

[35]   Mori T, Wang X, Aoki T, Lo EH. Downregulation of matrix metalloproteinase-9 and attenuation of edema via inhibition of ERK mitogen activated protein kinase in traumatic brain injury. J Neurotrauma 2002 Nov; 19(11): 1411-9.

[36]   Asahi M, Wang X, Mori T, et al. Effects of matrix metalloproteinase-9 gene knock-out on the proteolysis of blood-brain barrier and white matter components after cerebral ischemia. J Neurosci 2001 Oct 1; 21(19): 7724-32.

[37]   Zhu Y, Lee C, Shen F, Du R, Young WL, Yang GY. Angiopoietin-2 facilitates vascular endothelial growth factor-induced angiogenesis in the mature mouse brain. Stroke 2005 Jul; 36(7): 1533-7.

[38]   Mochizuki Y, Nakamura T, Kanetake H, Kanda S. Angiopoietin 2 stimulates migration and tube-like structure formation of murine brain capillary endothelial cells through c-Fes and c-Fyn. J Cell Sci 2002 Jan 1; 115(Pt 1): 175-83.

[39]   Lamalice L, Le Boeuf F, Huot J. Endothelial cell migration during angiogenesis. Circ Res 2007 Mar 30; 100(6): 782-94.

[40]   Kanda S, Miyata Y, Mochizuki Y, Matsuyama T, Kanetake H. Angiopoietin 1 is mitogenic for cultured endothelial cells. Cancer Res 2005 Aug 1; 65(15): 6820-7.

[41]   Peters KG, Kontos CD, Lin PC, et al. Functional significance of Tie2 signaling in the adult vasculature. Recent Prog Horm Res 2004; 59: 51-71.

[42]   Nagase T, Nagase M, Yoshimura K, Fujita T, Koshima I. Angiogenesis within the developing mouse neural tube is dependent on sonic hedgehog signaling: possible roles of motor neurons. Genes Cells 2005 Jun; 10(6): 595-604.

[43]   Vates GE, Hashimoto T, Young WL, Lawton MT. Angiogenesis in the brain during development: the effects of vascular endothelial growth factor and angiopoietin-2 in an animal model. J Neurosurg. 2005 Jul; 103(1): 136-45.

[44]   Nourhaghighi N, Teichert-Kuliszewska K, Davis J, Stewart DJ, Nag S. Altered expression of angiopoietins during blood-brain barrier breakdown and angiogenesis. Lab Invest 2003 Aug; 83(8): 1211-22.

[45]   Nag S, Papneja T, Venugopalan R, Stewart DJ. Increased angiopoietin2 expression is associated with endothelial apoptosis and blood-brain barrier breakdown. Lab Invest 2005 Oct; 85(10): 1189-98.

[46]   Zhu Y, Shwe Y, Du R, et al. Effects of angiopoietin-1 on vascular endothelial growth factor-induced angiogenesis in the mouse brain. Acta Neurochir Suppl 2006; 96: 438-43.

[47]   Dore-Duffy P, Wang X, Mehedi A, Kreipke CW, Rafols JA. Differential expression of capillary VEGF isoforms following traumatic brain injury. Neurol Res 2007 Jun; 29(4): 395-403.

[48]   Lindahl P, Johansson BR, Leveen P, Betsholtz C. Pericyte loss and microaneurysm formation in PDGF-B-deficient mice. Science 1997 Jul 11; 277(5323): 242-5.

[49]   Hellstrom M, Gerhardt H, Kalen M, et al. Lack of pericytes leads to endothelial hyperplasia and abnormal vascular morphogenesis. J Cell Biol 2001 Apr 30; 153(3): 543-53.

[50]   Kermani P, Hempstead B. Brain-derived neurotrophic factor: a newly described mediator of angiogenesis. Trends Cardiovasc Med 2007 May; 17(4): 140-3.

[51]   Kim H, Li Q, Hempstead BL, Madri JA. Paracrine and autocrine functions of brain-derived neurotrophic factor (BDNF) and nerve growth factor (NGF) in brain-derived endothelial cells. J Biol Chem 2004 Aug 6; 279(32): 33538-46.

[52]   Sobue K, Yamamoto N, Yoneda K, et al. Induction of blood-brain barrier properties in immortalized bovine brain endothelial cells by astrocytic factors. Neurosci Res 1999 Nov; 35(2): 155-64.

[53]   Tsuda S, Ohtsuru A, Yamashita S, Kanetake H, Kanda S. Role of c-Fyn in FGF-2-mediated tube-like structure formation by murine brain capillary endothelial cells. Biochem Biophys Res Commun 2002 Feb 1; 290(4): 1354-60.

[54]   Klint P, Kanda S, Kloog Y, Claesson-Welsh L. Contribution of Src and Ras pathways in FGF-2 induced endothelial cell differentiation. Oncogene 1999 Jun 3; 18(22): 3354-64.

[55]   Shono T, Kanetake H, Kanda S. The role of mitogen-activated protein kinase activation within focal adhesions in chemotaxis toward FGF-2 by murine brain capillary endothelial cells. Exp Cell Res 2001 Apr 1; 264(2): 275-83.

[56]   Shono T, Mochizuki Y, Kanetake H, Kanda S. Inhibition of FGF-2-mediated chemotaxis of murine brain capillary endothelial cells by cyclic RGDfV peptide through blocking the redistribution of c-Src into focal adhesions. Exp Cell Res 2001 Aug 15; 268(2): 169-78.

[57]   Kanda S, Miyata Y, Kanetake H, Smithgall TE. Fibroblast growth factor-2 induces the activation of Src through Fes, which regulates focal adhesion disassembly. Exp Cell Res 2006 Oct 1; 312(16): 3015-22.

[58]   Langford D, Hurford R, Hashimoto M, Digicaylioglu M, Masliah E. Signalling crosstalk in FGF2-mediated protection of endothelial cells from HIV-gp120. BMC Neurosci 2005; 6: 8.

[59]   Bendfeldt K, Radojevic V, Kapfhammer J, Nitsch C. Basic fibroblast growth factor modulates density of blood vessels and preserves tight junctions in organotypic cortical cultures of mice: a new in vitro model of the blood-brain barrier. J Neurosci 2007 Mar 21; 27(12): 3260-7.

[60]   Topel I, Stanarius A, Wolf G. Distribution of the endothelial constitutive nitric oxide synthase in the developing rat brain: an immunohistochemical study. Brain Res 1998 Mar 30; 788(1-2): 43-8.

[61]   Stanarius A, Topel I, Schulz S, Noack H, Wolf G. Immunocytochemistry of endothelial nitric oxide synthase in the rat brain: a light and electron microscopical study using the tyramide signal amplification technique. Acta Histochem 1997 Nov; 99(4): 411-29.

[62]   Zhang R, Wang L, Zhang L, et al. Nitric oxide enhances angiogenesis via the synthesis of vascular endothelial growth factor and cGMP after stroke in the rat. Circ Res 2003 Feb 21; 92(3): 308-13.

[63]   Zacharek A, Chen J, Zhang C, et al. Nitric oxide regulates Angiopoietin1/Tie2 expression after stroke. Neurosci Lett 2006 Aug 14; 404(1-2): 28-32.

[64]   Cui X, Chen J, Zacharek A, et al. Nitric oxide donor upregulation of stromal cell-derived factor-1/chemokine (CXC motif) receptor 4 enhances bone marrow stromal cell migration into ischemic brain after stroke. Stem Cells 2007 Nov; 25(11): 2777-85.

[65]   Salven P, Hattori K, Heissig B, Rafii S. Interleukin-1alpha promotes angiogenesis in vivo via VEGFR-2 pathway by inducing inflammatory cell VEGF synthesis and secretion. FASEB J 2002 Sep; 16(11): 1471-3.

[66]   Fan Y, Ye J, Shen F, et al. Interleukin-6 stimulates circulating blood-derived endothelial progenitor cell angiogenesis in vitro. J Cereb Blood Flow Metab 2008 Jan; 28(1): 90-8.

[67]   Li X, Dubey S, Varney ML, Dave BJ, Singh RK. IL-8 directly enhanced endothelial cell survival, proliferation, and matrix metalloproteinases production and regulated angiogenesis. J Immunol 2003 Mar 15; 170(6): 3369-76.

[68]   Fee D, Grzybicki D, Dobbs M, et al. Interleukin 6 promotes vasculogenesis of murine brain microvessel endothelial cells. Cytokine 2000 Jun; 12(6): 655-65.

[69]   Argaw AT, Zhang Y, Snyder BJ, et al. IL-1beta regulates blood-brain barrier permeability via reactivation of the hypoxia-angiogenesis program. J Immunol 2006 Oct 15; 177(8): 5574-84.

[70]   Chen Y, Pawlikowska L, Yao JS, et al. Interleukin-6 involvement in brain arteriovenous malformations. Ann Neurol 2006 Jan; 59(1): 72-80.

[71]   Chen Y, Fan Y, Poon KY, et al. MMP-9 expression is associated with leukocytic but not endothelial markers in brain arteriovenous malformations. Front Biosci 2006; 11: 3121-8.

[72]   Campbell IL, Abraham CR, Masliah E, et al. Neurologic disease induced in transgenic mice by cerebral overexpression of interleukin 6. Proc Natl Acad Sci USA 1993 Nov 1; 90(21): 10061-5.

[73]   Charalambous C, Pen LB, Su YS, Milan J, Chen TC, Hofman FM. Interleukin-8 differentially regulates migration of tumor-associated and normal human brain endothelial cells. Cancer Res 2005 Nov 15; 65(22): 10347-54.

[74]   Velazquez OC. Angiogenesis and vasculogenesis: inducing the growth of new blood vessels and wound healing by stimulation of bone marrow-derived progenitor cell mobilization and homing. J Vasc Surg 2007 Jun; (45 Suppl) A: A39-47.

[75]   Zhang ZG, Zhang L, Jiang Q, Chopp M. Bone marrow-derived endothelial progenitor cells participate in cerebral neovascularization after focal cerebral ischemia in the adult mouse. Circ Res 2002 Feb 22; 90(3): 284-8.

[76]   Iwata H, Sata M. Potential contribution of bone marrow-derived precursors to vascular repair and lesion formation: lessons from animal models of vascular diseases. Front Biosci 2007; 12: 4157-67.

[77]   Sunderkotter C, Steinbrink K, Goebeler M, Bhardwaj R, Sorg C. Macrophages and angiogenesis. J Leukoc Biol 1994 Mar; 55(3): 410-22.

[78]   Falcone DJ, McCaffrey TA, Haimovitz-Friedman A, Garcia M. Transforming growth factor-beta 1 stimulates macrophage urokinase expression and release of matrix-bound basic fibroblast growth factor. J Cell Physiol 1993 Jun; 155(3): 595-605.

[79]   Buschmann IR, Busch HJ, Mies G, Hossmann KA. Therapeutic induction of arteriogenesis in hypoperfused rat brain via granulocyte-macrophage colony-stimulating factor. Circulation 2003 Aug 5; 108(5): 610-5.

[80]   Harlan JM. Leukocyte-endothelial interactions. Blood. 1985 Mar; 65(3): 513-25.

[81]   Stumm RK, Rummel J, Junker V, et al. A dual role for the SDF-1/CXCR4 chemokine receptor system in adult brain: isoform-selective regulation of SDF-1 expression modulates CXCR4-dependent neuronal plasticity and cerebral leukocyte recruitment after focal ischemia. J Neurosci 2002 Jul 15; 22(14): 5865-78.

[82]   Hill WD, Hess DC, Martin-Studdard A, et al. SDF-1 (CXCL12) is upregulated in the ischemic penumbra following stroke: association with bone marrow cell homing to injury. J Neuropathol Exp Neurol 2004 Jan; 63(1): 84-96.

[83]   Tanaka R, Komine-Kobayashi M, Mochizuki H, et al. Migration of enhanced green fluorescent protein expressing

bone marrow-derived microglia/macrophage into the mouse brain following permanent focal ischemia. Neuroscience 2003; 117(3): 531-9.

[84]   Manoonkitiwongsa PS, Jackson-Friedman C, McMillan PJ, Schultz RL, Lyden PD. Angiogenesis after stroke is correlated with increased numbers of macrophages: the clean-up hypothesis. J Cereb Blood Flow Metab 2001 Oct; 21(10): 1223-31.

[85]   Yu SW, Friedman B, Cheng Q, Lyden PD. Stroke-evoked angiogenesis results in a transient population of microvessels. J Cereb Blood Flow Metab 2007 Apr; 27(4): 755-63.

[86]   Ding G, Jiang Q, Li L, Zhang L, *et al.* Angiogenesis detected after embolic stroke in rat brain using magnetic resonance T2*WI. Stroke 2008 May; 39(5): 1563-8.

[87]   Althaus J, Bernaudin M, Petit E, Toutain J, Touzani O, Rami A. Expression of the gene encoding the pro-apoptotic BNIP3 protein and stimulation of hypoxia-inducible factor-1alpha (HIF-1alpha) protein following focal cerebral ischemia in rats. Neurochem Int. 2006 Jun; 48(8): 687-95.

[88]   Marti HJ, Bernaudin M, Bellail A, *et al.* Hypoxia-induced vascular endothelial growth factor expression precedes neovascularization after cerebral ischemia. Am J Pathol 2000 Mar; 156(3): 965-76.

[89]   Lennmyr F, Ata KA, Funa K, Olsson Y, Terent A. Expression of vascular endothelial growth factor (VEGF) and its receptors (Flt-1 and Flk-1) following permanent and transient occlusion of the middle cerebral artery in the rat. J Neuropathol Exp Neurol 1998 Sep; 57(9): 874-82.

[90]   Wang RG, Zhu XZ. Expression of angiopoietin-2 and vascular endothelial growth factor in mice cerebral cortex after permanent focal cerebral ischemia. Acta Pharmacol Sin 2002 May; 23(5): 405-11.

[91]   Chen J, Zacharek A, Zhang C, *et al.* Endothelial nitric oxide synthase regulates brain-derived neurotrophic factor expression and neurogenesis after stroke in mice. J Neurosci 2005 Mar 2; 25(9): 2366-75.

[92]   Atochin DN, Wang A, Liu VW, *et al.* The phosphorylation state of eNOS modulates vascular reactivity and outcome of cerebral ischemia *in vivo*. J Clin Invest 2007 Jul; 117(7): 1961-7.

[93]   Zhang ZG, Zhang L, Tsang W, *et al.* Correlation of VEGF and angiopoietin expression with disruption of blood-brain barrier and angiogenesis after focal cerebral ischemia. J Cereb Blood Flow Metab 2002 Apr; 22(4): 379-92.

[94]   Lin TN, Nian GM, Chen SF, *et al.* Induction of Tie-1 and Tie-2 receptor protein expression after cerebral ischemia-reperfusion. J Cereb Blood Flow Metab 2001 Jun; 21(6): 690-701.

[95]   Zhu W, Khachi S, Hao Q, *et al.* Upregulation of EMMPRIN after permanent focal cerebral ischemia. Neurochem Int 2008 May; 52(6): 1086-91.

[96]   Zhao BQ, Tejima E, Lo EH. Neurovascular proteases in brain injury, hemorrhage and remodeling after stroke. Stroke 2007 Feb; 38(2 Suppl): 748-52.

[97]   Romanic AM, White RF, Arleth AJ, Ohlstein EH, Barone FC. Matrix metalloproteinase expression increases after cerebral focal ischemia in rats: inhibition of matrix metalloproteinase-9 reduces infarct size. Stroke 1998 May; 29(5): 1020-30.

[98]   Zhao BQ, Wang S, Kim HY, *et al.* Role of matrix metalloproteinases in delayed cortical responses after stroke. Nat Med 2006 Apr; 12(4): 441-5.

[99]   Lin TN, Te J, Lee M, Sun GY, Hsu CY. Induction of basic fibroblast growth factor (bFGF) expression following focal cerebral ischemia. Brain Res Mol Brain Res 1997 Oct 3; 49(1-2): 255-65.

[100]   Lin TN, Wang CK, Cheung WM, Hsu CY. Induction of angiopoietin and Tie receptor mRNA expression after cerebral ischemia-reperfusion. J Cereb Blood Flow Metab 2000 Feb; 20(2): 387-95.

[101]   Hayashi T, Wang XQ, Zhang HZ, *et al.* Induction of platelet derived-endothelial cell growth factor in the brain after ischemia. Neurol Res 2007 Jul; 29(5): 463-8.

[102]   Renner O, Tsimpas A, Kostin S, *et al.* Time- and cell type-specific induction of platelet-derived growth factor receptor-beta during cerebral ischemia. Brain Res Mol Brain Res 2003 May 12; 113(1-2): 44-51.

[103]   Krupinski J, Issa R, Bujny T, *et al.* A putative role for platelet-derived growth factor in angiogenesis and neuroprotection after ischemic stroke in humans. Stroke 1997 Mar; 28(3): 564-73.

[104]   Chopp M, Zhang ZG, Jiang Q. Neurogenesis, angiogenesis, and MRI indices of functional recovery from stroke. Stroke 2007 Feb; 38(2 Suppl): 827-31.

[105]   Issa R, Krupinski J, Bujny T, Kumar S, Kaluza J, Kumar P. Vascular endothelial growth factor and its receptor, KDR, in human brain tissue after ischemic stroke. Lab Invest 1999 Apr; 79(4): 417-25.

[106]   Slevin M, Krupinski J, Slowik A, Kumar P, Szczudlik A, Gaffney J Serial measurement of vascular endothelial growth factor and transforming growth factor-beta1 in serum of patients with acute ischemic stroke. Stroke 2000 Aug; 31(8): 1863-70.

[107]   Slevin M, Krupinski J, Slowik A, Rubio F, Szczudlik A, Gaffney J Activation of MAP kinase (ERK-1/ERK-2), tyrosine kinase and VEGF in the human brain following acute ischaemic stroke. Neuroreport. 2000 Aug 21; 11(12): 2759-64.

[108]   Issa R, AlQteishat A, Mitsios N, *et al.* Expression of basic fibroblast growth factor mRNA and protein in the human brain following ischaemic stroke. Angiogenesis 2005; 8(1): 53-62.

[109]   Krupinski J, Kumar P, Kumar S, Kaluza J Increased expression of TGF-beta 1 in brain tissue after ischemic stroke in humans. Stroke 1996 May; 27(5): 852-7.

[110]   Yip HK, Chang LT, Chang WN, *et al.* Level and value of circulating endothelial progenitor cells in patients after acute ischemic stroke. Stroke 2008 Jan; 39(1): 69-74.

[111]   Sobrino T, Hurtado O, Moro MA, *et al.* The increase of circulating endothelial progenitor cells after acute ischemic stroke is associated with good outcome. Stroke 2007 Oct; 38(10): 2759-64.

[112]   Al'Qteishat A, Gaffney J, Krupinski J, *et al.* Changes in hyaluronan production and metabolism following ischaemic stroke in man. Brain 2006 Aug; 129(Pt 8): 2158-76.

[113]   Rosell A, Ortega-Aznar A, Alvarez-Sabin J, *et al.* Increased brain expression of matrix metalloproteinase-9 after ischemic and hemorrhagic human stroke. Stroke 2006 Jun; 37(6): 1399-406.

[114]   Yuen CM, Chiu CA, Chang LT, *et al.* Level and value of interleukin-18 after acute ischemic stroke. Circ J 2007 Nov; 71(11): 1691-6.

[115]   Vila N, Castillo J, Davalos A, Esteve A, Planas AM, Chamorro A. Levels of anti-inflammatory cytokines and neurological worsening in acute ischemic stroke. Stroke 2003 Mar; 34(3): 671-5.

[116]   Kostulas N, Kivisakk P, Huang Y, Matusevicius D, Kostulas V, Link H. Ischemic stroke is associated with a systemic increase of blood mononuclear cells expressing interleukin-8 mRNA. Stroke 1998 Feb; 29(2): 462-6.

[117]   Smith CJ, Emsley HC, Gavin CM, *et al.* Peak plasma interleukin-6 and other peripheral markers of inflammation in the first week of ischaemic stroke correlate with brain infarct volume, stroke severity and long-term outcome. BMC Neurol 2004 Jan 15; 4: 2.

[118]   Vila N, Castillo J, Davalos A, Chamorro A. Proinflammatory cytokines and early neurological worsening in ischemic stroke. Stroke 2000 Oct; 31(10): 2325-9.

[119]   Rallidis LS, Vikelis M, Panagiotakos DB, *et al.* Inflammatory markers and in-hospital mortality in acute ischaemic stroke. Atherosclerosis 2006 Nov; 189(1): 193-7.

[120]   Tanne D, Haim M, Boyko V, *et al.* Soluble intercellular adhesion molecule-1 and risk of future ischemic stroke: a nested case-control study from the Bezafibrate Infarction Prevention (BIP) study cohort. Stroke 2002 Sep; 33(9): 2182-6.

[121]   Grau AJ, Boddy AW, Dukovic DA, *et al.* Leukocyte count as an independent predictor of recurrent ischemic events. Stroke 2004 May; 35(5): 1147-52.

[122]   Chen Y, Xu B, Arderiu G, *et al.* Retroviral delivery of homeobox D3 gene induces cerebral angiogenesis in mice. J Cereb Blood Flow Metab 2004 Nov; 24(11): 1280-7.

[123]   Shen F, Su H, Liu W, Kan YW, Young WL, Yang GY. Recombinant adeno-associated viral vector encoding human VEGF165 induces neomicrovessel formation in the adult mouse brain. Front Biosci 2006; 11: 3190-8.

[124]   Yang GY, Xu B, Hashimoto T, *et al.* Induction of focal angiogenesis through adenoviral vector mediated vascular endothelial cell growth factor gene transfer in the mature mouse brain. Angiogenesis 2003; 6(2): 151-8.

[125]   Harrigan MR, Ennis SR, Masada T, Keep RF. Intraventricular infusion of vascular endothelial growth factor promotes cerebral angiogenesis with minimal brain edema. Neurosurgery 2002 Mar; 50(3): 589-98.

[126]   Stiver SI, Tan X, Brown LF, Hedley-Whyte ET, Dvorak HF. VEGF-A angiogenesis induces a stable neovasculature

in adult murine brain. J Neuropathol Exp Neurol 2004 Aug; 63(8): 841-55.

[127]   Yoshimura S, Morishita R, Hayashi K, et al. Gene transfer of hepatocyte growth factor to subarachnoid space in cerebral hypoperfusion model. Hypertension 2002 May; 39(5): 1028-34.

[128]   Weis SM, Cheresh DA. Pathophysiological consequences of VEGF-induced vascular permeability. Nature 2005 Sep 22; 437(7058): 497-504.

[129]   Zhang ZG, Zhang L, Jiang Q, et al. VEGF enhances angiogenesis and promotes blood-brain barrier leakage in the ischemic brain. J Clin Invest 2000 Oct; 106(7): 829-38.

[130]   Pettersson A, Nagy JA, Brown LF, et al. Heterogeneity of the angiogenic response induced in different normal adult tissues by vascular permeability factor/vascular endothelial growth factor. Lab Invest 2000 Jan; 80(1): 99-115.

[131]   van Bruggen N, Thibodeaux H, Palmer JT, et al. VEGF antagonism reduces edema formation and tissue damage after ischemia/reperfusion injury in the mouse brain. J Clin Invest 1999 Dec; 104(11): 1613-20.

[132]   Kumai Y, Ooboshi H, Ibayashi S, et al. Postischemic gene transfer of soluble Flt-1 protects against brain ischemia with marked attenuation of blood-brain barrier permeability. J Cereb Blood Flow Metab 2007 Jun; 27(6): 1152-60.

[133]   Boudreau NJ, Varner JA. The homeobox transcription factor Hox D3 promotes integrin alpha5beta1 expression and function during angiogenesis. J Biol Chem 2004 Feb 6; 279(6): 4862-8.

[134]   Hansen SL, Myers CA, Charboneau A, Young DM, Boudreau N. HoxD3 accelerates wound healing in diabetic mice. Am J Pathol 2003 Dec; 163(6): 2421-31.

[135]   Lopez-Lopez C, LeRoith D, Torres-Aleman I. Insulin-like growth factor I is required for vessel remodeling in the adult brain. Proc Natl Acad Sci USA 2004 Jun 29; 101(26): 9833-8.

[136]   Zhu W, Fan Y, Frenzel T, et al. Insulin growth factor-1 gene transfer enhances neurovascular remodeling and improves long-term stroke outcome in mice. Stroke 2008 Apr; 39(4): 1254-61.

[137]   Ellsworth JL, Garcia R, Yu J, Kindy MS. Fibroblast growth factor-18 reduced infarct volumes and behavioral deficits after transient occlusion of the middle cerebral artery in rats. Stroke 2003 Jun; 34(6): 1507-12.

[138]   Morishita R, Aoki M, Hashiya N, et al. Therapeutic angiogenesis using hepatocyte growth factor (HGF). Curr Gene Ther 2004 Jun; 4(2): 199-206.

[139]   Shimamura M, Sato N, Oshima K, et al. Novel therapeutic strategy to treat brain ischemia: overexpression of hepatocyte growth factor gene reduced ischemic injury without cerebral edema in rat model. Circulation 2004 Jan 27; 109(3): 424-31.

[140]   Sugiura S, Kitagawa K, Tanaka S, et al. Adenovirus-mediated gene transfer of heparin-binding epidermal growth factor-like growth factor enhances neurogenesis and angiogenesis after focal cerebral ischemia in rats. Stroke 2005 Apr; 36(4): 859-64.

[141]   Sharma HS, Wiklund L, Badgaiyan RD, Mohanty S, Alm P. Intracerebral administration of neuronal nitric oxide synthase antiserum attenuates traumatic brain injury-induced blood-brain barrier permeability, brain edema formation, and sensory motor disturbances in the rat. Acta Neurochir Suppl 2006; 96: 288-94.

[142]   Rashid PA, Whitehurst A, Lawson N, Bath PM. Plasma nitric oxide (nitrate/nitrite) levels in acute stroke and their relationship with severity and outcome. J Stroke Cerebrovasc Dis 2003 Mar-Apr; 12(2): 82-7.

[143]   Gertz K, Priller J, Kronenberg G, et al. Physical activity improves long-term stroke outcome via endothelial nitric oxide synthase-dependent augmentation of neovascularization and cerebral blood flow. Circ Res 2006 Nov 10; 99(10): 1132-40.

[144]   Li L, Jiang Q, Zhang L, et al. Angiogenesis and improved cerebral blood flow in the ischemic boundary area detected by MRI after administration of sildenafil to rats with embolic stroke. Brain Res 2007 Feb 9; 1132(1): 185-92.

[145]   Rikitake Y, Kim HH, Huang Z, et al. Inhibition of Rho kinase (ROCK) leads to increased cerebral blood flow and stroke protection. Stroke 2005 Oct; 36(10): 2251-7.

[146]   Stamatovic SM, Keep RF, Mostarica-Stojkovic M, Andjelkovic AV. CCL2 regulates angiogenesis via activation of Ets-1 transcription factor. J Immunol 2006 Aug 15; 177(4): 2651-61.

[147]   Li Y, Lu Z, Keogh CL, Yu SP, Wei L. Erythropoietin-induced neurovascular protection, angiogenesis, and

cerebral blood flow restoration after focal ischemia in mice. J Cereb Blood Flow Metab 2007 May; 27(5): 1043-54.

[148]   Wang L, Zhang Z, Wang Y, Zhang R, Chopp M. Treatment of stroke with erythropoietin enhances neurogenesis and angiogenesis and improves neurological function in rats. Stroke 2004 Jul; 35(7): 1732-7.

[149]   Iwai M, Cao G, Yin W, Stetler RA, Liu J, Chen J Erythropoietin promotes neuronal replacement through revascularization and neurogenesis after neonatal hypoxia/ischemia in rats. Stroke 2007 Oct; 38(10): 2795-803.

[150]   Grasso G, Sfacteria A, Meli F, et al. The role of erythropoietin in neuroprotection: therapeutic perspectives. Drug News Perspect 2007 Jun; 20(5): 315-20.

[151]   Gibson CL, Bath PM, Murphy SP. G-CSF reduces infarct volume and improves functional outcome after transient focal cerebral ischemia in mice. J Cereb Blood Flow Metab 2005 Apr; 25(4): 431-9.

[152]   Gibson CL, Jones NC, Prior MJ, Bath PM, Murphy SP. G-CSF suppresses edema formation and reduces interleukin-1beta expression after cerebral ischemia in mice. J Neuropathol Exp Neurol 2005 Sep; 64(9): 763-9.

[153]   Lee ST, Chu K, Jung KH, et al. Granulocyte colony-stimulating factor enhances angiogenesis after focal cerebral ischemia. Brain Res 2005 Oct 5; 1058(1-2): 120-8.

[154]   Shyu WC, Lin SZ, Yang HI, et al. Functional recovery of stroke rats induced by granulocyte colony-stimulating factor-stimulated stem cells. Circulation 2004 Sep 28; 110(13): 1847-54.

[155]   Lu CZ, Xiao BG. Neuroprotection of G-CSF in cerebral ischemia. Front Biosci 2007; 12: 2869-75.

[156]   Lu CZ, Xiao BG. G-CSF and neuroprotection: a therapeutic perspective in cerebral ischaemia. Biochem Soc Trans 2006 Dec; 34(Pt 6): 1327-33.

[157]   Toth ZE, Leker RR, Shahar T, et al. The combination of granulocyte colony-stimulating factor and stem cell factor significantly increases the number of bone marrow-derived endothelial cells in brains of mice following cerebral ischemia. Blood 2008 Jun 15; 111(12): 5544-52.

[158]   Koch KC, Schaefer WM, Liehn EA, et al. Effect of catheter-based transendocardial delivery of stromal cell-derived factor 1alpha on left ventricular function and perfusion in a porcine model of myocardial infarction. Basic Res Cardiol 2006 Jan; 101(1): 69-77.

[159]   Hiasa K, Ishibashi M, Ohtani K, et al. Gene transfer of stromal cell-derived factor-1alpha enhances ischemic vasculogenesis and angiogenesis via vascular endothelial growth factor/endothelial nitric oxide synthase-related pathway: next-generation chemokine therapy for therapeutic neovascularization. Circulation 2004 May 25; 109(20): 2454-61.

[160]   Shyu WC, Lin SZ, Yen PS, et al. Stromal cell-derived factor-1 alpha promotes neuroprotection, angiogenesis, and mobilization/homing of bone marrow-derived cells in stroke rats. J Pharmacol Exp Ther 2008 Feb; 324(2): 834-49.

[161]   Jackson KA, Majka SM, Wang H, et al. Regeneration of ischemic cardiac muscle and vascular endothelium by adult stem cells. J Clin Invest 2001 Jun; 107(11): 1395-402.

[162]   Kocher AA, Schuster MD, Szabolcs MJ, et al. Neovascularization of ischemic myocardium by human bone-marrow-derived angioblasts prevents cardiomyocyte apoptosis, reduces remodeling and improves cardiac function. Nat Med 2001 Apr; 7(4): 430-6.

[163]   Levenberg S, Golub JS, Amit M, Itskovitz-Eldor J, Langer R. Endothelial cells derived from human embryonic stem cells. Proc Natl Acad Sci USA 2002 Apr 2; 99(7): 4391-6.

[164]   Strauer BE, Brehm M, Zeus T, et al. Repair of infarcted myocardium by autologous intracoronary mononuclear bone marrow cell transplantation in humans. Circulation 2002 Oct 8; 106(15): 1913-8.

[165]   Kokovay E, Li L, Cunningham LA. Angiogenic recruitment of pericytes from bone marrow after stroke. J Cereb Blood Flow Metab 2006 Apr; 26(4): 545-55.

[166]   Doetschman T, Shull M, Kier A, Coffin JD. Embryonic stem cell model systems for vascular morphogenesis and cardiac disorders. Hypertension 1993 Oct; 22(4): 618-29.

[167]   Ding DC, Shyu WC, Chiang MF, et al. Enhancement of neuroplasticity through upregulation of beta1-integrin in human umbilical cord-derived stromal cell implanted stroke model. Neurobiol Dis 2007 Sep; 27(3): 339-53.

[168]   Ukai R, Honmou O, Harada K, Houkin K, Hamada H, Kocsis JD. Mesenchymal stem cells derived from

peripheral blood protects against ischemia. J Neurotrauma 2007 Mar; 24(3): 508-20.

[169]   Shen LH, Li Y, Chen J, *et al.* Therapeutic benefit of bone marrow stromal cells administered 1 month after stroke. J Cereb Blood Flow Metab 2007 Jan; 27(1): 6-13.

[170]   Wu J, Sun Z, Sun HS, *et al.* Intravenously administered bone marrow cells migrate to damaged brain tissue and improve neural function in ischemic rats. Cell Transplant 2008; 16(10): 993-1005.

[171]   Chen J, Zhang ZG, Li Y, *et al.* Intravenous administration of human bone marrow stromal cells induces angiogenesis in the ischemic boundary zone after stroke in rats. Circ Res 2003 Apr 4; 92(6): 692-9.

[172]   Zacharek A, Chen J, Cui X, *et al.* Angiopoietin1/Tie2 and VEGF/Flk1 induced by MSC treatment amplifies angiogenesis and vascular stabilization after stroke. J Cereb Blood Flow Metab 2007 Oct; 27(10): 1684-91.

[173]   Onda T, Honmou O, Harada K, Houkin K, Hamada H, Kocsis JD. Therapeutic benefits by human mesenchymal stem cells (hMSCs) and Ang-1 gene-modified hMSCs after cerebral ischemia. J Cereb Blood Flow Metab 2008 Feb; 28(2): 329-40.

[174]   Kurozumi K, Nakamura K, Tamiya T, *et al.* BDNF gene-modified mesenchymal stem cells promote functional recovery and reduce infarct size in the rat middle cerebral artery occlusion model. Mol Ther 2004 Feb; 9(2): 189-97.

[175]   Ikeda N, Nonoguchi N, Zhao MZ, *et al.* Bone marrow stromal cells that enhanced fibroblast growth factor-2 secretion by herpes simplex virus vector improve

neurological outcome after transient focal cerebral ischemia in rats. Stroke 2005 Dec; 36(12): 2725-30.

[176]   Urbich C, Dimmeler S. Endothelial progenitor cells: characterization and role in vascular biology. Circ Res 2004 Aug 20; 95(4): 343-53.

[177]   Jia L, Takahashi M, Yoshioka T, Morimoto H, Ise H, Ikeda U. Therapeutic potential of endothelial progenitor cells for cardiovascular diseases. Curr Vasc Pharmacol 2006 Jan; 4(1): 59-65.

[178]   Khakoo AY, Finkel T. Endothelial progenitor cells. Annu Rev Med 2005; 56: 79-101.

[179]   Liew A, Barry F, O'Brien T. Endothelial progenitor cells: diagnostic and therapeutic considerations. Bioessays 2006 Mar; 28(3): 261-70.

[180]   Ghani U, Shuaib A, Salam A, *et al.* Endothelial progenitor cells during cerebrovascular disease. Stroke 2005 Jan; 36(1): 151-3.

[181]   Ohta T, Kikuta K, Imamura H, *et al.* Administration of ex vivo-expanded bone marrow-derived endothelial progenitor cells attenuates focal cerebral ischemia-reperfusion injury in rats. Neurosurgery 2006 Sep; 59(3): 679-86; discussion -86.

[182]   Li Z, Wu JC, Sheikh AY, *et al.* Differentiation, survival, and function of embryonic stem cell derived endothelial cells for ischemic heart disease. Circulation 2007 Sep 11; 116(11 Suppl): I46-54.

38 *Experimental Stroke, 2008, 1, 38-45*

Role of Matrix Metalloproteinases After Stroke: From Basic Research to Clinical Impact

Anna Rosell, Eng H. Lo and Xiaoying Wang*

Neuroprotection Research Laboratory, Departments of Radiology and Neurology, Massachusetts General Hospital, and Program in Neuroscience, Harvard Medical School, Barcelona, Spain; E-mail; WANGXI@helix.mgh.harvard.edu

Abstract: Matrix metalloproteinases (MMPs) comprise a family of zinc endopeptidases that play major roles in the physiology and pathology of the mammalian central nervous system (CNS). These proteinases are evolutionarily conserved as modulators of extracellular matrix during CNS development. After acute tissue injury such as that which occurs after stroke, MMPs become dysregulated and subsequently mediate acute neurovascular disruption and parenchymal destruction. Animal studies have demonstrated their participation in breakdown of neurovascular matrix and blood-brain barrier disruption with edema and/or hemorrhage. Moreover, perturbation of extracellular homeostasis triggered by MMPs may underlie processes responsible for the hemorrhagic complications of thrombolytic stroke therapy. Conversely, biphasic roles for some MMPs have been established since emerging data also suggest that some aspects of MMP activity during the delayed neuroinflammatory response may contribute to remodeling and stroke recovery.

INTRODUCTION

Nowadays, stroke remains a major cause of death and disability worldwide and its pathophysiology is highly complex. After the cerebral ischemic event, a cellular catastrophe occurs within the hypoxic tissue, leading in a few minutes to severe lesions at the infarction area that may extend through the surrounding tissue due to secondary cell loss. The initial vascular event rapidly leads to energy loss, which ultimately triggers a wide and intricately linked cascade of neuronal death pathways. Over the past decade, these molecular mechanisms have been thought to comprise excitotoxicity, oxidative stress and perhaps even programmed cell death signals such as apoptosis or autophagy [1]. But unfortunately, a decade of monotherapies focused on neuroprotection have not yielded successful treatments for stroke [2]; expanding the focus to include other cell types and extracellular matrix components [3,4]. In addition to these primarily *intra*-cellular events, an increasing emphasis on the importance of *inter*-cellular signalling is beginning to emerge, all cells in the so-called "neurovascular unit" will be affected, not just neurons [4, 5]. Neurovascular perturbations will lead to blood brain barrier (BBB) leakage, edema, hemorrhage, leukocyte infiltration, and progressive inflammatory reactions to brain injury over hours or even days after the initial stroke.

In this chapter, we will focus on the pathophysiologic actions of Matrix Metalloproteinases (MMPs) after cerebral ishcemia, because this family of diverse zinc endopeptidases can broadly target almost all components of the mammalian central nervous system (CNS) matrix. Is known that an uncontrolled MMP activity may be responsible for the degradation of extracellular matrix (ECM) and basal lamina (BL)

proteins such as laminin, fibronectin, collagen, proteoglycans and others [6,7]. Their baseline activity is need in many physiological processes such as morphogenesis, cell migration or ovulation but their dysregulation is involved in progression of diverse pathological conditions such as cancer, rheumatoid arthritis, periodontitis as well as brain injury and stroke [8].

MATRIX METALLOPROTEINASE FAMILY

As mentioned, matrix metalloproteinases comprise a family of zinc-dependent proteases involved in regulation of cell–matrix composition known for their ability to cleave one or several basal lamina and extracellular matrix components. Apart from being capable of degrading all kinds of extracellular matrix proteins, MMPs can also process a number of bioactive molecules. Since Xenopus collagenase was first identified over 40 years ago by Gros and Lapiere [9,10] more than 25 different secreted and cell surface-bound MMPs have been described. Although they are products of different genes, these endopeptidades share common structural (such as an amino-terminal propeptide and a catalytic and a hemopexin-like domain) and functional elements [11]. All members of the MMP family are produced in a latent form and become secreted or transmembrane-type proteins. The catalytic activity of the MMPs is regulated at multiple levels including transcription, secretion, activation and inhibition, being the last one accomplished by members of the TIMP (tissue inhibitor of metalloproteinases) family, which currently includes four proteins: TIMP-1, TIMP-2, TIMP-3, and TIMP-4 [11].

Kunlin Jin / Guo-Yuan Yang (Eds.)

Initially, MMPs were classified by their by descriptive names that were assigned based on limited knowledge of their preferred substrate specificities being named collagenases, gelatinases, stromelysins, and matrilysins. However, their substrate specificity is extensive since one single MMP can display distinct molecular interactions with other proteinases and substrates *in vivo* that make their biology unquestionably complex. For example, MMP-3, MMP-7, and MMP-10, members of the stromelysin subclass, can cleave many ECM components, including proteoglycans, fibronectin, collagens, and gelatins. The collagenases, MMP-1, MMP-8, and MMP-13, target primarily fibrillar, but also non fibrillar, collagens. The gelatinases, MMP- 2 and MMP-9, are also potent in their ability to cleave denatured collagens [12].

Regarding cerebral ischemia, extensive literature has demonstrated the implication of several MMPs in relation to brain injury, blood brain barrier permeability, hemorrhagic conversions or cell death, but also to matrix plasticity and tissue remodeling. In the following sections we will expose the role of this family of proteases after cerebral ischemia to carefully characterize the balance between multiphasic roles of MMPs after stroke.

MEDIATORS OF BRAIN INJURY

After ischemic stroke, some MMPs become dysregulated and the subsequent aberrant proteolysis of neurovascular matrix might lead to BBB leakage and cell death (Fig. **1**). The mechanisms of MMP–mediated brain injury are diverse: by direct degradation of brain matrix-substrates or indirectly through activation of other bioactive molecules.

Dysregulation in acute ischemic stroke

The standard hypothesis postulates that some MMPs play a central pathologic role in stroke by degrading

ECM substrates that are essential for normal signaling and homeostasis within the neurovascular unit. As we will discuss, many groups have demonstrated that in experimental models of cerebral ischemia and in human stroke, several MMPs are rapidly increased in ischemic brain.

Two early studies published in 1997 [13,14] demonstrated for the first time that MMP-9 and MMP-2 are elevated in the ischemic human brain. More recent data confirmed the presence of high MMP-9 levels not only in infarcttissue but also in the peri-infarct areas, perhaps suggesting a role for MMPs in the process of infarct growth [15]. Similar findings have also been reported for peri-hematoma tissue from patients that suffered from hemorrhagic stroke [15]. Importantly, MMP-9 levels seem to peak within infarcts that undergo hemorrhagic conversion, correlating with enhanced erythrocyte extravasation and neutrophil infiltration surrounding the affected capillaries, together with severe collagen IV degradation in the basal lamina [16]. These human studies are consistent with animal model data showing microvascular basal lamina injury and loss of collagen type IV, which can be reversed with hypothermic treatments that reduce enzymatic activity of MMP-2 and MMP-9 in ischemia-reperfusion rat models [17,18]. Therefore, the implication of these two MMPs in the pathogenesis of stroke has been unequivocally demonstrated although their source and modulation is still under discussion as we will examine.

While most of the stroke literature is filled with MMP-2 and MMP-9 data, other MMP members may play important roles as well. For example, MMP-3 (also named stromelysin-1) can be activated after ischemia-reperfusion in rat brain, causing the cleavage of the cerebral matrix agrin [19]. MMP-3 also contributes to BBB opening during neuroinflammation after intracerebral LPS injection in mice [20]. Correspondingly, MMP-3 knockout mice

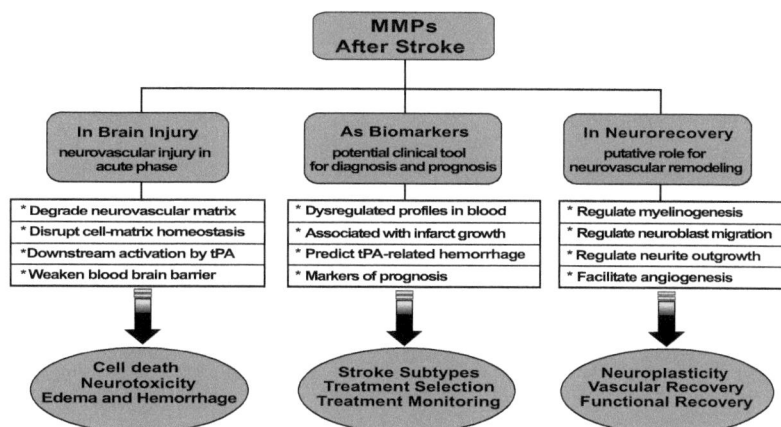

Fig. (1). Diagram representing the multiphasic roles of MMPs after stroke. Acute effects involve BBB damage and brain cell death while delayed actions involve neurovascular remodeling and neurovasculogenesis that may contribute to stroke recovery. Biomarker monitoring might be a potential tool for diagnosis and prognosis of stroke.

showed less degradation of tight junctions proteins (occludin, claudin-5, laminin-alpha-1) together with reduced neutrophil infiltration, compared to wild-type animals [20]. Finally, a recent investigation suggested a role for MMP-3 in the intracranial bleeding that occurs after thrombotic middle cerebral artery occlusion in mice [21]. The authors demonstrated that MMP-3 expression was significantly elevated in ischemic tissue, and MMP-3 knockout mice treated with t-PA had significantly reduced hemorrhagic transformation compared to t-PA-treated wild-type mice. Altogether, it is likely that MMPs function in a network-like fashion with upstream and downstream proteases being closely coupled.

In spite of the strong data implicating MMPs in stroke, the cellular source of this protease remains to be fully defined. MMPs can be synthesized by resident brain cells or peripheral cells recruited to injured brain from the blood stream during the neuroinflammatory response. Elevated MMPs from brain endothelial cells, astrocytes or neurons mediate neurovascular damage and extend infarct volumes. In some studies, this endogenous brain MMP-response clearly dominates compared to inflammatory components [22,23]. In contrast, other studies suggest that invading neutrophils comprise a significant source of MMP-9 that degrade basal lamina and lead to BBB breakdown after transient focal cerebral ischemia [24,25]. In fact, chimeric mice lacking leukocytic MMP-9 present similar lesions as MMP-9 knockouts but not those chimeric animals lacking MMP-9 in brain cells [25]. A recent study in human stroke brain tissue demonstrated that leukocytic MMP-9 is co-localized with collagen IV proteolysis in basal lamina, which in turn appeared to correspond with areas of MMP-9-positive neutrophil infiltration in infarcted and hemorrhagic areas [16]. Therefore, we might hypothesize that endogenous MMP-9 from brain resident cells might mostly contribute to primary neuronal cell death and infarct establishment while leukocyte-derived MMP-9 might contribute to infarct progression and hemorrhagic conversions. A better understanding of the temporal sequencing of these events may allow us to better target our MMP inhibition strategies in stroke.

Therefore, current knowledge suggests that decoupling of this putative MMP network may occur but future studies, perhaps using protein arrays, may be required to assess not just MMP-2, -3 and -9, but all family members to truly "fingerprint" the role that the proteases play in acute neurovascular injury.

Mechanisms of hemorrhagic transformation

Fundamentally, hemorrhagic transformation in cerebral ischemia occurs after an increase in permeability within the BBB. This secondary but threatening complication further damages the entire neurovascular unit, which comprises the extracellular matrix,

endothelial cells, astrocytes, neurons, and pericytes. In fact in some patients, a large and symptomatic intracranial hemorrhage (ICH) can occur, significantly worsening neurological outcome and increasing mortality rate up to 40%. Thus, neurovascular injury in this context can significantly extend parenchymal injury into irreversible infarction and pan-necrosis [4]. The underlying pathways of ischemia, HT, and neurovascular compromise are highly complex and diverse triggered by proteolysis, oxidative stress, and leukocyte infiltration but here we will shortly describe MMP implication to hemorrhagic conversions.

At the neurovascular interface, proteolysis of the matrix is a major contributor to intracranial hemorrhage. Degradation of essential components such as laminin, fibronectin, collagens, or proteoglycans, destabilizes structural support for the BBB, producing leakage and breakdown. Although many proteases are expressed in the brain under normal and ischemic conditions, both animal and human studies suggest that the MMP family and the tissue plasminogen activator (tPA) system play a central role.

As described in the previous section, in the past decade, many groups have demonstrated that MMPs such as MMP-2, MMP-3, and MMP-9, are rapidly increased in the ischemic brain, and these responses are closely related to infarct extension, neurological outcome, or hemorrhagic conversion [15, 19, 26, 27] but a specific role has been proposed for MMP-9 as a triggering protease for HT. Animal models have demonstrated that MMP-9 and MMP-3 increase after thrombolysis [21, 28], and pharmacological or genetic inhibition of MMP-9 significantly decreases the risk of hemorrhagic complications after thrombolysis [29, 30]. As mentioned, microvascular basal lamina injury and loss of collagen type IV can be reversed with hypothermic treatments that reduce enzymatic activity of MMP-2 and MMP-9 in ischemia-reperfusion rat models [17]. These results are consistent with human studies showing that MMP-9 peaks in areas that undergo hemorrhagic conversion, correlating with enhanced erythrocyte extravasation, neutrophil infiltration, and severe collagen IV degradation in the basal lamina [16].

t-PA interactions

Tissue Plasminogen Activator (tPA) is a serine protease that catalyses the conversion of plasminogen to plasmin. Thrombolysis, treatment to achieve artery recanalitzation in ischemic stroke, can be accomplished with the administration of tPA, the only Food and Drug Administration (FDA)-approved drug for this disease [31]. Then, in the properly selected set of patients, thrombolysis with tPA rescues brain tissue. The primary action of tPA occurs inside the blood vessel to rescue compromised brain tissue if blood flow is successfully restored by early thrombolytic reperfusion. Besides clot lysis, tPA may have pleiotropic actions in the brain and might be potentially neurotoxic and may also trigger important protease actions on the neurovascular unit, some of which would be responsible for mediating HT in the ischemic brain [32].

Although unequivocal human data are lacking, findings from animal models suggest that possibly deleterious consequences of tPA reperfusion may develop because tPA is more than just a clot buster [33]. Animal models attribute BBB injury to protease effects of pleiotropic actions of tPA, including activation of apoptosis [34], cleavage of the N-methyl-D-aspartate (NMDA) NR1 subunit [35], or activation of other extracellular proteases [36]. Specifically, tPA may also target brain extracellular matrix by activation of other extracellular proteases such as those in the MMP family [3]. An interesting hypothesis is that t-PA might in fact amplify MMP-9 responses after stroke. It has been demonstrated in cell culture systems that t-PA up-regulates MMP-9 through low-density lipoprotein receptor-related protein (LRP) signaling [36]. *In vivo* models show that thrombolytic therapy with t-PA augments MMP-9 levels in ischemic brain tissue [28] as well as the peripheral circulation in rats [37]. But not only exogenous tPA can activate proteolytic-cascades within the ischemic brain, recent data suggests that endogenous tPA contributes to hippocampal injury after cerebral ischemia, and these pathophysiologic pathways may involve links to aberrant activation of caspases and MMPs [38]. In this study, tPA deficient mice were protected against transient global cerebral ischemia.

Insofar as MMP-9 may degrade critical neurovascular matrix in microvessels, this tPA-MMP-9 hypothesis might explain some of the clinical complications of hemorrhagic transformation that currently limit the wide-spread use of thrombolytic stroke therapy. Reperfusion of ischemic brain is clearly beneficial, but a deeper understanding of how tPA also affects neurovascular matrix may reveal new approaches to further improve tPA thrombolysis.

Acute MMP inhibition

So far, we have described detrimental actions of some MMPs in the acute phase of stroke, but, can we target these MMP responses for pharmacologic benefit in stroke?

Several experimental studies have reported that various hydroxymate-based compounds might serve as adequate MMP inhibitors in rodent models of stroke. Batimastat or BB-94 significantly reduced infarct size in a murine model of cerebral ischemia [29]. Similarly, BB-94 also prevented hippocampal neuronal death after transient global cerebral ischemia in mice [39]. In experimental rat models of embolic stroke, BB-94 and BB-1101 were able to decrease hemorrhagic transformation [30], and ameliorate mortality after delayed t-PA thrombolysis. Inhibition of MMPs also seems to rescue BBB integrity after focal cerebral ischemia and lipopolysaccharide-induced neuroinflammation [40,41]. From a mechanistic and cellular standpoint, the promise of using MMP inhibitors for neuroprotection is based on the potential ability of this approach to prevent anoikis-like cell death [42,43]. Of course, these data remain highly preliminary. Translating animal model findings into effective stroke therapies is extremely difficult, and there is a great distance between experimental compounds and clinical reality. Nevertheless, if MMP pathways of neurovascular pathophysiology are fully established, one can envision alternate pharmacologic approaches as MMP inhibitors in human patients.

Acute inhibition of MMP activity by genetic modifications, hydroxymate inhibitors, or monoclonal antibodies all seemed to effectively reduce edema, infarct size and hemorrhagic events [21,30,29,40]. However, the long-term effects of MMP inhibition remain to be fully characterized. A recently published paper suggests that some caution may be warranted. Sood *et al.* [44] showed in a rodent ischemic stroke model that early administration of the hydroxymate MMP inhibitor BB-1101 successfully reduced acute BBB leakage, but ended up impairing long-term functional recovery in these animals. These MMP-remodelling actions in the chronic phase of stroke will be further analysed since multiphasic roles of these proteases might require an extremely fine regulation of potential MMP inhibition.

CLINICAL STROKE BIOMARKERS

Because tissue access in the stroke patient is confined to the post-mortem brain, a large number of MMP human-studies have been conducted in blood, which further offers the possibility of obtaining time-course data during stroke evolution. However, the use of peripheral blood to assess MMP levels has been somehow criticized due to the imprecise understanding of the true source of these MMPs. Nevertheless, peripheral blood MMP studies in stroke patients have increasingly become a promising clinical tool comprising potential biomarkers for diagnosis and prognosis (Fig. 1).

To date, MMP-9 has been the most studied MMP in the blood stream. High levels of this protease have been found in patients with ischemic and hemorrhagic strokes, compared to healthy individuals [45,46]. More importantly, acute MMP-9 levels have been related to infarct size, poor neurological outcome and hemorrhagic transformation complications [45,47,48]. MMP-9 levels assessed at hospital entry have been identified as predictors of the infarct volume measured with diffusion-weighted MRI [49] and these biomarkers are further correlated with stroke lesion growth, even with the application of thrombolytic therapy [50]. An interesting finding in this regard is the relationship between MMP-9 biomarker levels and t-PA administration. An initial study suggested that compared to other therapies such as hypothermia, MMP-9 levels were especially elevated in patients that received t-PA [51]. A more recent study confirmed that blood MMP-9 levels in stroke patients treated with t-PA were significantly higher than those in untreated patients [52]. Consistent with the hypothesis of deleterious MMP actions during ischemic stroke, hyperacute MMP-9 blood levels emerged as a powerful predictor of further hemorrhagic complications after t-PA thrombolysis [53].

For other MMP family members, the results have been more variable. While some laboratories have documented high MMP-2 serum levels after ischemic stroke, others have reported decreased MMP-2 levels compared with non-stroke controls [45,48]. And in some studies, MMP-2 did not appear to have a consistent correlation with neurological status [45], subtype of hemorrhage [53] or infarct growth [50]. Similar variations have been reported for MMP-13. Some investigations proposed that MMP-13 is an independent predictor of infarct growth at 24 hours after stroke onset [50]. But others could not detect clear differences in MMP-13 blood levels one day after stroke compared to controls [51]. Besides proteases, mammalian CNS also contains endogenous tissue inhibitors of metalloproteinases (TIMPs). In general, measurements of various TIMPs (including TIMP1 and TIMP2) in blood suggest that imbalances between protease and inhibitor might be present after stroke [48,51,52]. But the specificity of TIMPs as independent stroke biomarkers remain to be fully elucidated.

Although less frequent, hemorrhagic stroke is a devastating cerebrovascular event with high rates of mortality. Compared to ischemic strokes, the use of MMPs as biomarkers in cerebral hemorrhage is less studied. Several studies suggest that similar elevations in MMP-2, -3, and -9 along with imbalances in TIMPs are indeed present after intracerebral hemorrhage (ICH) [46]. However the temporal profile of these responses may be quite different. In this study and another [54], MMP-9 was found to be related to perihematomal edema volume and neurological worsening, while MMP-3 was strongly related with mortality [46]. Another group investigated subarachnoid hemorrhage, and found that MMP-2 levels were decreased whereas MMP-9 levels were increased, compared to control subjects [55].

The potential validity of using these MMP assays as stroke biomarkers may ultimately require further mechanistic investigations in animal models. But these types of studies are relatively rare, in part because it is difficult to perform repeated blood draws in small rodents over long periods of time. One rigorous study comparing brain and blood MMP-9 levels was performed by Koh and colleagues in a middle cerebral artery occlusion ischemic model in rats. This study suggested that early increases in MMP-9 occurred in blood, whereas brain MMP-9 levels showed a more delayed elevation over time [56]. More recently, another study examining the utility of minocycline as an MMP inhibitor in rat embolic stroke models showed that t-PA treatment was associated with augmented MMP-9 levels in blood. And the ability of minocycline to protect against tPA-associated hemorrhagic transformation was correlated with improvements in MMP-9 biomarker levels [37].

Taken together, the experimental and clinical data are promising. Blood MMPs appear to correlate with MRI and neurological outcomes and combination therapies to inhibit MMPs appear to ameliorate some of the tPA-associated alterations in this putative biomarker. Can MMPs truly become useful biomarkers to help us jump from bench to bedside? Although the concept is exciting, the approach remains still speculative at the present time. But no doubt, monitoring MMPs in blood could become a promising tool to guide clinicians in the diagnosis and prognosis of stroke, much in the same vein as current neuroimaging or neurosonology techniques.

NEUROVASCULAR REMODELING AFTER STROKE

In the brain, MMPs are expressed during development and contribute to morphogenesis of the CNS. MMPs affect cell-cell and cell-matrix interactions by cleavage of extracellular matrix proteins and regulation of the intercellular microenvironment and may modulate bioavailable levels of various growth factors.

In this section, we will explore the emerging hypothesis that in contrast to acute pathology, proteases as MMPs might contribute to beneficial remodeling during stroke recovery. Apart from the discussed MMP activity on ECM and basal lamina substrates, this proteolytic activity may also modulate levels of various growth factors by processing pro-form precursors or by liberating active molecules from matrix-hidden compartments. For example, MMP-9's ability to mobilize VEGF from the ECM can activate quiescent vasculature, thus switching on the vascular system to ramp up angiogenesis in both normal and neoplasic tissues [57].

Other authors have demonstrated regeneration roles for MMPs in the injured CNS. A discrete expression of some MMPs can have beneficial roles in remyelination [58]. In a lysolecithin-induced demyelination toxic model, MMP-9 knockout mice were impaired in myelin reformation [58]. The corresponding rescue experiment demonstrated that MMP-9 expressed locally around a demyelinating lesion of the spinal cord facilitated remyelination. While acute MMP inhibition improved locomotor recovery, extended treatment failed, consistent with the idea that delayed remodeling requires MMP activity in the CNS. Recently, MMP-2 has been shown to participate actively in wound healing and the promotion of functional recovery in the spinal cord [59]. Between 7 and 14 days after injury, MMP-2 increased in reactive astrocytes surrounding the lesion, and locomotion was impaired in mice deficient for MMP-2, associated with reduced white matter sparing. Finally, the beneficial role for MMP-9 in hippocampal synaptic physiology, plasticity, and memory has been demonstrated by Nagy and colleagues [60]. The broad spectrum MMP inhibitor GM6001 interferes with long term potentiation and MMP-9 knockout mice also show impairments in long term potentiation and learning. Once again, the rescue experiment worked, i.e. additional treatment with exogenous recombinant MMP-9 to the null-mutant slices completely restored the deficiencies in long term potentiation. Taken together, these data are consistent with the idea that MMPs comprise key molecules for promoting the remodeling of ischemic brain via angiogenesis, vasculogenesis or neurogenesis (Fig. **1**).

Coupling neurogenic responses

The subventricular zone (SVZ) of the lateral ventricles and the subgranular zone (SGZ) of the hippocampus are critical structures for neurogenesis in adult brain. Increased neurogenesis can be triggered by the CNS insults such as stroke, trauma and seizure [61-63]. Stroke leads to the expansion of SVZ and produces BrdU-labeled immature cells and DCX-positive neural precursors in the SVZ [64,65]. Although what initiates and promotes endogenous neurogenesis has not been fully understood, upregulation of stem cells and growth factors are likely to affect stroke-induced neurogenesis [65,66]. Implantation of stem cells can improve functional recovery in experimental stroke [67]. Newly generated neural precursors migrate toward infarcted areas, where they differentiate and express markers of neostriatal spiny neurons near damaged areas [64]. Several lines of evidence appear to support the idea that MMPs may play a role in neuroblast migration. During postnatal development, MMP-9 is associated with granule cell migration in the cerebellum [68], and migration of oligodendrocyte progenitors requires MMPs [69]. By removing insulin-like growth factor binding protein 6 (IGFBP-6) and controlling the bioavailability of IGF-1, MMPs participates in regulate myelinogenesis during brain development [70]. Mice deficient in MMP-9 show continued demyelination after injury, perhaps because of failure in clearing injury-induced deposits of NG2 proteoglycan [58]. At 2 weeks after stroke in mice, MMP-9 was enhanced in the SVZ and was colocalized with BrdU and DCX-positive neuroblast cells [66]. Furthermore, inhibition of MMPs reduced the extension of neuroblast signals that extended from the SVZ into the damaged striatum. These data indicate that MMPs may contribute to endogenous repair mechanisms by helping the migration of neuroblasts after stroke.

Insofar as newborn neurons and vascular components can be activated during stroke recovery, the multiple stimuli involved remain to be fully elucidated. This potential microenvironment has been termed the neurovascular niche [71], which proposes that angiogenesis and neurogenesis are linked thorough specific growth factors such as SDF-1 or Ang-1. The link with MMPs in this scenario involves the fact that MMP-9 is known to liberate soluble c-kit ligands following SDF-1 upregulation [72]. Recruitment of stem and progenitor cells from the bone marrow niche requires MMP-9 mediated release of kit-ligand [72]. Other authors have demonstrated that vascular endothelial cells secrete growth factors and chemokines, which may support the survival of newly formed neurons in recovering brain. Administration of human cord blood-derived CD34$^+$ cells following stroke induced neovascularization in the peri-infarct cortex and increased neuroblast migration to the damaged cortex [73]. Data such as these provides a direct link between therapeutic neovascularization after stroke and neuronal regeneration. Wang and colleagues [74] demonstrated that intraperitoneal injection of erythropoietin during 7 consecutive days after ischemia improved angiogenesis and neurogenesis in the stroke boundary. The activation of these endothelial precursor cells were correlated with increased secretion of MMP-2 and MMP-9. The link between these protease and cytokine mechanisms are supported by the finding that conditioned medium from these preparations stimulated migration of neural progenitor cells from SVZ neurospheres, while treatment with a MMP inhibitor abolished neural progenitor cell migration enhanced by EPO-treated brain endothelial mouse cells.

As described in the earlier sections, numerous studies in experimental animal stroke models suggest that MMP inhibitors might present a feasible therapeutic approach for stroke. But what happens if they are involved in delayed remodeling after stroke. A recent published paper showed that at 7 and 14 days after focal cerebral ischemia, these same peri-infarct areas lit up with increased MMP-9 signals that colocalized with NeuN-positive and GFAP-positive cells. Delayed treatment with MMP inhibitors at one week after stroke increased ischemic brain injury and impaired functional recovery [75]. Taken together these findings suggest that MMPs might indeed participate in some forms of neurovascular remodeling after stroke.

The idea that neurovascular plasticity contributes to stroke recovery can be a powerful new concept for stroke therapy. Obviously, the therapeutic time window for interventions based on promoting recovery would be much larger than those for targeting acute stroke per se. Clearly, the cellular microenvironment and the MMPs that modulate the ECM would comprise critical checkpoints that regulate these processes. What remains to be fully defined are the inter-cellular signals that allow MMPs to interact with these substrates of stroke recovery.

CONCLUSIONS

Extensive data from molecular, cellular and whole animal models and humans support a deleterious role for MMPs in acute stroke. These mechanistic findings are now increasingly validated by biomarker measurements in human stroke patients. Nevertheless, emerging data now suggest that MMPs play complex and multiphasic roles after stroke and brain injury. During delayed phases of stroke recovery, MMPs may interact with ECM and growth factor or cytokine substrates to modulate neurovascular plasticity. The challenge will be to define spatial and temporal controls that allow one to target acute MMP dysregulation and ameliorate neurovascular pathophysiology without interfering with endogenous nerovasculogenesis and brain tissue repair. Endogenous MMP responses, perhaps as part of a broader inflammatory and remodelling response, may turn out to be key mediators in stroke recovery. An important goal as we move forward will be to carefully define the balance between biphasic roles of MMPs after stroke in acute and chronic phases. Pharmacologic targeting will have to optimize acute inhibition of deleterious MMP actions without compromising the beneficial effects of matrix plasticity during stroke recovery.

REFERENCES

[1] Lo EH, Dalkara T, Moskowitz MA. Mechanisms, challenges and opportunities in stroke. Nat Rev Neurosci 2003; 4(5): 399-415.

[2] Young AR, Ali C, Duretête A, Vivien D. Neuroprotection and stroke: time for a compromise. J Neurochem 2007; 103(4): 1302-9.

[3] Lo EH, Wang X, Cuzner ML. Extracellular proteolysis in brain injury and inflammation: role for plasminogen activators and matrix metalloproteinases. J Neurosci Res. 2002; 69(1): 1-9.

[4] Lee SR, Wang X, Tsuji K, Lo EH. Extracellular proteolytic pathophysiology in the neurovascular unit after stroke. Neurol Res 2004; 26(8): 854-61.

[5] Hawkins BT, Davis TP. The blood-brain barrier/neurovascular unit in health and disease. Pharmacol Rev 2005; 57(2): 173-85.

[6] Nagase H, Visse R, Murphy G. Structure and function of matrix metalloproteinases and TIMPs. Cardiovasc Res 2006; 69(3): 562-73.

[7] Galis ZS, Khatri JJ. Matrix metalloproteinases in vascular remodeling and atherogenesis: the good, the bad, and the ugly. Circ Res 2002; 90(3): 251-62.

[8] Lemaître V, D'Armiento J. Matrix metalloproteinases in development and disease.Birth Defects Res C Embryo Today 2006; 78(1): 1-10.

[9] Gross J, Lapiere CM. Collagenolytic activity in amphibian tissues: a tissue culture assay. Proc Natl Acad Sci USA 1962; 48: 1014-22.

[10] Gross J. How tadpoles lose their tails: path to discovery of the first matrix metalloproteinase. Matrix Biol 2004; 23(1): 3-13.

[11] Massova I, Kotra LP, Fridman R, Mobashery S. Matrix metalloproteinases: structures, evolution, and diversification. FASEB J 1998; 12(12): 1075-95.

[12] Hulboy DL, Rudolph LA, Matrisian LM. Matrix metalloproteinases as mediators of reproductive function. Mol Hum Reprod 1997; 3(1): 27-45.

[13] Anthony DC, Ferguson B, Matyzak MK, Miller KM, Esiri MM, Perry VH. Differential matrix metalloproteinase expression in cases of multiple sclerosis and stroke. Neuropathol Appl Neurobiol 1997; 23(5): 406-15.

[14] Clark AW, Krekoski CA, Bou SS, Chapman KR, Edwards DR. Increased gelatinase A (MMP-2) and gelatinase B (MMP-9) activities in human brain after focal ischemia. Neurosci Lett 1997; 28; 238(1-2): 53-6.

[15] Rosell A, Ortega-Aznar A, Alvarez-Sabín J, et al. Increased brain expression of matrix metalloproteinase-9 after ischemic and hemorrhagic human stroke. Stroke 2006; 37(6): 1399-406.

[16] Rosell A, Cuadrado E, Ortega-Aznar A, Hernández-Guillamon M, Lo EH, Montaner J. MMP-9-positive neutrophil infiltration is associated to blood-brain barrier breakdown and basal lamina type IV collagen degradation during hemorrhagic transformation after human ischemic stroke. Stroke 2008; 39(4): 1121-6.

[17] Hamann GF, Burggraf D, Martens HK, et al. Mild to moderate hypothermia prevents microvascular basal lamina antigen loss in experimental focal cerebral ischemia. Stroke 2004; 35(3): 764-9.

[18] Hamann GF, Liebetrau M, Martens H, et al. Microvascular basal lamina injury after experimental focal cerebral ischemia and reperfusion in the rat. J Cereb Blood Flow Metab 2002; 22(5): 526-33.

[19] Solé S, Petegnief V, Gorina R, Chamorro A, Planas AM. Activation of matrix metalloproteinase-3 and agrin cleavage in cerebral ischemia/reperfusion. J Neuropathol Exp Neurol 2004; 63(4): 338-49.

[20] Gurney KJ, Estrada EY, Rosenberg GA. Blood-brain barrier disruption by stromelysin-1 facilitates neutrophil infiltration in neuroinflammation. Neurobiol Dis 2006; 23(1): 87-96.

[21] Suzuki Y, Nagai N, Umemura K, Collen D, Lijnen HR. Stromelysin-1 (MMP-3) is critical for intracranial bleeding after t-PA treatment of stroke in mice. J Thromb Haemost 2007; 5(8): 1732-9.

[22] Maier CM, Hsieh L, Yu F, Bracci P, Chan PH. Matrix metalloproteinase-9 and myeloperoxidase expression: quantitative analysis by antigen immunohistochemistry in a model of transient focal cerebral ischemia. Stroke 2004; 35(5): 1169-74.

[23] Harris AK, Ergul A, Kozak A, Machado LS, Johnson MH, Fagan SC. Effect of neutrophil depletion on gelatinase expression, edema formation and hemorrhagic transformation after focal ischemic stroke. BMC Neurosci 2005; 6: 49.

[24] Justicia C, Panés J, Solé S, et al. Neutrophil infiltration increases matrix metalloproteinase-9 in the ischemic brain after occlusion/reperfusion of the middle cerebral artery in rats. J Cereb Blood Flow Metab 2003; 23(12): 1430-40.

[25] Gidday JM, Gasche YG, Copin JC, et al. Leukocyte-derived matrix metalloproteinase-9 mediates blood-brain barrier breakdown and is proinflammatory after transient focal cerebral ischemia. Am J Physiol Heart Circ Physiol 2005; 289(2): H558-68.

[26] Planas AM, Solé S, Justicia C. Expression and activation of matrix metalloproteinase-2 and -9 in rat brain after transient focal cerebral ischemia. Neurobiol Dis 2001; 8(5): 834-46.

[27] Rosenberg GA, Navratil M, Barone F, Feuerstein G. Proteolytic cascade enzymes increase in focal cerebral ischemia in rat. J Cereb Blood Flow Metab 1996; 16(3): 360-6.

[28] Tsuji K, Aoki T, Tejima E, et al. Tissue plasminogen activator promotes matrix metalloproteinase-9 upregulation after focal cerebral ischemia. Stroke 2005; 36(9): 1954-9.

[29] Asahi M, Asahi K, Wang X, Lo EH. Reduction of tissue plasminogen activator-induced hemorrhage and brain injury by free radical spin trapping after embolic focal cerebral ischemia in rats. J Cereb Blood Flow Metab 2000; 20(3): 452-7.

[30] Sumii T, Lo EH. Involvement of matrix metalloproteinase in thrombolysis-associated hemorrhagic transformation after embolic focal ischemia in rats. Stroke 2002, 33: 831-6.

[31] National Institute of Neurological Disorders and Stroke rt-PA stroke study group. N Engl J Med 1995; 333(24): 1581-7.

[32] Indyk JA, Chen ZL, Tsirka SE, Strickland S. Laminin chain expression suggests that laminin-10 is a major isoform in the mouse hippocampus and is degraded by the tissue plasminogen activator/plasmin protease cascade during excitotoxic injury. Neuroscience 2003; 116(2): 359-71.

[33] Kaur J, Zhao Z, Klein GM, Lo EH, Buchan AM. The neurotoxicity of tissue plasminogen activator? J Cereb Blood Flow Metab 2004; 24(9): 945-63.

[34] Liu D, Cheng T, Guo H, et al. Tissue plasminogen activator neurovascular toxicity is controlled by activated protein C. Nat Med 2004; 10(12): 1379-83.

[35] Nicole O, Docagne F, Ali C, et al. The proteolytic activity of tissue-plasminogen activator enhances NMDA receptor-mediated signaling. Nat Med 2001; 7(1): 59-64.

[36] Wang X, Lee SR, Arai K, et al. Lipoprotein receptor-mediated induction of matrix metalloproteinase by tissue plasminogen activator. Nat Med 2003; 9(10): 1313-7.

[37] Murata Y, Rosell A, Scannevin RH, Rhodes KJ, Wang X, Lo EH. Extension of the thrombolytic time window with minocycline in experimental stroke. Stroke 2008; 39(12): 3372-7.

[38] Lee SR, Lok J, Rosell A, *et al.* Reduction of hippocampal cell death and proteolytic responses in tissue plasminogen activator knockout mice after transient global cerebral ischemia. Neuroscience 2007; 150(1): 50-7.

[39] Lee SR, Tsuji K, Lee SR, Lo EH. Role of matrix metalloproteinases in delayed neuronal damage after transient global cerebral ischemia. J Neurosci 2004; 24(3): 671-8.

[40] Pfefferkorn T, Rosenberg GA. Closure of the blood-brain barrier by matrix metalloproteinase inhibition reduces rtPA-mediated mortality in cerebral ischemia with delayed reperfusion. Stroke 2003; 34(8): 2025–30.

[41] Rosenberg GA, Estrada EY, Mobashery S. Effect of synthetic matrix metalloproteinase inhibitors on lipopolysaccharide-induced blood-brain barrier opening in rodents: Differences in response based on strains and solvents. Brain Res 2007; 1133(1): 186-92.

[42] Gu Z, Cui J, Brown S, *et al.* A highly specific inhibitor of matrix metalloproteinase-9 rescues laminin from proteolysis and neurons from apoptosis in transient focal cerebral ischemia. J Neurosci 2005; 25(27): 6401-8.

[43] Gu Z, Kaul M, Yan B, *et al.* S-nitrosylation of matrix metalloproteinases: signaling pathway to neuronal cell death. Science 2002; 297(5584): 1186-1190.

[44] Sood RR, Taheri S, Candelario-Jalil E, Estrada EY, Rosenberg GA. Early beneficial effect of matrix metalloproteinase inhibition on blood-brain barrier permeability as measured by magnetic resonance imaging countered by impaired long-term recovery after stroke in rat brain. J Cereb Blood Flow Metab 2008; 28(2): 431-8.

[45] Montaner J, Alvarez-Sabín J, Molina C, *et al.* Matrix metalloproteinase expression after human cardioembolic stroke: temporal profile and relation to neurological impairment. Stroke 2001; 32(8): 1759-66.

[46] Alvarez-Sabín J, Delgado P, Abilleira S, *et al.* Temporal profile of matrix metalloproteinases and their inhibitors after spontaneous intracerebral hemorrhage: relationship to clinical and radiological outcome. Stroke 2004; 35(6): 1316-22.

[47] Montaner J, Alvarez-Sabín J, Molina CA, *et al.* Matrix metalloproteinase expression is related to hemorrhagic transformation after cardioembolic stroke. Stroke 2001; 32(12): 2762-7.

[48] Vukasovic I, Tesija-Kuna A, Topic E, Supanc V, Demarin V, Petrovcic M. Matrix metalloproteinases and their inhibitors in different acute stroke subtypes. Clin Chem Lab Med 2006; 44(4): 428-34.

[49] Montaner J, Rovira A, Molina CA, *et al.* Plasmatic level of neuroinflammatory markers predict the extent of diffusion-weighted image lesions in hyperacute stroke. J Cereb Blood Flow Metab 2003; 23(12): 1403-7.

[50] Rosell A, Alvarez-Sabín J, Arenillas JF, *et al.* A matrix metalloproteinase protein array reveals a strong relation between MMP-9 and MMP-13 with diffusion-weighted image lesion increase in human stroke. Stroke 2005; 36(7): 1415-20.

[51] Horstmann S, Kalb P, Koziol J, Gardner H, Wagner S. Profiles of matrix metalloproteinases, their inhibitors, and laminin in stroke patients: influence of different therapies. Stroke 2003; 34(9): 2165-70.

[52] Ning M, Furie KL, Koroshetz WJ, *et al.* Association between tPA therapy and raised early matrix metalloproteinase-9 in acute stroke. Neurology 2006; 66(10): 1550-5.

[53] Montaner J, Molina CA, Monasterio J, *et al.* Matrix metalloproteinase-9 pretreatment level predicts intracranial hemorrhagic complications after thrombolysis in human stroke. Circulation 2003; 107(4): 598–603.

[54] Abilleira S, Montaner J, Molina CA, Monasterio J, Castillo J, Alvarez-Sabin J. Matrix metalloproteinase-9 concentration after spontaneous intracerebral hemorrhage. J Neurosurg 2003; 99(1): 65-70.

[55] Horstmann S, Su Y, Koziol J, Meyding-Lamade U, Nagel S, Wagner S. MMP-2 and MMP-9 levels in peripheral blood after subarachnoid hemorrhage. J Neurol Sci 2006; 251(1-2): 82-6.

[56] Koh SH, Chang DI, Kim HT, *et al.* Effect of 3-aminobenzamide, PARP inhibitor, on matrix metalloproteinase-9 level in plasma and brain of ischemic stroke model. Toxicology 2005; 214(1-2): 131-9.

[57] Bergers G, Brekken R, McMahon G, *et al.* Matrix metalloproteinase-9 triggers the angiogenic switch during carcinogenesis. Nat Cell Biol 2000; 2(10): 737-44.

[58] Larsen PH, Wells JE, Stallcup WB, Opdenakker G, Yong VW. Matrix metalloproteinase-9 facilitates remyelination in part by processing the inhibitory NG2 proteoglycan. J Neurosci 2003; 23(35): 11127-35.

[59] Hsu JY, McKeon R, Goussev S, Werb Z, Lee JU, Trivedi A, Noble-Haeusslein LJ. Matrix metalloproteinase-2 facilitates wound healing events that promote functional recovery after spinal cord injury. J Neurosci 2006; 26(39): 9841-50.

[60] Nagy V, Bozdagi O, Matynia A, *et al.* Matrix metalloproteinase-9 is required for hippocampal late-phase long-term potentiation and memory. J Neurosci 2006; 26(7): 1923-34.

[61] Arvidsson A, Collin T, Kirik D, Kokaia Z, Lindvall O. Neuronal replacement from endogenous precursors in the adult brain after stroke. Nat Med 2002; 8(9): 963-70.

[62] Chirumamilla S, Sun D, Bullock MR, Colello RJ. Traumatic brain injury induced cell proliferation in the adult mammalian central nervous system. J Neurotrauma 2002; 19(6): 693-703.

[63] Gray WP, May K, Sundström LE. Seizure induced dentate neurogenesis does not diminish with age in rats. Neurosci Lett 2002; 330(3): 235-8.

[64] Parent JM, Vexler ZS, Gong C, Derugin N, Ferriero DM. Rat forebrain neurogenesis and striatal neuron replacement after focal stroke. Ann Neurol 2002; 52(6): 802-13.

[65] Thored P, Arvidsson A, Cacci E, *et al.* Persistent production of neurons from adult brain stem cells during recovery after stroke. Stem Cells 2006; 24(3): 739-47.

[66] Nakatomi H, Kuriu T, Okabe S, *et al.* Regeneration of hippocampal pyramidal neurons after ischemic brain injury by recruitment of endogenous neural progenitors. Cell 2002; 110(4): 429-41.

[67] Zhang ZG, Jiang Q, Zhang R, *et al.* Magnetic resonance imaging and neurosphere therapy of stroke in rat. Ann Neurol 2003; 53(2): 259-63.

[68] Vaillant C, Meissirel C, Mutin M, Belin MF, Lund LR, Thomasset N. MMP-9 deficiency affects axonal outgrowth, migration, and apoptosis in the developing cerebellum. Mol Cell Neurosci 2003; 24(2): 395-408.

[69] Yong VW. Metalloproteinases: mediators of pathology and regeneration in the CNS. Nat Rev Neurosci 2005; 6(12): 931-44.

[70] Larsen PH, DaSilva AG, Conant K, Yong VW. Myelin formation during development of the CNS is delayed in matrix metalloproteinase-9 and -12 null mice. J Neurosci 2006; 26(8): 2207-14.

[71] Ohab JJ, Fleming S, Blesch A, Carmichael ST. A neurovascular niche for neurogenesis after stroke. J Neurosci 2006; 26(50): 13007-16.

[72] Heissig B, Hattori K, Dias S, *et al.* Recruitment of stem and progenitor cells from the bone marrow niche requires MMP-9 mediated release of kit-ligand. Cell 2002; 109(5): 625-37.

[73] Taguchi A, Soma T, Tanaka H, *et al.* Administration of CD34+ cells after stroke enhances neurogenesis via angiogenesis in a mouse model. J Clin Invest 2004; 114(3): 330-8.

[74] Wang L, Zhang ZG, Zhang RL, *et al.* Matrix metalloproteinase 2 (MMP2) and MMP9 secreted by erythropoietin-activated endothelial cells promote neural progenitor cell migration. J Neurosci 2006; 26(22): 5996-6003.

[75] Zhao BQ, Wang S, Kim HY, *et al.* Role of matrix metalloproteinases in delayed cortical responses after stroke. Nat Med 2006; 12(4): 441-5.

Blood Brain Barrier Dysfunction and the Endothelin System in Cerebral Ischemia

Samuel W. Cramer[1] **, Lin Li**[1] **and Dandan Sun**[*]

[1]*Dept. of Neurosurgery,* [2]*Neuroscience Training Program, Univ. of Wisconsin School of Medicine and Public Health, Madison, WI 53792, USA; E-mail: sun@neurosurg.wisc.edu*

Abstract: The blood brain barrier (BBB) is the central homeostatic controller of the brain environment and plays an important role in disease. Disruption of normal BBB functionality is a significant event in the pathogenesis of cerebral ischemia. Therefore, strategies that attenuate BBB disruption during cerebral ischemia and reperfusion represent viable therapeutic approaches capable of decrease the severity of ischemic injury, including reducing the risk of hemorrhage and edema formation. The endothelin (ET) system comprises three peptides (ET-1, ET-2, and ET-3) and two receptor sub-types (ET$_A$ and ET$_B$) [1,2]. This system is involved in a diverse array of physiological process. The ET system is also plays an integral role in BBB dysfunction through the modulation of ion transporters, water channels, and the recruitment of various cellular mediators of the inflammatory response. Because of this involvement, the ET system represents a possible therapeutic target for the treatment of cerebral ischemia. This review examines the interplay between the BBB and the ET system in cerebral ischemia.

INTRODUCTION

The blood brain barrier (BBB) is a specialized structure which functions to regulate the entry of small molecules into the microenvironment surrounding the neurons of the brain. Beyond this more traditional view, the BBB is increasingly understood to be a dynamic structural interface between the blood and brain, capable of modulating the interaction between these two physiologically discrete regions. As the central homeostatic controller of the brain environment, the BBB plays an important role in many neuropathologies.

The specialized nature of the BBB offers a particular challenge in both understanding the mechanisms of neuropathologies (such as stroke) and the delivery of drugs across the BBB to treat brain injury. Stroke describes a range of conditions caused by blockage or hemorrhage of blood vessels supplying the brain. Disruption of cerebral blood flow in the ischemic brain regions is a leading cause of stroke [3]. Among the many physiological perturbations characteristic to cerebral ischemia, a few are: depletion of essential nutrients and oxygen; increased BBB permeability; loss of ionic homeostasis; edema formation; as well as immediate and delayed cell death. Because of the diverse mechanisms involved in ischemia-reperfusion injury, many potential therapeutic targets exist. One possible approach would be to target the endothelin (ET) system because of its influence in a number of physiological processes, many of which may exacerbate injury caused by cerebral ischemia. Consequently, this review will provide a broad overview of the BBB and the ET system followed by a discussion of the interplay between the BBB and ET in cerebral ischemia.

ORGANIZATION AND STRUCTURE OF THE BBB

The apical portion of the BBB is formed by cerebral endothelial cells (CECs) which form a continuous lining of the cerebral microvasculature [4-6]. The basement membrane, pericytes, and smooth muscle cells are found below the CEC layer. Greater than 99 % of the basolateral portion of this structure is then enveloped by astrocytic end-feet [6]. Given the integrated nature of the BBB, it is not surprising that its optimal function is highly dependent on the dynamic interaction between astrocytes, pericytes, neurons, and CECs [4].

The absence of fenestrations and a small number of pinocytic vesicles are unique attributes of CECs which distinguish them from the endothelial cells found outside of the brain [7]. Some of the other characteristics exhibited by brain microvascular CECs include: tight junction complexes between CECs which act to cement neighboring CECs into a continuous, tile-like network lining the cerebral-vasculature and thus restricts the permeability of water-soluble molecules across the BBB; selective carrier- and receptor-mediated uptake and transport of nutrients from the blood to the brain interstitial fluid; a high density of mitochondria; and the presence of efflux transport proteins [4-6].

Pericytes are flat connective tissue cells found in the basal lamina. Their primary function is to provide structural support to the capillary walls [4]. CECs and pericytes form in close proximity and studies have indicated that they are capable of intercommunication *via* gap junctions. Pericytes are believed to be capable of modulating CEC proliferation, migration, differentiation and survival [6]. The CEC basement membrane facilitates physical interactions between pericytes and CECs [8]. The extracellular matrix (ECM) of the basement membrane is composed of versican, chondroitin heparin sulfate proteoglycans, collagens, laminin, fibronectin, entactin, and thrombospondin [7]. Multiple intracellular signaling pathways are mediated by cell-ECM interactions and are necessary to maintain proper neurovascular homeostasis. For example, the ECM is involved in CEC tight junction maintenance [6].

Astrocytes play an integral part in BBB formation and function. They are capable of modulating the specializations of the BBB such as tight junction formation, gap junctional area, and expression of various transporters [4,6]. Astrocytes are instrumental in the regulation of brain water homeostasis *via* the expression of aquaporin water channels in their end-feet [8]. They also mediate signaling between neurons and the vascular unit, regulating local perfusion rates in response to neuronal activity [4,5,8].

BBB IN PATHOPHYSIOLOGY OF ISCHEMIC STROKE

Disruption of normal BBB functionality is a significant event in the patholophysiology of ischemia reperfusion injury. Perturbations in the BBB's ability to maintain the selectively permeable barrier between blood and brain result in the unregulated passage of small molecules, fibrinogen and plasma into the brain parenchyma [5]. Migration of pericytes away from brain microvessels, the release of inflammatory mediators (bradykinin, histamine), cytokines (interleukins and tumor necrosis factor), excitatory amino acids, nitric oxide, and activated matrix metalloproteinases (MMPs) are among some of the events involved in ischemia-reperfusion-mediated changes in BBB structure and function [5,7]. Failure in BBB integrity leads to vasogenic edema and hemorrhage and is one of the pathological consequences of ischemic injury [5,7]. Strategies that attenuate BBB disruption during ischemia and reperfusion are known to decrease the severity of injury, including the risk of hemorrhage and edema formation. Decreasing the damage and disruption of the BBB is also neuroprotective [5,9]. Consequently, reducing BBB dysfunction post ischemia would be one aspect of an effective stroke therapy.

ET SYSTEM

The ET family is composed of three 21 amino acid peptides known as ET-1, ET-2, and ET-3, each of which is the product of a different gene [1,2]. ET-2 and ET-3 differ from ET-1 by two and six amino acids, respectively [1,2]. The three ETs are not circulating hormones under ordinary physiological conditions. Instead they act as paracrine and autocrine factors throughout the body. This conclusion is based on the observation that under normal conditions circulating plasma concentrations of ET-1 are approximately 1 pM and plasma levels of ET-2 and

ET-3 are even lower while both ET receptors exhibit affinities for their respective ligands in the nanomolar range [2]. ET-1 is understood to be the most potent vasoconstrictor yet discovered [10]. Each of the ET variants is the product of a unique, two-step biochemical pathway which involves the cleavage of the precursor peptides, which are approximately 200 amino acid residues long, by furin-like endopeptidases to form biologically inactive products known as big ETs [1]. These big ETs are further processed by membrane-bound zinc metalloproteases known as endothelin-converting enzymes which produce the final, mature ET product [1,2]. ET-1 is synthesized by endothelial cells, airway epithelial cells, macrophages, fibroblasts, cardiomyocytes, brain neurons as well as other cell types [2]. Expression of ET-2 is most prominent in the epithelial cells of the intestine and ET-3 is expressed by brain neurons, epithelial cells of the renal tubules, and intestinal epithelial cells [2]. In the central nervous system (CNS), all three ETs are expressed throughout the brain in neurons, endothelial cells, and in astrocytes [1]. Two subtypes of ET receptors, ET_A and ET_B, have been described [2]. These receptors exhibit similar structural characteristics such as seven transmembrane domains and the activation of G protein mediated signaling cascades when activated [1,2]. ET_A and ET_B exhibit differential affinities for the three ET ligands. ET_A has nanomolar affinities for ET-1 and ET-2, and an approximately two orders of magnitude lower affinity for ET-3. In contrast, ET_B has equal nanomolar affinities for all three ET peptide variants [2]. ET_A and ET_B are expressed in a wide range of tissue types, many of which simultaneously express both receptors. ET_A is found in smooth muscle cells, cardiomyocytes, hepatocytes, brain neurons, melanocytes, osteoblasts, adipocytes, and assorted reproductive tract cells [2]. ET_B is expressed on all of these cell types as well as being expressed in endothelial cells and renal collecting-duct cells [2]. Many factors have been identified which influence the expression of ET_A and ET_B. ET_B protein expression is up-regulated in response to tumor necrosis factor-alpha and fibroblast growth factor in endothelial cells. In smooth muscle cells, insulin and nitric oxide have been shown to increase the expression of ET_A [2].

ET IN CEREBRAL ISCHEMIA

In human cerebral arteries, ET_A and ET_B mediate opposing responses when activated. ET_A receptor activation, because of their high abundance on smooth muscle cells, results in a contractile effect in cerebral arteries, whereas when ET_B receptors are activated they largely mediate vasodialation [1,11]. Interestingly, when signaled to do so, CECs release ET primarily on the basolateral side, toward the brain parenchyma, and not the apical side toward the cerebralvascular lumen [2]. In the brain, ET_A receptors have been detected in vascular smooth muscle, neurons, CECs, and cultured astrocytes (mRNA); while ET_B receptors have been localized in neurons, astrocytes, microglia, ependyma, CECs, and vascular smooth muscle cells [12,13]. These findings highlight the diverse signaling possibilities of the endothelin system in the brain. Multiple studies have been conducted in humans to investigate plasma levels of ET-1 following ischemic stroke. The results have been conflicting, with some indicating that ET-1 plasma levels are elevated following ischemic stroke [14-16], while others have failed to observe a significant change in ET-1 levels during this period [17,18]. However, ET-1 is significantly elevated in the cerebral spinal fluid of stroke patients during the period following stroke onset [17]. In this study, elevation in ET-1 was correlated with cortical infarct volume. Concomitant with cerebral spinal fluid sampling, plasma ET-1 levels were also measured and found not to be significantly different from control levels [17]. Despite the incongruities between some of the previous findings, it appears plausible that ET-1 levels are elevated in both cerebral spinal fluid and plasma post ischemia. Based on the observation that ET-1 levels are elevated post ischemia in humans, together with studies using animal models (for example, the observation that over-expression of ET-1 in mouse CECs exacerbates cerebral damage following ischemia) indicates that ET-1 plays a role in the pathogenesis of ischemia-reperfusion injury [19]. Using immunocytochemistry and electron microscopy, the localization of ET-1, ET-2, and ET-3 was investigated following global ischemia in rats [20]. This study found that following ischemia, the most intense ET immunoreactivity was localized to perivascular astrocytic end-feet. Furthermore, high levels of ET immunoreactivity was observed in microglia and macrophages found in close proximity to the cerebralvasculature. Expression of ET_A and ET_B may also be influenced by ischemia/reperfusion injury. In rats subject to middle cerebral artery occlusion (MCAO) followed by reperfusion, ET_A and ET_B mRNA was found to be significantly increased in middle cerebral arteries subject to occlusion versus non-occluded middle cerebral arteries [11]. Similarly, significant up-regulation of both ET_A and ET_B mRNA has been observed in the ipsilateral cerebral hemisphere of rats following permanent MCAO [21]. Pharmacological blockade of both ET_A and ET_B (using the $ET_{A/B}$ inhibitor TAK-044) during MCAO has also been shown to improve neurological function in rats [22]. Interestingly, selective antagonism of the ET_B receptor with BQ-788 during focal ischemia has been shown to result in increased infarct volume [23]. This may be due in part to the ET_B receptor's implicated role in the clearance of ET-1 from the blood stream which would thereby hasten the reduction of circulating ET-1 levels [24]. Blocking ET_B receptors, therefore, may increase the circulatory half-life of ET-1, allowing it to mediated greater reductions in cerebral perfusion rates and activate other targets which may lead to greater injury.

During experimental focal ischemia, the specific antagonism of ET_A is able to reduce the severity of brain injury [25-27]. The therapeutic effects of ET_A antagonism during ischemia reperfusion observed in these studies were largely ascribed to improved cerebral profession rates resulting from reduced vasoconstriction of the cerebral microvasculature. This likely plays a role, however, inhibition of ET_A receptors during reperfusion post ischemia has also been shown to be neuroprotective without affecting cerebral blood flow rates [26,28]. Thus, the role of the ET system in ischemia reperfusion injury may be more diverse than the modulation of cerebral profusion.

ET MEDIATED BBB DYSFUNCTION IN CEREBRAL ISCHEMIA

Studies suggest ET-1 is capable of increasing the permeability of the BBB which has been shown to contribute to cerebral edema formation resulting from ischemia-reperfusion injury [29]. For example, transgenic mice engineered to over-express ET-1 in astrocytes or CECs show heightened susceptibility to cerebral ischemia [19,30]. In the case where ET-1 was overexpressed in astrocytes, the injury was characterized by increased BBB permeability and increased edema following transient MCAO compared to wild-type mice [30].

Application of S-0139, a specific ET_A receptor antagonist, during post MCAO reperfusion was significantly effective in reducing brain edema formation, infarction volume, and albumin extravasation (a measure of BBB permeability) in rats [25]. This study implicates the specific involvement of the ET_A receptor pathway in the observed BBB disruption following ischemia. However, the specific mechanisms for these observed therapeutic effects of ET_A receptor blockade remain to be elucidated in their entirety.

CEREBRAL ISCHEMIA AND ET'S CONTRIBUTION TO BBB DYSRUPTION

MMPs are members of a group of Zn^{2+}- and Ca^{2+}-dependent endopeptidases. Expression of MMPs is low in most tissues during normal physiological conditions and is induced when ECM remodeling is required [31]. MMPs play an important role in tissue repair following injury. However, MMPs have been shown to contribute to BBB disruption following ischemia [32]. Regulation of MMPs is predominately done by a family of endogenous inhibitors known as tissue inhibitor of matrix metalloproteinases (TIMPs) [32]. Induction of both MMPs (specifically, MMP-2 and MMP-9) and TIMPs has been shown to occur following focal ischemia [5]. Members of both the MMP and TIMP families may be regulated, in part, by the endothelin system [32]. Evidence for this is provided by a study where intracerebral-ventricular administration of the ET_B specific agonist $Ala^{1,3,11,15}$-ET-1 was shown to induce the up-regulation of

TIMP-1 and TIMP-3 mRNA in many different regions of the brain [32]. This study also suggests that reactive astrocytes are the primary source for the increased production of TIMP-1 and TIMP-3 mRNA. ET-1 is capable of modulating the expression of MMPs and ECM in smooth muscle cells and fibroblasts. Additionally, ET-1 can stimulate the release of MMPs from macrophages and can stimulate a chemotactic response from human neutrophils and monocytes [33]. Evidence indicates that following ischemic injury, CNS tissue experiences an initial wave of neutrophils followed by infiltration of monocytes [34]. Recruitment of these leukocytes is a double edged-sword, as they are both capable of repairing tissue injury and further exacerbating it through the production of proteases, reactive oxygen species, and lipid-derived mediators [35]. ET-1 has been shown (through the activation of the ET_A receptor) to directly induce the production of monocyte chemoattractant factor-1 mRNA in cultured human brain derived endothelial cells [35]. This ET-1 induced upregulation of monocyte chemoattractant factor-1 may be involved in the observed microglia accumulation and macrophage transmigration (across the CEC layer) in response to ischemic injury and, thus, be responsible, in part, for the physical disruption of the BBB following ischemic injury [35]. Another study investigated the relationship between ET-1 and the production of the highly potent neutrophil chemotactic factor interleukin-8, which is an effective mediator of neutrophil migration and extravasation [34]. The results indicate that ET-1 directly induces an increase in the transcription and subsequent expression of interleukin-8 in cultured human brain derived endothelial cells [34].

BBB TRANSPORTER/CHANNEL EX-PRESSION AND ACTIVITY POST ISCHMIA: ET'S ROLE

In the period immediately following the onset of ischemic stroke, brain edema begins in the absence of any physical disruption of the BBB [36]. This process is thought to result from the secretion of Na+, Cl-, and water from the blood to the brain, with physical deterioration of the BBB not occurring until approximately four to six hours post ischemia onset [36,37]. The activity of Na+ transporters on the luminal membrane of BBB endothelial cells, coincident with the activity of Na+/K+-ATPase and Cl- efflux pathways, play a central role in the early development of brain edema following ischemia onset [36]. Early edema formation may be influenced by the actions of the endothelin system. In cultured rat brain endothelial cells, activation of the ETA receptor by either ET-1 or ET-3 (though ET-1 did so with higher potency than ET-3) was shown to increase the rate of K+ uptake [37]. Using pharmacological methods, the authors showed that the increase in K+ uptake was mediated by both the Na+/K+-ATPase and Na+-K+-Cl- cotransporter systems. Furthermore, the

stimulated activity of these transporter systems resulted from ETA mediated activation of protein kinase C [37]. Subtle differences in the relationship between the ET system and K+ uptake and efflux were reported when studied in cultured human brain endothelial cells. With this system, it was found that ET-1 but not ET-3 was capable of stimulating the activity of both the Na+/K+-ATPase and Na+-K+-Cl-cotransporter [38]. This study also reported that ET-1 is involved in stimulating the uptake of Ca2+. All observed changes in ion transport elicited by ET-1 were found to be mediated through activation of the ETA receptors coupled to the phospholipase C system. The ET system has also been demonstrated to be capable of modulating the activity (as measured by Na+ uptake rate) of the Na+/H+ exchanger in cultured rat brain capillary endothelial cells [39]. The change in activity of the Na+/H+ exchanger occurred via the activation of the ETA receptor by the binding of either ET-1 or ET-3, with both peptides stimulating Na+ uptake with similar potencies. The ETA receptor mediated this activity change in a protein kinase C independent manner [39]. Transgenic mice with constitutively over-expressed astrocytic ET-1 experience significantly more brain water accumulation following transient MCAO than their wild-type counterparts. In these ET-1 over-expressing mice, it was observed that aquaporin 4 expression was increased in astrocytic end-feet following transient MCAO [30]. Given the role of aquaporin 4 in cerebral water homeostasis, and the near complete envelopment of cerebral microvessels by astrocytic end-feet, these changes may augment edema formation by facilitating the transmigration of water from the blood vessels to the brain.

CONCLUSIONS

Cerebral ischemia causes a complex series of events which ultimately leads to immediate and delayed brain cell death. Currently, there are very few therapeutic options available for the treatment of this common neuropathology. However, because of the complex nature of cerebral ischemia and the multitude of events which contribute to the overall brain injury, there appear to be many possible therapeutic targets though the most effective treatment will almost certainly involve a multivalent approach. The ET system represents one possible target due to its demonstrated role in BBB dysfunction during cerebral ischemia.

There are many changes in the ET system in response to cerebral ischemia. ET-1 is released, and transcription of both ET_A and ET_B mRNA is increased in the brain. Furthermore, inhibition of the ET_A receptor during cerebral ischemia attenuates brain injury. Different mechanisms have emerged as routes by which the ET system is capable of exacerbating cerebral ischemic injury. The most investigated contribution to ischemic stroke injury is ET-1 induced vasoconstriction and subsequent reduction in cerebral blood flow *via* smooth muscle ET_A receptor activation. The ET system is also directly involved in BBB dysfunction, a hallmark of cerebral ischemia, through the modulation of ion transporters, water channels, and the recruitment of various cellular mediators of the inflammatory response.

Though progress has been made in elucidating mechanisms of the ET system's involvement cerebral ischemia, many questions remain. Much of the work has focused on the vasoactive properties of the ET system and on ET's role in BBB dyshomeostasis, whereas little attention has been given to the possible involvement of the ET system in other brain regions.

REFERENCES

[1]   Schinelli S. Pharmacology and physiopathology of the brain endothelin system: an overview. Curr Med Chem 2006; 13(6): 627-38.

[2]   Kedzierski RM, Yanagisawa M. Endothelin system: the double-edged sword in health and disease. Annu Rev Pharmacol Toxicol 2001; 41: 851-76.

[3]   Lo EH, Dalkara T, Moskowitz MA. Mechanisms, challenges and opportunities in stroke. Nat Rev Neurosci 2003; 4(5): 399-415.

[4]   Banerjee S, Bhat MA. Neuron-glial interactions in blood-brain barrier formation. Annu Rev Neurosci 2007; 30: 235-58.

[5]   Takahashi M, Macdonald RL. Vascular aspects of neuroprotection. Neurol Res 2004; 26(8): 862-9.

[6]   Persidsky Y, Ramirez SH, Haorah J, Kanmogne GD. Blood-brain barrier: structural components and function under physiologic and pathologic conditions. J Neuroimmune Pharmacol 2006; 1(3): 223-36.

[7]   Kaur C, Ling EA. Blood brain barrier in hypoxic-ischemic conditions. Curr Neurovasc Res 2008; 5(1): 71-81.

[8]   Lok J, Gupta P, Guo S, Kim WJ, Whalen MJ, van Leyen K *et al.* Cell-cell signaling in the neurovascular unit. Neurochem Res 2007; 32(12): 2032-45.

[9]   Davis W, Mahale S, Carranza A, Cox B, Hayes K, Jimenez D *et al.* Exercise pre-conditioning ameliorates blood-brain barrier dysfunction in stroke by enhancing basal lamina. Neurol Res 2007; 29(4): 382-7.

[10]   Yanagisawa M, Kurihara H, Kimura S, Goto K, Masaki T. A novel peptide vasoconstrictor, endothelin, is produced by vascular endothelium and modulates smooth muscle Ca2+ channels. J Hypertens Suppl 1988; 6(4): S188-91.

[11]   Stenman E, Malmsjo M, Uddman E, Gido G, Wieloch T, Edvinsson L. Cerebral ischemia upregulates vascular endothelin ET(B) receptors in rat. Stroke 2002; 33(9): 2311-6.

[12]   Kallakuri S, Kreipke CW, Rossi N, Rafols JA, Petrov T. Spatial alterations in endothelin receptor expression are temporally associated with the altered microcirculation after brain trauma. Neurol Res 2007; 29(4): 362-8.

[13]   Ehrenreich H, Costa T, Clouse KA, Pluta RM, Ogino Y, Coligan JE *et al.* Thrombin is a regulator of astrocytic endothelin-1. Brain Res 1993; 600(2): 201-7.

[14]   Brondani R, Rieder CR, Valente D, Araujo LF, Clausell N. Levels of vascular cell adhesion molecule-1 and endothelin-1 in ischemic stroke: a longitudinal prospective study. Clin Biochem 2007; 40(3-4): 282-4.

[15]   Ziv I, Fleminger G, Djaldetti R, Achiron A, Melamed E, Sokolovsky M. Increased plasma endothelin-1 in acute ischemic stroke. Stroke 1992; 23(7): 1014-6.

[16]   Alioglu Z, Orem A, Bulbul I, Boz C, Ozmenoglu M, Vanizor B. Evaluation of plasma endothelin-1 levels in patients with cerebral infarction. Angiology 2002; 53(1): 77-82.

[17]   Lampl Y, Fleminger G, Gilad R, Galron R, Sarova-Pinhas I, Sokolovsky M. Endothelin in cerebrospinal fluid and plasma of patients in the early stage of ischemic stroke. Stroke 1997; 28(10): 1951-5.

[18]   Haapaniemi E, Tatlisumak T, Hamel K, Soinne L, Lanni C, Opgenorth TJ *et al.* Plasma endothelin-1 levels neither increase nor correlate with neurological scores, stroke risk factors, or outcome in patients with ischemic stroke. Stroke 2000; 31(3): 720-5.

[19]   Leung JW, Ho MC, Lo AC, Chung SS, Chung SK. Endothelial cell-specific over-expression of endothelin-1 leads to more severe cerebral damage following transient middle cerebral artery occlusion. J Cardiovasc Pharmacol 2004; 44 Suppl 1: S293-300.

[20]   Gajkowska B, Mossakowski MJ. Localization of endothelin in the blood-brain interphase in rat hippocampus after global cerebral ischemia. Folia Neuropathol 1995; 33(4): 221-30.

[21]   Loo LS, Ng YK, Zhu YZ, Lee HS, Wong PT. Cortical expression of endothelin receptor subtypes A and B following middle cerebral artery occlusion in rats. Neuroscience 2002; 112(4): 993-1000.

[22]   Briyal S, Gulati A, Gupta YK. Effect of combination of endothelin receptor antagonist (TAK-044) and aspirin in middle cerebral artery occlusion model of acute ischemic stroke in rats. Methods Find Exp Clin Pharmacol 2007; 29(4): 257-63.

[23]   Chuquet J, Benchenane K, Toutain J, MacKenzie ET, Roussel S, Touzani O. Selective blockade of endothelin-B receptors exacerbates ischemic brain damage in the rat. Stroke 2002; 33(12): 3019-25.

[24]   Plumpton C, Ferro CJ, Haynes WG, Webb DJ, Davenport AP. The increase in human plasma immunoreactive endothelin but not big endothelin-1 or its C-terminal fragment induced by systemic administration of the endothelin antagonist TAK-044. Br J Pharmacol 1996; 119(2): 311-4.

[25]   Matsuo Y, Mihara S, Ninomiya M, Fujimoto M. Protective effect of endothelin type A receptor antagonist on brain edema and injury after transient middle cerebral artery occlusion in rats. Stroke 2001; 32(9): 2143-8.

[26]   Zhang Y, Belayev L, Zhao W, Irving EA, Busto R, Ginsberg MD. A selective endothelin ET(A) receptor antagonist, SB 234551, improves cerebral perfusion following permanent focal cerebral ischemia in rats. Brain Res 2005; 1045(1-2): 150-6.

[27]   Dawson DA, Sugano H, McCarron RM, Hallenbeck JM, Spatz M. Endothelin receptor antagonist preserves microvascular perfusion and reduces ischemic brain damage following permanent focal ischemia. Neurochem Res 1999; 24(12): 1499-1505.

[28]   Hauck EF, Hoffmann JF, Heimann A, Kempski O. EndothelinA receptor antagonist BSF-208075 causes immune modulation and neuroprotection after stroke in gerbils. Brain Res 2007; 1157: 138-45.

[29]   Miller RD, Monsul NT, Vender JR, Lehmann JC. NMDA- and endothelin-1-induced increases in blood-brain barrier permeability quantitated with Lucifer yellow. J Neurol Sci 1996; 136(1-2): 37-40.

[30]   Lo AC, Chen AY, Hung VK, Yaw LP, Fung MK, Ho MC *et al.* Endothelin-1 overexpression leads to further water accumulation and brain edema after middle cerebral artery occlusion via aquaporin 4 expression in astrocytic end-feet. J Cereb Blood Flow Metab 2005; 25(8): 998-1011.

[31]   Gasche Y, Soccal PM, Kanemitsu M, Copin JC. Matrix metalloproteinases and diseases of the central nervous system with a special emphasis on ischemic brain. Front Biosci 2006; 11: 1289-301.

[32]   Koyama Y, Baba A, Matsuda T. Intracerebroventricular administration of an endothelin ETB receptor agonist increases expression of tissue inhibitor of matrix metalloproteinase-1 and -3 in rat brain. Neuroscience 2007; 147(3): 620-30.

[33]   Abraham D, Ponticos M, Nagase H. Connective tissue remodeling: cross-talk between endothelins and matrix metalloproteinases. Curr Vasc Pharmacol 2005; 3(4): 369-79.

[34]   Hofman FM, Chen P, Jeyaseelan R, Incardona F, Fisher M, Zidovetzki R. Endothelin-1 induces production of the neutrophil chemotactic factor interleukin-8 by human brain-derived endothelial cells. Blood 1998; 92(9): 3064-72.

[35]   Chen P, Shibata M, Zidovetzki R, Fisher M, Zlokovic BV, Hofman FM. Endothelin-1 and monocyte chemoattractant protein-1 modulation in ischemia and human brain-derived endothelial cell cultures. J Neuroimmunol 2001; 116(1): 62-73.

[36]   Brillault J, Lam TI, Rutkowsky JM, Foroutan S, O'Donnell ME. Hypoxia effects on cell volume and ion uptake of cerebral microvascular endothelial cells. Am J Physiol Cell Physiol 2008; 294(1): C88-96.

[37]   Kawai N, Yamamoto T, Yamamoto H, McCarron RM, Spatz M. Endothelin 1 stimulates Na+,K(+)-ATPase and Na(+)-K(+)-Cl- cotransport through ETA receptors and protein kinase C-dependent pathway in cerebral capillary endothelium. J Neurochem 1995; 65(4): 1588-96.

[38]   Spatz M, Kawai N, Bembry J, Lenz F, McCarron RM. Human brain capillary endothelium: modulation of K+ efflux and K+, Ca2+ uptake by endothelin. Neurochem Res; 1998; 23(8): 1125-32.

[39]   Kawai N, McCarron RM, Spatz M. Endothelins stimulate sodium uptake into rat brain capillary endothelial cells through endothelin A-like receptors. Neurosci Lett 1995; 190(2): 85-8.

Research Progress of Hypothermia: Selective Intra-arterial Infusion and Regional Brain Cooling in Acute Stroke Therapy

Yuchuan Ding[1,*] and Justin Charles Clark[2]

[1]*Department of Neurosurgery, the University of Texas Health Science Center at San Antonio, USA;*
E-mail: dingy2@uthscsa.edu

[2]*Department of Neurosurgery, the Barrow Neurological Institute, Phoenix, AZ, USA*

Abstract: In the United States, stroke is the 3rd leading cause of death, behind diseases of the heart and cancer, and the number 1 cause of disability. Basic research on stroke has been extensive, but clinically effective therapies are still lacking. Recombinant tissue plasminogen activator (tPA) is the only drug approved by the Food and Drug Administration (FDA) for selected patients (3%) with ischemic stroke. The benefit of this thrombolytic therapy is largely limited by it's selection criteria and its side effects. An area of stroke research that holds much promise is regional brain cooling. The neuroprotective effect of hypothermia has long been recognized. Currently used whole body cooling for brain injury treatment from stroke was abandoned because of management problems, severe side effects and delayed onset of cerebral hypothermia. Recent studies in a rat stroke model have utilized a unique technique to infuse the microvasculature in the ischemic territory prior to reperfusion with cold saline, leading to a improved outcomes in this animal model. Translating the research done with combined intra-arterial revascularization and local brain cooling to the clinical realm could advance the treatment of stroke beyond the levels achieved by current therapies.

THERAPEUTIC WINDOW IN ACUTE ISCHEMIC STROKE

Stroke is the third leading cause of death and the leading cause of serious, long-term disability in many developed countries. More than 700,000 strokes occur annually in the United States, with an impact of more than $50 billion in health care expenditures and lost productivity [1]. Basic research on stroke has been extensive, but previous therapeutic approaches have been unsuccessful. Clinically, there are no effective therapeutic tools for ameliorating brain damage caused by ischemia and subsequent reperfusion from stroke. In fact, no agents have successfully completed phase III development as neuroprotectants against stroke. Among the agent-classes under consideration are calcium channel blockers, glutamate receptor antagonists, GABA receptor agonists, antioxidants/radical scavengers, phospholipid precursors, nitric oxide signal-transduction down-regulators and leukocyte inhibitors; as well as therapies such as hemodilution [2].

Ischemic stroke is responsible for approximately 70-80% of all strokes, and is usually caused by clots or particles that plug an artery [3]. Cerebral infarction may ensue within minutes of a critical reduction in cerebral blood flow. It has been reported that the middle cerebral artery (MCA) is the most common site of obstruction in ischemic stroke. Up to 78% of patients with acute stroke due to MCA occlusion die or become severely disabled [3, 4]. The ischemic crisis caused by obstruction of the artery initiates a cascade of intracellular events within the affected cells, which eventually leads to cellular death. Thus, the early reestablishment of tissue perfusion seems to be a logical first step in the treatment of acute ischemic stroke.

Until recently, the only FDA (U.S. Food and Drug Administration) approved treatment for recanalization therapy in acute ischemic stroke has been intravenous (IV) recombinant tissue plasminogen activator (tPA) delivered within the first 3 hours of stroke onset. The NINDS–tPA trials demonstrated that treatment within 3 hours from symptom onset benefited patients with stroke, despite an increased risk of symptomatic hemorrhage [5, 6]. Unfortunately, the majority of individuals experiencing a stroke do not present for medical attention within the first 3 hours of symptom onset. Sadly, after nearly a decade of experience, only 1-3% of patients with stroke in the United States currently receive IV tPA [7].

Recently, local intra-arterial (IA) thrombolysis using recombinant prourokinase has also been found to improve outcome in patients with acute M1 or M2 segment occlusions of the MCA [8, 9]. IA delivery of thrombolytic agents into occluded MCA segments within 6 hours of symptom onset in the Prolyse in Acute Cerebral Thromboembolism (PROACT) II trial, resulted in a recanalization rate of 66% [8]. Overall, the recanalization rates with IA reported in the literature are higher than IV thrombolysis. However, the FDA still requests an additional study because of the borderline statistical significance of the overall results.

Unfortunately, the degree of recanalization after a stroke does not always correlate with the patient's clinical outcome. Although recanalization is successful in many cases, the outcome remains poor, consistent with a reperfusion injury [10-12]. Treatment approaches based on recanalization as a primary outcome measure have therefore drawn criticism. Recanalization may result in a variety of outcomes including neurological improvement, no clinical change, reperfusion hemorrhage, or massive cerebral edema, resulting in neurological worsening or death, depending on timing, depth, and duration of ischemia [13]. While arterial reopening is indeed important, the final outcome of the patient's clinical status is paramount. Clearly, improvements in interventions that will prevent brain damage and lengthen the therapeutic window for treating stroke are imperative. Specifically, there exists a need to develop a new therapy for stroke that will allow us to increase the narrow 3-6 hour therapeutic time window that presently exists, as well as decrease the poor clinical outcome experienced currently after recanalizaton.

HYPOTHERMIA IS A POWERFUL NEUROPROTECTANT

1. Therapeutic effect of hypothermia

Data have been accumulated to suggest that "non-drug" approaches toward stroke therapy, such as therapeutic hypothermia, caffeinol, normobaric hyperoxia, glucose regulation, albumin, and magnesium, might provide new opportunities to treat stroke [14]. The importance of these alternate and sometimes complementary methods is growing as noted by the willingness of the NINDS, through its key 'Specialized Program of Translational Research in Acute Stroke' (SPOTRIAS) initiative, to fund several trials of therapeutics, including hypothermia.

Induced hypothermia is one of the best studied and most highly effective forms of neuroprotection. Multiple groups have demonstrated the remarkable benefit of mild or moderate (30-34°C) hypothermia in limiting the damage of global and focal ischemia in animal models and clinical studies [15-23]. The mechanisms of neuroprotection conferred by brain cooling in stroke therapy are multifactorial and synergistic [15-18, 21-25]. It has been shown that hypothermia decreases energy metabolism via reduced cerebral metabolic rates of glucose and oxygen, as well as reduced ATP breakdown in the mammalian central nervous system [26]. Hypothermia reduces glutamate release and intracellular calcium rises after ischemia [27], and directly inhibits calcium-mediated effects on calcium/calmodulin kinase [28, 29]. Intra-ischemic hypothermia prevents neuronal cell death after cerebral ischemia and reperfusion by reducing both apoptosis and necrosis [30-33]. Hypothermia also has significant effects on reducing the production of hydroxyl radicals and suppressing nitric oxide and peroxynitrite formation against ischemic insult [34, 35], leading to inhibition of apoptosis [36].

Additionally, it has been well recognized [37-40] that hypothermia provides protection against stroke-induced inflammatory responses, since Chopp and his colleagues first demonstrated a reduction in neutrophil infiltration after focal ischemia/reperfusion injury [19]. The reduction of ischemic injury and leukocyte infiltration has been correlated with a diminished over-expression of ICAM-1 mRNA, which normally occurs in the wake of an ischemic stroke [41, 42]. A recent study demonstrated that hypothermia induces increases in cerebral galanin concentrations, leading to ischemic neuroprotection in the rat brain [43]. Galanin has been suggested to serve as a neurotropic and/or regenerative factor in the nervous system.

As discussed above, stroke is a complex pathological process involving multiple pathways that are active during the entire ischemic and post-ischemic period. No single treatment is likely to be completely effective in ischemic stroke therapy; rather, it will be through the prevention, limitation or reversal at multiple deleterious sites along the ischemic stroke cascade that this disease will be treated. Hypothermia, which exhibits multiple and synergistic salutary effects on stroke-mediated cell death, has the potential to play an important role in the treatment of this condition.

2. Limitation of hypothermia in stroke therapy

Classical techniques for inducing therapeutic hypothermia are achieved by whole-body surface cooling with the use of cooling blankets, alcohol applied to exposed skin, or ice bags to groin, axilla, and neck. These approaches require intensive efforts from the medical and nursing staff for induction, as well as maintenance of the target temperature. In addition, these approaches take as long as 3 to 7 hours for cooling to the target body core temperature of 32-34°C [44, 45]. Further, surface cooling is associated with severe complications, such as pneumonia (40%) [46], impaired immune function, decreased cardiac output, cardiac arrhythmias [47, 48] and thrombocytopenia [49].

Very recent technological developments on the induction and maintenance of systemic therapeutic hypothermia is the use of a special heat-exchange catheter that is placed in the inferior vena cava [50]. This new high-tech device cools the ischemic tissue *indirectly* by thermal conduction of heat flow from the ischemic tissue to the cooled healthy tissue, since the blood vessel that supplies the infarcted region is occluded [51, 52]. Although this system may be able to accelerate the cooling rate as compared to the classical surface cooling methods, thermal conduction is a relatively slow physical process. In addition, the incidence of adverse effects for surface cooling (see above) is also a disadvantage of this procedure. Regarding a regional cooling method by the cooling cap and helmet, theoretical analyses [53-55] and empirical measurements [56, 57] suggest that such cooling systems are effective in reducing the temperature in the superficial cerebral region, but not in deep brain structure, such as the basal ganglia. The clinical outcome from these therapies is not promising. An effective intra- or post-ischemic mechanism for inducing cerebral hypothermia without reducing body core temperature is highly desirable.

Since most patients who suffer a stroke do not reach treatment until hours after the onset of symptoms, delayed intra-ischemic or post-ischemic intervention is an important issue in stroke therapy. Some clinical studies have suggested that the neuroprotective properties of mild or moderate hypothermia in acute ischemic stroke can only be achieved by either earlier initiation of brain cooling after onset of stroke, or by prolonged hypothermic setting for up to 48 to 72 hours [44, 46, 58, 59]. Many studies in animal models with global and focal transient cerebral ischemia have demonstrated the effectiveness of postischemic hypothermia [15, 41, 60-65], but prolonged application of postischemic hypothermia seems to be necessary to achieve significant and

persistent neuroprotection [15, 39, 66-69]. Furthermore, it is likely that mild post-ischemic hypothermia simply delays neuronal damage in ischemia [39, 70].

Taken together, results from previous studies suggest that intra- or post- ischemic hypothermia produces powerful neuroprotection against cerebral ischemia/reperfusion injury, and that the more clinically relevant post-ischemic hypothermia requires a prolonged application time to achieve significant and persistent neuroprotection. Thus, an enhanced procedure of post-ischemic hypothermia for short duration would be beneficial.

INTRA-ARTERIAL INFUSION AND SELECTIVE BRAIN HYPOTHERMIA

1. Intra-arterial revascularization in acute stroke

As mentioned above, the application of intra-arterial thrombolytic therapy by means of a microcatheter has

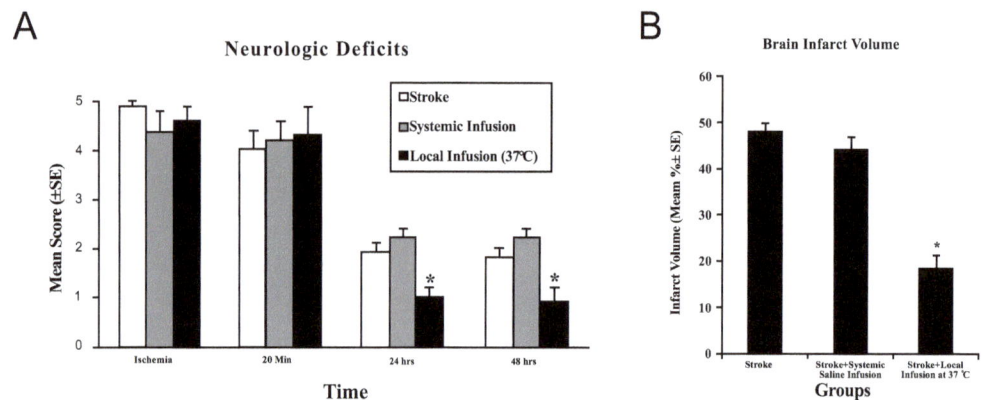

Fig. (1). Graph of neurological scores indicating outcomes of ischemic animals in stroke, stroke with systemic infusion, stroke with local infusion groups (A). The severity of the deficits was comparable during ischemia and early reperfusion (20 minutes). Neurological outcome was further improved in animals receiving local infusions at 24 and 48 hours after reperfusion, respectively (p<0.001, indicated by •). Infarct volume in the same ischemic rat groups is also shown (stroke, stroke with systemic infusion, stroke with local infusion of saline) (B). A significantly (p<0.001, indicated by •) reduced infarct volume was found in ischemic rats with a local saline infusion, compared to that in rats without the infusion.

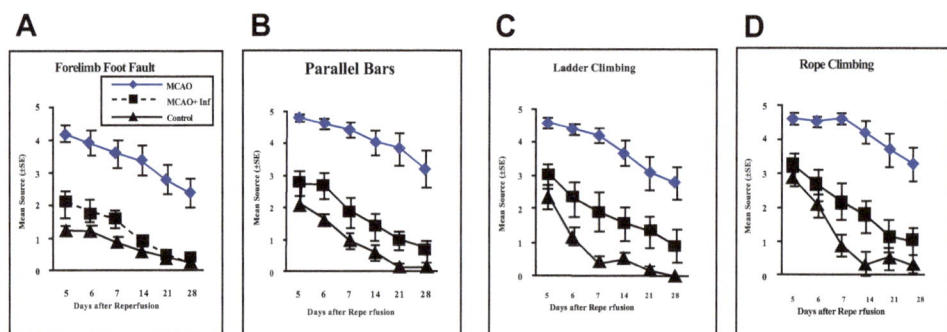

Fig. (2). Graphs depicting motor performance, including forelimb foot faults (A), parallel bars crossing (B), rope climbing (C), and ladder climbing (D). In all tests, the performance of the animals that underwent MCA occlusion (MCAO) without local infusion were significantly worse (p<0.001) than the scores in the ischemic rats that received infusion (MCAO-Inf) and control animals, up to 28 days after reperfusion. There was no significant difference between rats that had suffered stroke treated with infusion and control animals.

been used successfully in human stroke to revascularize acutely occluded cerebral vessels, such as the MCA. These therapies work via either mechanical disruption or suction of the clot, as well as by delivering thrombolytic drugs [5, 8, 71-79], or by using a combination of these techniques [80, 81]. During these procedures, an infusion microcatheter, guided to the site of the lesion via the guide catheter over a microguidewire, is advanced distally to the site of occlusion and gradually pulled back through the clot to permit infusion of thrombolytic drugs distal to, within, and proximal to the occluded segment. Microcatheters placed in the MCA have been continuously flushed with heparinized saline to prevent clot propagation on the distal catheter tip.

2. Therapeutic potential of local MCA infusion of saline

It has been widely reported that if reperfusion of ischemic tissue is not initiated early enough, it can lead to extensive secondary cell injury and death [82-88]. During reperfusion, blood flow and oxygen supply exacerbate tissue damage by augmenting the accumulation of inflammatory cells, leading to the overproduction of oxygen free radicals and microvascular dysfunction [83-102].

Removal of biochemical byproducts and toxic mediators, such as cytokines, free fatty acids and adverse mechanical and rheological events, which accumulate in the ischemic territory, could potentially

Changes of CBF during and after MCA occlusion

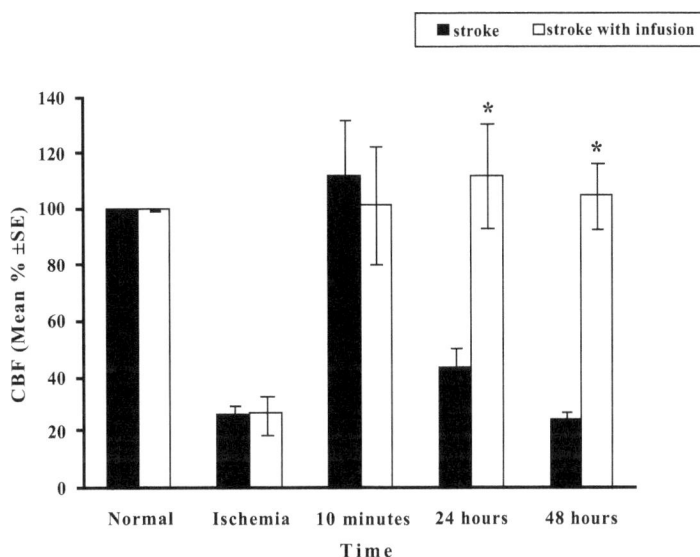

Fig. (3). Changes of cerebral blood flow (CBF) during ischemia and reperfusion between the ischemic rats with and without local infusion. The degree of cortical perfusion during ischemia was substantially decreased in all animals. Although the local CBF in these animals consistently attained pre-ischemic levels within 10 minutes after onset of reperfusion in the two groups of ischemic rats with or without local infusion, CBF was significantly reduced (p<0.001, indicated by ∗) at 24 and 48 hours after reperfusion in the non-infused rats, compared to a relative normal perfusion in the saline-infused rats.

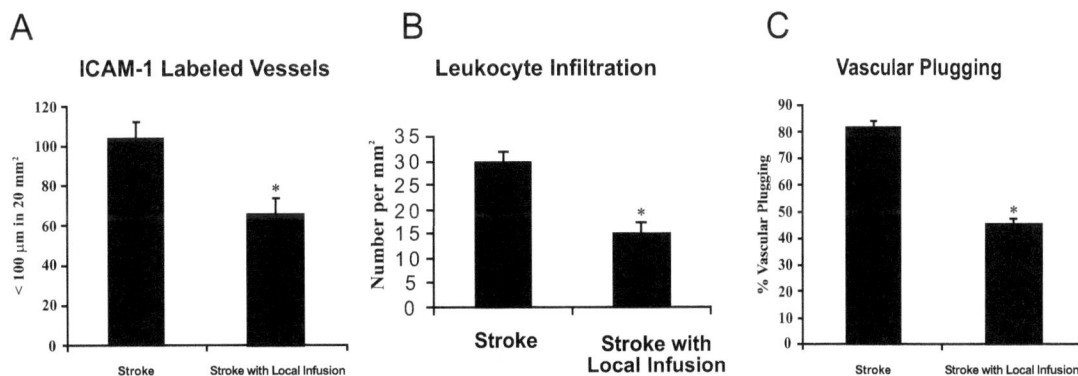

Fig. (4). Inflammatory events and vascular plugging were compared between ischemic groups with or without local saline infusion 48 hours after ischemia and reperfusion. Quantitative analysis of ICAM-1 immuno-labeled microvessels demonstrated that the number of ICAM-1 positive vessels in the local infusion group was significantly (p<0.05, indicated by ∗) reduced by 37%, from 104±8 to 66±5, per 20 mm^2 of lesion region (**A**). When the numbers of leukocytes in preoptic, striatal and cortical lesions were compared, a 50% reduction was associated with pre-reperfusion infusion, with the average number of leukocytes/mm^2 infiltrated into infarcted regions being significantly (p<0.01, indicated by ∗) reduced from 30±2/mm^2 in infused to 15±2/mm^2 in non-infused groups (**B**). In the infarct region, the percentage of plugged vessels was significantly (p<0.01, indicated by ∗) reduced by 44%, from 81±3% in ischemic animals without local infusion to 45±2% with local infusion (**C**).

minimize the reperfusion injury. In a previous study [103], we used a novel intraluminal hollow filament to "flush" the occluded area prior to establishing reperfusion. The salutary effects conferred by intra-arterial "flushing" of saline may involve more than one mechanism of ischemia/reperfusion injury [104]. This treatment significantly reduced neurological deficits and infarct volume (Fig. **1**) and improved functional outcome (Fig. **2**).

Flushing of saline into ischemic territory preserved adequate blood flow during reperfusion (Fig. **3**). The benefits of vascular infusion include removal of biochemical byproducts and toxic mediators, such as cytokines and adhesion molecules, which accumulate in the ischemic territory [105], and of adverse mechanical and rheological events [106]. We observed that the improvements in cerebral microcirculation correlated to a significant (p<0.001) reduction in endothelial expression of ICAM-1, vascular-parenchymal infiltration of inflammatory

leukocytes (61%), and microvascular plugging (45%) (Fig. **4**). Further study was undertaken to investigate if flushing the ischemic territory prior to reperfusion could reduce the overexpression of inflammatory cytokines during reperfusion. A significant overexpression (9-26 fold) of the genes encoding TNF-α and IL-1β in ischemic rats was found during early reperfusion at 6 and 12 hours in ischemic rats without flushing (Fig. **5**). This increase was significantly reduced at both 6 and 12 hours post-reperfusion as a result of saline flushing. In addition, we investigated whether flushing of ischemic territory could reduce expression of matrix metalloproteinases (MMP), especially, gelatinase MMP-2 and MMP-9, during reperfusion, leading to reduced disruption of microvascular integrity [107]. MMP-2 and MMP-9 are believed to contribute to remodeling of the extracellular matrix (ECM) of the blood brain barrier (BBB) by breaking down the major basal lamina components including collagen IV, laminin, and fibronectin, leading to BBB disruption

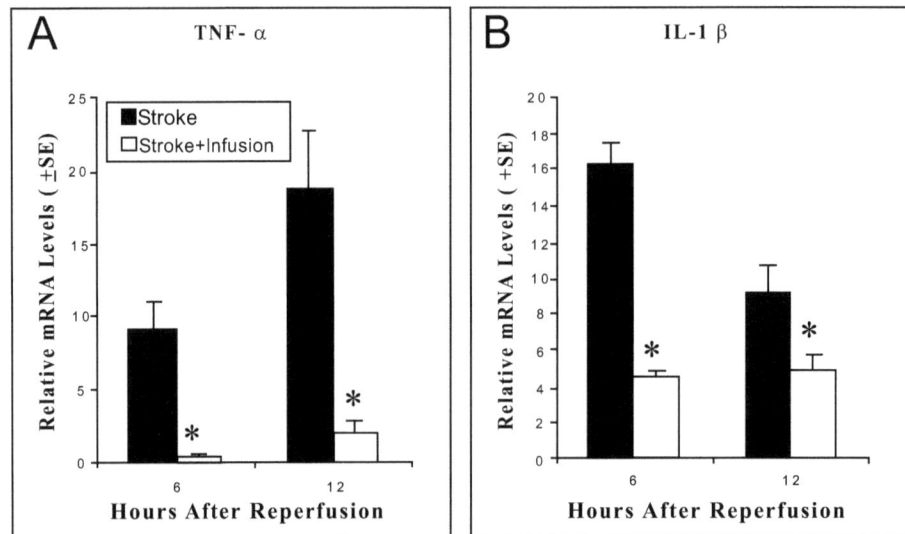

Fig. (5). Graphs depicting changes in the relative levels of mRNA encoding TNF-α (**A**) and IL-1β (**B**) during early reperfusion at 6 and 12 hours in the ischemic groups with or without local saline infusion prior to reperfusion. The mRNA levels for the control group were arbitrarily assigned as 1.0 ± 0.0 to serve as reference (not shown). A significantly (p<0.05) increased relative level of TNF-α and IL-1β mRNA was observed in ischemic rats without brain infusion during reperfusion at 6 and 12 hours. This increase was significantly reduced by local infusion (p<0.05, indicated by *).

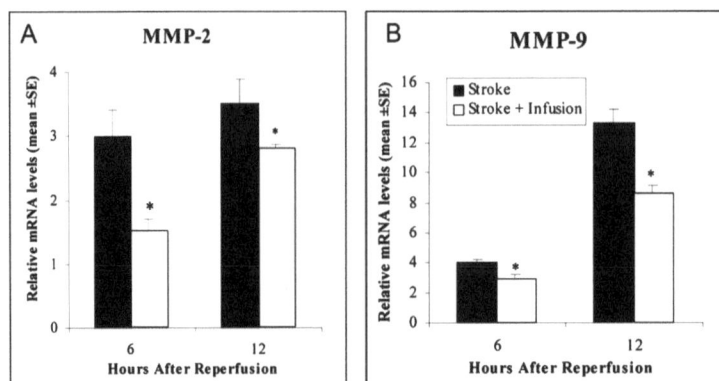

Fig. (6). Graphs depicting changes of relative levels of mRNA encoding MMP-2 (**A**) and MMP-9 (**B**) during early reperfusion at 6 and 12 hours in two ischemic groups with or without brain saline infusion. A significant (p<0.01, indicated by *) reduction was induced by the cerebral flushing procedure in ischemic rats during reperfusion at 6 and 12 hours, as compared to ischemic rats without brain infusion.

[108, 109]. Brain edema was reduced by 19±4%, and overexpression of the mRNA encoding MMP-2 and -9 found in ischemic rats was significantly (p<0.05) ameliorated as a result of saline flushing (Fig. **6**).

The mechanism through which intra-arterial saline infusion confers its neuroprotection is thought to be via its ability to interfere with a series of injurious events, which are triggered by ischemia and potentiated by reperfusion; thereby preventing the potentially multifactorial interactions between ischemically damaged tissue and reestablished blood flow and oxygenation. This therapy has the potential to lengthen the therapeutic window for recanalization after stroke and improve clinical outcomes in ischemic stroke patients.

3. Highly selective brain hypothermia in ischemic territory

A few studies have introduced the concept of selective cooling, in which the target organ, rather than whole body, is selected as a therapeutic end-point for hypothermia [25]. Cold carotid artery perfusion with temperature-decreased blood, localized cerebral ventricular perfusion with a hypothermic solution, and head surface cooling have all been tried clinically or experimentally for selective brain cooling and neuroprotection [24, 68, 110, 111]. Also, a single bolus high-volume (100 ml/kg) flush of cold saline (4^{0}C) into the abdominal aorta given 2 minutes after the onset of cardiac arrest rapidly induces moderate-to-deep cerebral hypothermia and results in survival without functional and histological brain damage,

even after 30 minute of no blood flow in dog [112]. Additionally, regional infusion of the crossclamped infrarenal rabbit aorta with hypothermic saline and adenosine (8°C, 30 ml/kg, for 10 minutes) improved behavioral and histological outcome in postischemic spinal cord injury [113]. The model of infusing microvasculature in the ischemic territory could provide a powerful tool for brain hypothermia in stroke therapy, by which highly selective brain regions, especially in ischemic territories, could be cooled [114].

In a transient focal ischemic stroke induced by MCA occlusion for 3 hours, the potential of cold saline infusion in inducing regional hypothermia was tested through the hollow filament inserted into the MCA in rat stroke model [114, 115]. The ischemic territory was locally infused with 6 ml of cold (20°C) saline for 10 minutes prior to withdrawal of the filament and reperfusion (for 48 hours). The cold saline infusion rapidly and significantly reduced mean temperature in the MCA supplied territory in cerebral cortex from 37.2±0.1°C to 33.4±0.4°C [$F_{(8, 48)}$ = 35.88, p<0.01], and in the striatum from 37.5±0.2°C to 33.9±0.4°C [$F_{(8, 48)}$ = 26.66, p<0.01]. The significantly (p<0.01) reduced cortical and striatal temperatures remained for up to 60 minutes after the onset of reperfusion. In the ischemic rats perfused locally with saline at body temperature (37°C), brain temperature remained normal during ischemia and reperfusion [in the cortex, 37.3±0.3°C, $F_{(8, 32)}$ = 1.99, p>0.05, and in the striatum, 37.5±0.2°C, $F_{(8, 32)}$ = 0.31, p>0.05]. In ischemic rats that received the same amount of cold saline systemically through a femoral artery, a mild hypothermia was induced in cortex (35.3±0.2°C, $F_{(8, 48)}$

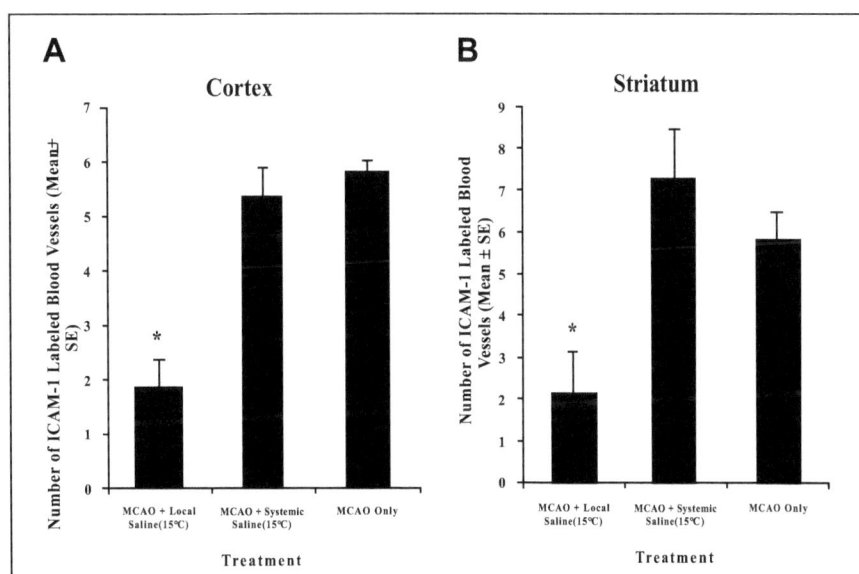

Fig. (7). Graph depicting the magnitude of the inflammatory injury after stroke (3-hour MCA occlusion followed by 48-hour reperfusion) in 3 different stroke groups with local cold infusion, systemic cold infusion, and no infusion. Significant (p<0.001, indicated by∗) reductions in the concentration of ICAM-1 positive vessels per 0.025mm^2 within cortical (**A**) and striatal (**B**) regions were found in rats with local brain cooling, in contrast to control ischemic rats with systemic cold infusion or without infusion.

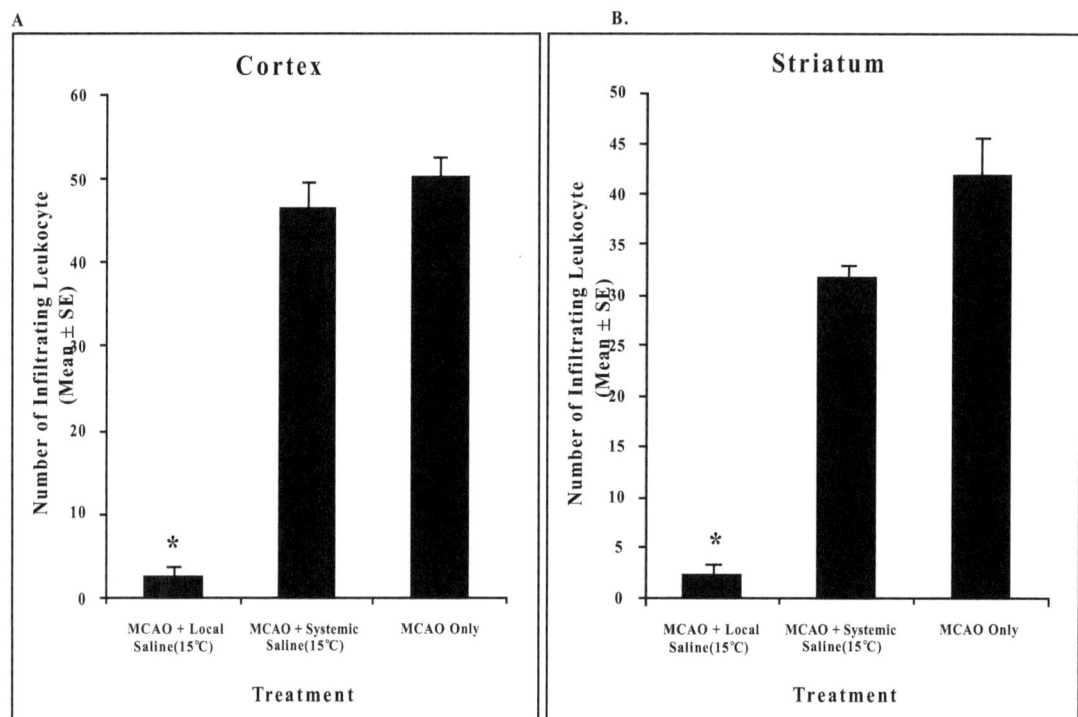

Fig. (8). Graph of the numbers of infiltrating leukocytes in ischemic animals with 3-hour MCA occlusion. After 48 hours of reperfusion, a significant (p<0.01, indicated by *) decrease in leukocyte infiltration was revealed in the local brain cooling group, showing a largely reduced number of infiltrating leukocytes in ischemic cortex (**A**) and striatum (**B**), as compared to that in other ischemic animal groups without local brain cooling.

= 13.21, p<0.01) but not in striatum (36.8±0.2°C, $F_{(8, 48)}$ = 1.48, p>0.05). The reduced cortical temperature returned to normal within 5 minutes. In the ischemic groups with either local or systemic cold saline, the body temperature measured from the rectum was slightly reduced but remained above 36°C, and soon returned to normal levels. K-ANOVA (Kruskal-Wallis test) revealed that ischemic animals with local cold saline (20°C) infusion had significantly decreased deficits compared to stroke without infusion or with systemic cold infusion at 20 minute and 24 through 48 hours after reperfusion. Comparison of infarction within the territory of the occluded MCA including the cortex and striatum indicates that a local cooling infusion significantly (P<0.001) reduced infarct volume by about 90%. Motor functional performance determined by different tasks, such as forelimb foot fault placing, parallel bar traversing, rope climbing and ladder climbing, was significantly (p<0.01) improved with local brain cooling infusion at day 14 and 28 after reperfusion. The therapeutic mechanisms underlying local brain cooling involved a reduction in stroke-mediated inflammatory injury. Brain cooling infusion significantly (p<0.01) reduced endothelial ICAM-1 expression (Fig. **7**) and inflammatory leukocyte infiltration (Fig. **8**) in ischemic cortex and striatum.

Recently, local IA perfusion with coolant to induce regional hypothermia in stroke patients has been theoretically proposed in 3 different studies [51, 53, 116]. Due to the fact that the cold liquid is

transported through the microvasculature and distributed throughout the parenchyma, the heat exchange is extremely effective, leading to rapid tissue cooling. Theoretically, cooling in localized cerebral infarction having a mass of 300 g is 30-times faster than classic surface cooling and 10-20 times faster than endovascular cooling via an endovascular catheter placed in the inferior vena cava.

Both the rate and volume of infusion in the local infusion model is a critical issue that may affect this therapy's feasibility and safety in clinical settings. The previous studies suggest that a brief (10 minutes) local infusion of cold saline can effectively and quickly induce regional brain hypothermia. This post-ischemic hypothermia for short duration (up to 60 minutes rather than prolonged 48 to 72 hours as mentioned above) significantly ameliorates brain injury from stroke in rats. This local hypothermic procedure enhances neuroprotection induced by local infusion in stroke. Six ml of cold saline (15-20°C) infusion at speed of 0.6 ml per minute produces stronger neuroprotection (90% infarct volume reduction in 3 hour MCA occlusion vs. 70% infarct volume reduction in 2 hour MCA occlusion) as compared to 10 ml of warm saline infusion (37°C) at speed of 3 ml per minute. These findings together suggest that both fast infusion with large volume (which might be due to removing accumulated toxins and biochemical byproducts) and slow cooling infusion produce profound neuroprotection. However, the slow infusion with less solution volume may be more realistic and safer in clinical settings.

The temperature of the infused solution is another major issue in the local infusion procedure. The remarkable benefit of mild or moderate (30-34°C) hypothermia has been well-documented as one of the most powerful neuroprotective strategies in cerebral ischemia both experimentally and clinically [15-18]. The coolant temperature of 15-20°C are determined based on previous findings that neuroprotection can be achieved without causing significant brain edema. In our study on ischemic rats, cold saline infusion at 5°C caused death with severe cerebral edema (7 out of 13) at around 24 hours of reperfusion although the animals had a promising recovery at early reperfusion. Furthermore, studies on hypothermic preservation of harvested organs for transplantation indicated that cold (4°C) crystalloid perfusion could potentially cause hypothermic cell swelling and functional failure [117-119].

Solution type is also a critical issue in selective cooling infusion. Previous research supports the potential benefits of bolus administration of hypertonic solution, which reduces both the presence of proinflammatory mediators (cytokines and adhesion molecules) and the adhesion of polymorphonuclear cells to the cerebral microvasculature, as well as improves microcirculation in septic and hemorrhagic shock [120-126]. Extensive studies have demonstrated that various concentrations of hypertonic saline (2.7, 3, 5, 7.5, 23.5%) provide therapeutic effects in cerebral ischemia/reperfusion injury [127-130]. Studies have further demonstrated that the addition of 2% to 6% Dextran to hypertonic saline solution enhances its neuroprotective effects by decreasing microvessel permeability [131, 132]. These solutions may also reduce hypothermia-induced cell swelling and tissue edema, especially when a lower temperature (15-20°C) infusion is used to induce a more intense degree of hypothermia. Clinically, hypertonic solutions (hypertonic saline or/and hypertonic saline dextran) in various concentrations have been used in patients with intracranial pathologies, including stroke and hemorrhagic shock [120, 121, 131, 133, 134]. Reduced cerebral ischemia and improved cerebral oxygen delivery induced by the use of hypertonic solution are attributable to multifactorial effects. In addition to enhancement of cerebral perfusion pressure and increase in intravascular volume and therefore maintenance of adequate cardiac output and blood pressure, a hypertonic solution can effectively reduce ICP and cerebral edema. Hypertonic solutions may decrease hydraulic permeability in activated and highly permeable endothelium by increasing intravascular osmotic pressure, resulting in dehydration of the cerebrovascular endothelium.

There are some concerns that rapid changes in serum sodium concentration induced by too-high dose and/or rate of hypertonic solution may cause heart failure, lung edema, and electrolyte abnormalities (Qureshi and Suarez 2000). However, 7.2-23% of saline has been safely administered in patients, without such side effects [129, 135-137].

CLINICAL RELEVANCE

1. Intra-arterial revascularization and local brain cooling in acute stroke

IA thrombolytic therapy by means of a microcatheter has been used successfully to reopen acute occlusion of cerebral vessels, such as the MCA, either by mechanical disruption or removal of the clot, as well as to deliver thrombolytic drugs in human stroke [7, 8, 72-78, 80, 138]. These studies using IA catheterization suggest that local infusion of coolant into the ischemic territory prior to reperfusion is feasible in clinical practice. From a physical point of view [51], the previous theoretical and experimental research showed that localized infusion and hypothermia in brain tissue jeopardized by ischemia is possible with the aid of a combined guiding/micro-catheter set-up that is used routinely in interventional neuroradiology in the treatment of acute stroke. The instruments and experience necessary to perform the proposed local infusion and hypothermia are available in each Department of Neuroradiology or Neurosurgery. The logistics of actually performing perfusion in the human are relatively simple as this is a normal part of performing endovascular interventions for many neuroendovascular surgeons (Ringer et al., 2001). A great variety of endovascular tools exist for delivering medications and devices to intracranial vessels. Therefore, it is expected that this new therapy could be easily added to an angiography suite.

It is our hope that future studies will determined the ideal hypothermic level, duration of cooling, adequate infusion volume and speed for maximal benefit and minimum adverse affects, in order to identify which treatments have the highest therapeutic potential in clinical settings.

2. Selective intra-arterial infusion and "cocktail" therapy

The above studies have suggested the feasibility in using highly selective hypothermia induced by cerebral IA infusion in acute stroke therapy. In addition, the procedure of intra-arterial infusion and selective brain hypothermia could be used in acute stroke treatment, possibly in combination with IA thrombolysis or mechanical disruption of clots by means of a microcatheter. The intra-arterial infusion technique would also allow delivery of high concentrations of protective agents into the ischemic area. Most recently, a local infusion model has been used for super-selective MCA infusion of MK-801, a putative neuroprotectant, in rats [139]. The administration of a low dose of MK-801 (0.3 mg/kg body weight) resulted in a significantly smaller infarct volume than systemic application. This super-selective MCA infusion is a valuable tool for the selective delivery of this drug, which would enhance drug uptake into cerebral ischemic tissue, as well as for infusion of super-oxygenated solution and for other "non-drug" natural agents (eg, albumin, magnesium) [14]. It may also be useful for gene transfer, or application of stem cells. Therefore, in addition to brain cooling infusions, various combinations of neuroprotective agents could be regionally administered, and the ultimate neuroprotective concept of a "cocktail" could be devised.

REFERENCES

[1] Levy EI, Sauvageau E, Hanel RA, Parikh R, Hopkins LN. Am J Neuroradiol 2006; 27: 2069-72.

[2] Ginsberg MD. Neuropharmacology 2008.

[3] Overgaard K. Cerebrovasc Brain Metab Rev 1994; 6: 257-86.

[4] Samama MM, Desnoyers PC, Conard J, Bousser MG. Thromb Haemost 1997; 78: 173-9.

[5] The National Institute of Neurological Disorders and Stroke rt-PA Stroke Study Group. Tissue plasminogen activator for acute ischemic stroke. N Engl J Med 1995; 333: 1581-7.

[6] Saver JL. Arch Neurol 2004; 61: 1066-70.

[7] Kim D, Jahan R, Starkman S, et al. Am J Neuroradiol 2006; 27: 2048-52.

[8] Furlan A, Higashida R, Wechsler L, et al. JAMA 1999; 282: 2003-11.

[9] Arnold M, Schroth G, Nedeltchev K, et al. Stroke 2002; 33: 1828-33.

[10] Cruz-Flores S, Thompson DW, Boiser JR. J Neuroimaging 2001; 11: 447-51.

[11] Wardlaw JM, del Zoppo GJ, Yamaguchi T, Berge E. Cochrane Database Syst Rev 2003; CD000213.

[12] Koudstaal PJ, Stibbe J, Vermeulen M. BMJ 1988; 297: 1571-4.

[13] Wechsler LR. Stroke 2006; 37: 1341-2.

[14] Singhal AB, Lo EH. Stroke 2008; 39: 289-91.

[15] Colbourne F, Sutherland G, Corbett D. Mol Neurobiol 1997; 14: 171-201.

[16] Barone FC, Feuerstein GZ, White RF. Neurosci Biobehav Rev 1997; 21: 31-44.

[17] Kataoka K, Yanase H. Neurosci Res 1998; 32: 103-17.

[18] Corbett D, Thornhill J. Brain Pathol 2000; 10: 145-52.

[19] Chen H, Chopp M, Vande LA, Dereski MO, Garcia JH, Welch KM. J Neurol Sci 1992; 107: 191-8.

[20] Holzer M, Bernard SA, Hachimi-Idrissi S, Roine RO, Sterz F, Mullner M. Crit Care Med 2005; 33: 414-8.

[21] Liu L, Yenari MA. Front Biosci 2007; 12: 816-25.

[22] Hemmen TM, Lyden PD. Stroke 2007; 38: 794-9.

[23] Hoesch RE, Geocadin RG. Neurologist 2007; 13: 331-42.

[24] Busto R, Ginsberg MD. In: Cerebrovascular Disease Pathophysiology, Diagnosis, and Management. Ginsberg MD, Bogousslavsky J, Eds. Malden, Massachusetts: Blackwell Science.1998, pp. 287-307.

[25] Ginsberg MD, Busto R. Stroke 1998; 29: 529-34.

[26] Erecinska M, Thoresen M, Silver IA. J Cereb Blood Flow Metab 2003; 23: 513-30.

[27] Nakashima K, Todd MM. Stroke 1996; 27: 913-8.

[28] Takata T, Nabetani M, Okada Y. Neurosci Lett 1997; 227: 41-4.

[29] Hu BR, Kamme F, Wieloch T. Neuroscience 1995; 68: 1003-16.

[30] Ohmura A, Nakajima W, Ishida A, et al. Brain Dev 2005; 27: 517-26.

[31] Zhu C, Wang X, Xu F, et al. Eur J Neurosci 2006; 23: 387-93.

[32] Zhu C, Wang X, Cheng X, et al. Brain Res 2004; 996: 67-75.

[33] Eberspacher E, Werner C, Engelhard K, et al. Acta Anaesthesiol Scand 2005; 49: 477-87.

[34] McManus T, Sadgrove M, Pringle AK, Chad JE, Sundstrom LE. J Neurochem 2004; 91: 327-36.

[35] Horiguchi T, Shimizu K, Ogino M, Suga S, Inamasu J, Kawase T. J Neurotrauma 2003; 20: 511-20.

[36] Van HA, Hachimi-Idrissi S, Sarre S, Ebinger G, Michotte Y. Eur J Neurosci 2005; 22: 1327-37.

[37] Toyoda T, Suzuki S, Kassell NF, Lee KS. Neurosurgery 1996; 39: 1200-05.

[38] Ishikawa M, Sekizuka E, Sato S, et al. Stroke 1999; 30: 1679-86.

[39] Inamasu J, Suga S, Sato S, et al. J Neuroimmunol 2000; 109: 66-74.

[40] Maier CM, Ahern K, Cheng ML, Lee JE, Yenari MA, Steinberg GK. Stroke 1998; 29: 2171-80.

[41] Kawai N, Okauchi M, Morisaki K, Nagao S. Stroke 2000; 31: 1982-9.

[42] Wang G, Deng H, Maier C, Sun G, Yenari M. Neuroscience 2002; 114: 1081.

[43] Theodorsson A, Holm L, Theodorsson E. Neuropeptides 2008; 42: 79-87.

[44] Kammersgaard LP, Rasmussen BH, Jorgensen HS, Reith J, Weber U, Olsen TS. Stroke 2000; 31: 2251-6.

[45] Schwab S, Georgiadis D, Berrouschot J, Schellinger PD, Graffagnino C, Mayer SA. Stroke 2001; 32: 2033-5.

[46] Schwab S, Schwarz S, Spranger M, Keller E, Bertram M, Hacke W. Stroke 1998; 29: 2461-6.

[47] Feigin V, Anderson N, Gunn A, Rodgers A, Anderson C. Lancet Neurol 2003; 2: 529.

[48] Labiche LA, Grotta JC. NeuroRx 2004; 1: 46-70.

[49] Bernard SA, MacC JB, Buist M. Crit Care 1999; 3: 167-72.

[50] Steinberg GK, Ogilvy CS, Shuer LM, et al. Neurosurgery 2004; 55: 307-14.

[51] Slotboom J, Kiefer C, Brekenfeld C, et al. Neuroradiology 2004; 46: 923-34.

[52] De Georgia MA, Krieger DW, bou-Chebl A, et al. Neurology 2004; 63: 312-317.

[53] Diao C, Zhu L, Wang H. Ann Biomed Eng 2003; 31: 346-53.

[54] Nelson DA, Nunneley SA. Eur J Appl Physiol Occup Physiol 1998; 78: 353-9.

[55] Van Leeuwen GM, Hand JW, Lagendijk JJ, Azzopardi DV, Edwards AD. Pediatr Res 2000; 48: 351-6.

[56] Corbett R, Laptook A, Gee J, Garcia D, Silmon S, Tollefsbol G. J Neurochem 1998; 71: 1205-14.

[57] Mellergard P. Neurosurgery 1992; 31: 671-7.

[58] Steiner T, Friede T, Aschoff A, Schellinger PD, Schwab S, Hacke W. Stroke 2001; 32: 2833-5.

[59] Schwab S, Schwarz S, Aschoff A, Keller E, Hacke W. Acta Neurochir Suppl (Wien) 1998; 71: 131-4.

[60] Xue D, Huang ZG, Smith KE, Buchan AM. Brain Res 1992; 587: 66-72.

[61] Zhang RL, Chopp M, Chen H, Garcia JH, Zhang ZG. Stroke 1993; 24: 1235-40.

[62] Zhang ZG, Chopp M, Chen H. J Neurol Sci 1993; 117: 240-4.

[63] Yanamoto H, Hong SC, Soleau S, Kassell NF, Lee KS. Brain Res 1996; 718: 207-11.

[64]   Maier CM, Sun GH, Kunis D, Yenari MA, Steinberg GK. J Neurosurg 2001; 94: 90-6.

[65]   Colbourne F, Sutherland GR, Auer RN. J Neurosci Methods 1996; 67: 185-90.

[66]   Colbourne F, Corbett D. J Neurosci 1995; 15: 7250-60.

[67]   Yanamoto H, Nagata I, Nakahara I, Tohnai N, Zhang Z, Kikuchi H. Stroke 1999; 30: 2720-6.

[68]   Huh PW, Belayev L, Zhao W, Koch S, Busto R, Ginsberg MD. J Neurosurg 2000; 92: 91-9.

[69]   Kollmar R, Schabitz WR, Heiland S, et al. Stroke 2002; 33: 1899-904.

[70]   Dietrich WD, Busto R, Alonso O, Globus MY, Ginsberg MD. J Cereb Blood Flow Metab 1993; 13: 541-9.

[71]   Ringer AJ, Tomsick TA. Neurol Res 2002; 24 Suppl 1, S43-6.

[72]   Barnwell SL, Clark WM, Nguyen TT, Neill OR, Wynn ML, Coull BM. Am J Neuroradiol 1994; 15: 1817-22.

[73]   Balousek PA, Knowles HJ, Higashida RT, del Zoppo GJ. Curr Opin Cardiol 1996; 11: 550-7.

[74]   Bucker A, Schmitz R, Vorwerk D, Gunther RW. J Vasc Interv Radiol 1996; 7: 445-9.

[75]   Broderick JP. Semin Neurol 1998; 18: 471-84.

[76]   Lewandowski CA, Frankel M, Tomsick TA, et al. Stroke 1999; 30: 2598-605.

[77]   Ueda T, Sakaki S, Nochide I, Kumon Y, Kohno K, Ohta S. Stroke 1998; 29: 2568-74.

[78]   Takis C, Kwan ES, Pessin MS, Jacobs DH, Caplan LR. Am J Neuroradiol 1997; 18: 1661-8.

[79]   Qureshi AI, Ali Z, Suri MF, et al. Neurosurgery 2001; 49: 1-48.

[80]   Ringer AJ, Qureshi AI, Fessler RD, Guterman LR, Hopkins LN. Neurosurgery 2001; 48: 1282-8.

[81]   Qureshi AI, Siddiqui AM, Suri MF, et al. Neurosurgery 2002; 51: 1319-27.

[82]   Hallenbeck JM, Dutka AJ. Arch Neurol 1990; 47: 45-1254.

[83]   Zivin JA. Neurology 1998; 50: 599-603.

[84]   Ginsberg MD. Cerebrovasc Brain Metab Rev 1990; 2: 58-93.

[85]   Siesjo BK. J Neurosurg 1992; 77: 169-84.

[86]   Siesjo BK. J Neurosurg 1992; 77: 337-54.

[87]   Aronowski J, Strong R, Grotta JC. J Cereb Blood Flow Metab 1997; 17: 1048-56.

[88]   Clark RK, Lee EV, White RF, Jonak ZL, Feuerstein GZ, Barone FC. Brain Res Bull 1994; 35: 387-92.

[89]   Korthuis RJ, Granger DN, Townsley MI, Taylor AE. Circ Res 1985; 57: 599-609.

[90]   McCord JM. N Engl J Med 1985; 312: 159-63.

[91]   Schmidley JW. Stroke 1990; 21: 1086-90.

[92]   Jean WC, Spellman SR, Nussbaum ES, Low WC. Neurosurgery 1998; 43: 1382-96.

[93]   Watson BD. Cell Mol Neurobiol 1998; 18: 581-98.

[94]   DeGraba TJ. Neurology 1998; 51, S62-8.

[95]   Becker KJ. Curr Opin Neurol 1998; 11: 45-9.

[96]   Hall ED. In: Miller LP, Eds. Stroke Therapy. Basic, Preclinical, and Clinical Directions. San Diego, CA: Metabasis Therapeutics, Inc.1999, pp. 245-270.

[97]   Kato H, Kogure K. Cell Mol Neurobiol 1999; 19: 93-108.

[98]   Barone FC, Feuerstein GZ. J Cereb Blood Flow Metab 1999; 19: 819-34.

[99]   Dirnagl U, Iadecola C, Moskowitz MA. Trends Neurosci 1999; 22: 391-7.

[100]   Emerich DF, Bartus RT. In: Miller LP, Eds. Stroke Therapy: Basic, Preclinical, and Clinical Directions. Wiley-Liss, Inc.1999, pp. 195-218.

[101]   White BC, Sullivan JM, DeGracia DJ, J Neurol Sci 2000; 179: 1-33.

[102]   Kiessling M, Hossmann KA. Brain Pathology 1994; 4: 21-22.

[103]   Ding Y, Yao B, Zhou Y, Park H, McAllister JP, II, Diaz FG. J Neurosurg 2002; 96: 310-9.

[104]   Ding Y, Li J, Rafols JA, Phillis JW, Diaz FG. Stroke 2002; 33: 2492-8.

[105]   Ding Y, Young C, Li J, et al. Neurosci Lett 2003; 353: 173-6.

[106]   Liu S, Connor J, Peterson S, Shuttleworth CW, Liu KJ. J Cereb Blood Flow Metab 2002; 22: 1222-30.

[107]   Ding YH, Li J, Rafols JA, Ding Y. Neurosci Lett 2004; 372: 35-9.

[108]   Hosomi N, Ban CR, Naya T, et al. J Cereb Blood Flow Metab 2005; 25: 959-67.

[109]   Mun-Bryce S, Rosenberg GA. J Cereb Blood Flow Metab 1998; 18: 1163-72.

[110]   Ooboshi H, Ibayashi S, Takano K, et al. Brain Res 2000; 884: 23-30.

[111]   Kuluz JW, Gregory GA, Yu AC, Chang Y. Stroke 1992; 23: 1792-6.

[112]   Behringer W, Prueckner S, Kentner R, et al. Anesthesiology 2000; 93: 1491-9.

[113]   Herold JA, Kron IL, Langenburg SE, et al. J Thorac Cardiovasc Surg 1994; 107: 536-41.

[114]   Ding Y, Li J, Luan X, et al. Neurosurgery 2004; 54: 956-64.

[115]   Luan X, Li J, McAllister JP, Diaz FG, Clark JC, Fessler RD, Ding Y. Acta Neuropathol 2004; 107: 227-34.

[116]   Konstas AA, Neimark MA, Laine AF, Pile-Spellman J. J Appl Physiol 2007; 102: 1329-40.

[117]   Serna DL, Powell LL, Kahwaji C, et al. ASAIO J 2000; 46: 547-52.

[118]   Ferrera R, Michel P, Hadour G, Chiari P, Chambers D, Rodriguez C. J Heart Lung Transplant 2000; 19: 792-800.

[119]   Hauet T, Mothes D, Goujon JM, Carretier M, Eugene M. J Pharmacol Exp Ther 2001; 297: 946-52.

[120]   Oliveira RP, Velasco I, Soriano F, Friedman G. Crit Care 2002; 6: 418-23.

[121]   Pascual JL, Khwaja KA, Chaudhury P, Christou NV. J Trauma 2003; 54, S133-40.

[122]   Eversole RR, Smith SL, Beuving LJ, Hall ED. Circ Shock 1993; 40: 125-31.

[123]   Pascual JL, Khwaja KA, Ferri LE, et al. J Trauma 2003; 54: 121-30.

[124]   Pascual JL, Ferri LE, Seely AJ, et al. Ann Surg 2002; 236: 634-42.

[125]   Corso CO, Okamoto S, Leiderer R, Messmer K. J Surg Res 1998; 80: 210-20.

[126]   Angle N, Hoyt DB, Coimbra R, et al. hock 1998; 9: 164-70.

[127]   Hamaguchi S, Okuda Y, Kitajima T, Masawa N. Can J Anaesth 2002; 49: 745-8.

[128]   Tseng MY, Al R, Pickard JD, Rasulo FA, Kirkpatrick PJ. Stroke 2003; 34: 1389-96.

[129]   Schwarz S, Georgiadis D, Aschoff A, Schwab S. Stroke 2002; 33: 136-40.

[130]   Qureshi AI, Suarez JI, Bhardwaj A, et al. Crit Care Med 1998; 26: 440-6.

[131]   Victorino GP, Newton CR, Curran B. Shock 2003; 19: 183-6.

[132]   Victorino GP, Newton CR, Curran B. J Surg Res 2002; 104: 101-5.

[133]   Victorino GP, Newton CR, Curran B. J Surg Res 2003; 112: 79-83.

[134]   Suarez JI. Stroke 2003; 34: 1396-1397.

[135]   Mazhar R, Samenesco A, Royston D, Rees A. J Thorac Cardiovasc Surg 1998; 115: 178-89.

[136]   Murphy JT, Horton JW, Purdue GF, Hunt JL. Arch Surg 1999; 134: 1091-7.

[137]   Jarvela K, Kaukinen S. Eur J Anaesthesiol 2001; 18: 100-7.

[138]   Becker KJ, Brott TG. Stroke 2005; 36: 400-3.

[139]   Woitzik J, Schilling L. J Neurosurg 2007; 106: 872-8.

Experimental Stroke, 2008, 1, 63-73

Stem Cell Transplantation and Cerebral Ischemia

Christine L. Keogh,[1] **Shan Ping Yu**[1,2] **and Ling Wei**[1,2,*]

[1]*Department of Pathology and Laboratory Medicine, Medical University of South Carolina, Charleston, SC 29464, USA; Tel: 404-712-8661; E-mail: lwei7@emory.edu*
[2]*Department of Anesthesiology, Emory University School of Medicine, Atlanta, GA 30322, USA*

Abstract: Stroke is caused by a partial or full blockage of the blood supply to certain part of the brain and afflicts both young and old. Stroke can be either hemorrhagic or ischemic in nature and can also result from a permanent blockage or a transient occlusion of one or several arteries. The transient stroke may additionally involve reperfusion injury. Currently, the only effective means of stroke treatment is early administration of tissue plasminogen activator (tPA), which has a small window of opportunity (within 3 hours after the onset of stroke). Thus development of new therapies especially the delayed treatments many hours and even days after stroke is very much needed. One treatment approach that has recently garnered a lot of attention is stem cell transplantation. Much of neuroscience research focuses on the analysis and characterization of both the endogenous response of stem cell proliferation and migration following an ischemic insult as well as the effects of exogenous stem cell transplantation. Studies have identified endogenous stem cell niches in the adult and the neonatal rodent brain and many groups have tried to harness the ability of the host to regenerate damaged tissue following stroke. This chapter will briefly review endogenous stem cell experimentation and cover recent advancements in exogenous stem cell transplantation.

INTRODUCTION

Both methods of stem cell therapy, enhancement of the endogenous host stem cell response and exogenous transplantation, share common goals. These therapies aim to protect against cell death that is caused by ischemia and to increase regeneration, with the ultimate goal of functional recovery of the patient. Neuroprotection, angiogenesis, and neurogenesis are popular areas of study within the neuroscience field. A number of obstacles, however, exist for both therapies. Studies are examining whether the endogenous response is sufficient for functional recovery, and there are a number of groups using a variety of approaches to increase the endogenous response. On the other hand, exogenous cell transplants must survive long-term, differentiate according to the local microenvironmental cues, and

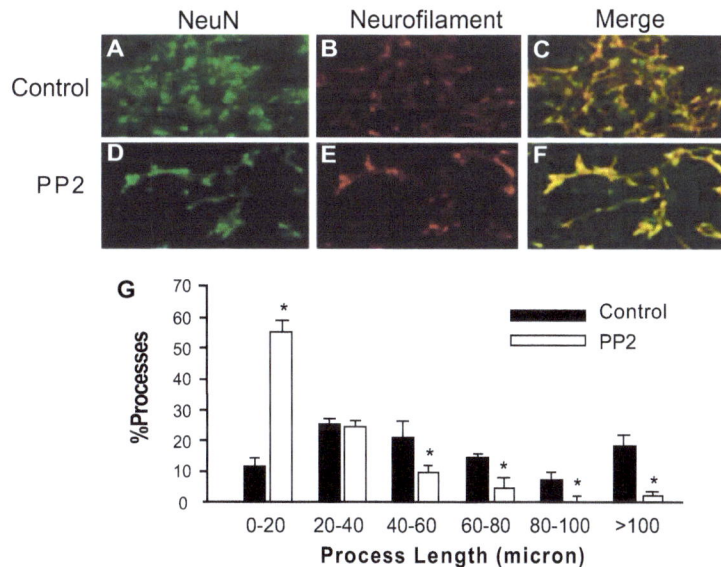

Fig. (1). The role of Src kinases on neurite development during ES cell neuronal differentiation

RA-induced ES cells were plated on PDL-laminin coated dishes with or without PP2 and morphology was examined. **A** to **F**. Four days after RA-induction, differentiating ES cells were stained with NenN (green) and neurofilament (red) for identification of neuron-like cells and neurite outgrowth. ES cell-derived neuronal cells showed a complex network of branched processes (top row). The Src family kinase inhibitor PP2 (10 µM) added in the culture medium reduced the number of processes and disrupted the neurite extension (bottom row). **C**. Quantitative data were generated by image analysis to compare process lengths of differentiated neuron-like cells. Cells cultured in the presence of PP2 had reduced average lengths of neurites; ~60% of processes counted in this group were less than 20 µm; a large distribution of longer process was seen with control cells on the right of the graph. Six non-overlapping fields were counted for each of 3 experiments per group. *. $P < 0.05$ compared with controls.

integrate into the host tissue, making functional connections while not resulting in a deleterious situation such as tumorigenesis. Other exogenous studies are aiming to increase the mobilization of endogenous cells by the application of various growth factors and other molecules [1-3]. Recently, transplantation using adult stem cells or bone marrow-derived stem cells has been extensively explore in order to avoid ethical obstacles and gain some unique advantages such as the reduced inflammatory responses with autografts of bone marrow mesenchymal stem cells (BMSCs) [4].

THE MOLECULAR MECHANISM OF NEURONAL DIFFERENTIATION OF EMBRYONIC STEM CELLS

Mouse embryonic stem (ES) cells can be induced to differentiate down a neural lineage by the retinoic acid (RA) protocol [5]. *In vitro* mouse ES cells have been shown to express NMDA receptor subunits in an age-appropriate dependent pattern of expression and generally exhibit an excitotoxic response that mimics *in vivo* CNS responses [6]. ES cells that are directed toward a neural lineage can differentiate into neurons, oligodendrocytes, astrocytes, and perhaps other supporting cells of the CNS. In our investigation, we have identified specific signaling pathways in the neural differentiation of ES cells [7]. ES cell derived neuron-like cells expressed neurofilament, synaptophysin, glutamate receptors, NMDA and kainate currents, became vulnerable to excitotoxicity, and formed functional excitatory synapses (Fig. **1**). These developmental events were blocked or attenuated when cells were grown in the presence of Src family kinase inhibitor, PP2 (Fig. **1**). However, there was no change in the expression of GABAergic specific protein GAD67 during PP2 treatment.

In a consequent investigation, we showed that activation of the mitogen-activated protein kinase (MAPK) pathway is involved in cell survival, differentiation, and growth during neural development [8]. The MAPK family consists of three major groups: extracellular signal-regulated kinase (ERK), c-Jun N-terminal kinase (JNK)/stress-activated protein kinase (SAPK), and p38. Among these three, ERK has various functions in the development of the nervous system [9]. Recent studies using cell lines and primary neuronal cultures have showed that ERK is involved in proliferation, differentiation, and cell survival [10-13]. Our data demonstrates that the ERK-STAT3 pathway is required for the development of ES cell-derived neurons *in vitro*. We tested the hypothesis that ERK 1/2 phosphorylation is an early signaling event required for the neuronal differentiation of ES cells. Cultured mouse ES cells were treated with the RA protocol to generate neurally induced progenitor cells. Western blot analysis showed a dramatic increase in ERK 1/2 phosphorylation (p-ERK 1/2) 1-5 days after the RA induction, which was attenuated in the presence of the p-ERK ½-specific

inhibitor UO126. Phospho-ERK 1/2 inhibition significantly reduced the number of NeuN-positive cells and the expression of associated cytoskeletal proteins. In differentiating ES cells, there was increased nuclear translocation of STAT3 and decreased protein expression levels of glial cell line-derived neurotrophic factor (GDNF), brain-derived neurotrophic factor (BDNF) and nerve growth factor (NGF). The STAT3 translocation was attenuated by UO126. These data indicate that ERK 1/2 phosphorylation is a key event required for early neuronal differentiation and survival of ES cells [8].

STEM CELL TRANSPLANTATION AS A POTENTIAL THERAPY FOR ISCHEMIC STROKE

The idea behind exogenous cell transplantation goes beyond just that of cell replacement. Cerebral ischemia results in a cavity that is devoid of any real functioning tissue, which is surrounded by an area subjected to delayed cell death (penumbra) where scarring and attempts at regeneration occur. The transplanted cells not only fill this ischemic core and must survive and integrate, but they also may secrete protective and proliferative factors that will, in turn, promote the survival and regeneration of the endogenous host tissue, which has been called the 'paracrine effect' [14]. These exogenous cells must rely on themselves as well as cues from the host tissue microenvironment to migrate to the necessary area, differentiate into the appropriate cell type, and make synaptic connections.

STEM CELLS FOR TRANSPLANTATION THERAPY

Among different stem cells, BMSCs exhibit a unique advantage of autograft application, which greatly eliminates the concerns of graft rejection and ethical issues that are commonly associated with transplantation of many other stem cells. Previous investigations showed that intravenously injected BMSCs can pass through the blood brain barrer and translocate into or "homing to" the brain ischemic regions [15]. Those cells are being evaluated in human clinical trials for efficacy in treating genetic diseases of bone, to speed hematopoietic recovery after bone marrow transplantation and treat the severe graft-versus-host disease (GVHD) [10]. In the past few years, BMSCs have also been reported to exhibit a broad degree of plasticity commensurate with other adult stem cell populations, they can differentiate *in vitro* and *in vivo* into non-mesodermal cell types such as neurons and astrocytes [16]. Cells derived from BMSCs or stromal cells can also differentiate into mesodermal, endodermal and ectodermal cell types. BMSCs have been reported to promote repair and regeneration of nervous tissue within the central and peripheral nervous systems, although the mechanism by which this occurs remains undetermined. As a

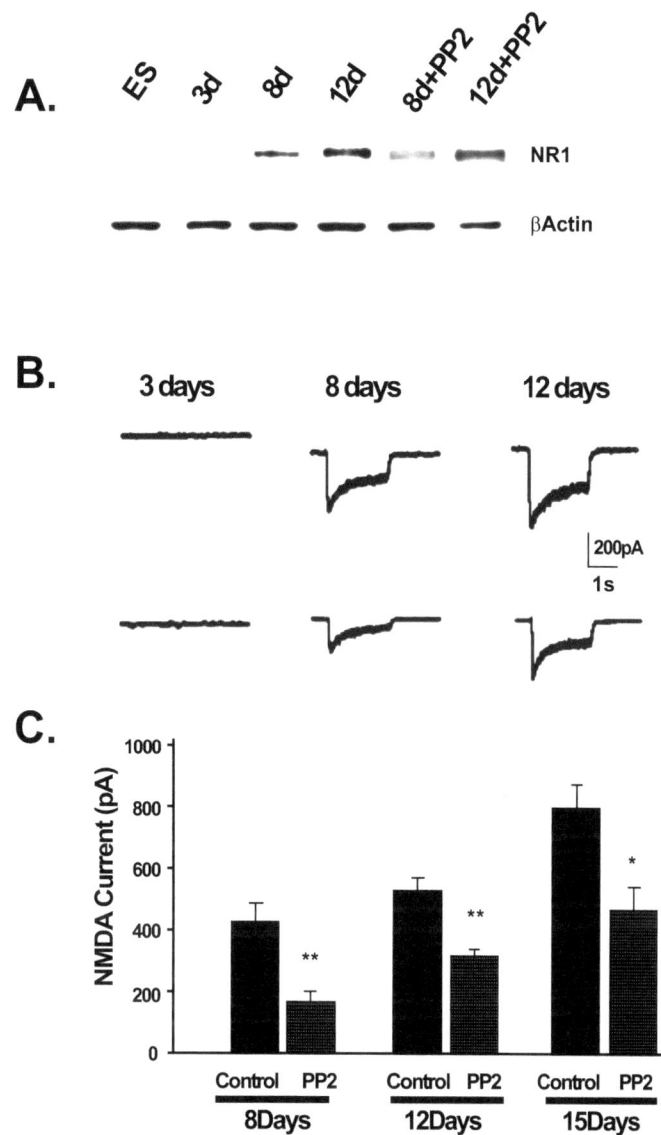

Fig. (2). Effects of inhibiting the activity of Src family kinases on the expression and function of NMDA receptors in differentiating ES cells A. Western blot analysis was performed to determine the time course of NR1 expression during neural differentiation of ES cells. Expression of the essential NR1 subunit emerged 8 days in differentiation and increased at 12 days. Application of PP2 (10 µM) into the culture medium significantly attenuated the NMDA receptor expression. B. Whole-cell recording at the holding potential of –70 mV could not detect any membrane current in response to local NMDA (100 µM) application, consistent with the lack of the receptor expression at day 4. Coincident with NR1 expression, whole-cell NMDA currents were recorded in cells 8 days in differentiation. Corresponding to the higher expression of NMDA receptors, the current grew larger at 12 days. Supporting a diminished NMDA receptor expression, noticeably smaller NMDA current was recorded in cells cultured with 10 µM PP2. During whole-cell recording, PP2 was not added to the recording solutions, excluding a possible direct effect of PP2 on NMDA receptors. C. Quantified data show attenuated NMDA currents at each time point tested from 8 to 15 days in differentiation. N ≥ 7 cells. *. P < 0.05 compared with controls.

possible mechanism, BMSCs may act as trophic mediators and can secrete several growth factors. These secreted factors can provide the host tissue with trophic supports, reduce apoptosis of the injured tissue, and stimulate endogenous regenerative activities [17-33].

When transplanted into irradiated mice, EGFP-marked hematopoietic stem cells differentiated into parenchymal microglial and perivascular cells in the brain, and their numbers increased following brain ischemia induced by middle cerebral artery (MCA) occlusion. However, only few transplanted cells were found to be NeuN-positive neuronal cells [4]. Another similar study determined that bone marrow-derived cells were both endothelial cell- and NeuN-positive at 7 and 14 days after stroke [34]. The administration of human BMSCs intravenously into rats following ischemia resulted into an increase in angiogenesis in the penumbra, which was associated with an increase in vascular endothelial growth factor (VEGF) and VEGFR2 levels in the brain [29]. BMSCs have also been associated with a decrease in endogenous apoptosis and an increase in endogenous cellular proliferation, therefore acting primarily as a cell therapy and secondarily as an endogenous stem cell enhancement technique [29]. Conversely, human BMSCs grafted into the penumbra of the cortex resulted in animals that exhibited significant improvement in limb placement tests, yet the morphology of the transplanted cells did not mimic endogenous cells, inferring that the BMSCs were not functional. This is an example of the 'paracrine' effect of transplanted cells that provide trophic or growth support to host cells [35]. Mouse BMSCs transplanted into the striatum following adult MCAO resulted in restoration of cerebral blood flow (CBF) and blood brain barrier (BBB) to near normal levels as determined by laser Doppler and Evans blue assay [36]. This phenomenon was associated with an increase in neurotrophic factor expression in the areas of transplantation and restored CBF.

Human umbilical cord blood (hUCB) contains large numbers of hematopoietic colony-forming cells that can be induced to express neuronal and glial cell lineage markers [37]. Use of autologous stem cells such as peripheral blood hematopoietic stem cells mobilized from the bone marrow can be mobilized by G-CSF.

Intracerebral peripheral blood hematopoietic stem cell (CD34+) (PBSC) transplantation after chronic cerebral ischemia differentiated into GFAP+ neurons, and vascular endothelial cells, enhanced neuroplastic effects, increased local CBF, and improved neurological function [37]. A significant increase in VEGF and SDF-1 was observed in the peri-infarct areas when compared to vehicle control [38].

Neural precursor cells (NPCs), derived from donor rats that expressed human placental alkaline phosphatase for stable and reliable graft tracking, were evaluated following transplantation into the normal developing and adult brain and spinal cord [39]. These cells were lineage-restricted to neuronal and glial fate. The study, which assessed the fate of the transplanted cells up to 15 months *in vivo*, determined that the cells grafted similarly to endogenous cells and differentiated into neurons, oligodendrocytes and astrocytes. These cells also formed synapses and no abnormal cell growth was found [39].

Genetic modification prior to transplantation is one method aiming to enhance the therapeutic potential of exogenous cells. Intravenous administration of human BMSCs and cells that were modified with angiopoeitin-1 (Ang-1), a potent angiogenic factor,

following adult rat MCAO resulted in an increase in angiogenesis, blood flow, and improved functional outcome. The Ang-1-modified cells resulted in only a modest improvement when compared to the unmodified cells [40]. Hippocampal progenitors transfected with NGF that were transplanted after traumatic brain injury resulted in improved neuromotor function and spatial learning behavior and was associated with a decrease in hippocampal cell death [41].

An exciting new type of stem cell that avoids both immune system and ethical concerns altogether is the inducible pluripotent stem cell (iPS). The initial study added 4 genes (Oct3/4, Sox2, c-myc, and Klf4) to mouse tail cells and produced iPS cells that resembled embryonic stem (ES) cells both morphologically and functionally [42]. Another group has since created iPS cells by overexpressing 3 of the 4 genes, omitting c-myc, a well established proto-oncogene [43]. Mouse cells from a skin biopsy were also reprogrammed to a pluripotent state to generate mouse-induced iPS cells. These cells were directed to differentiate to a certain lineage, hematopoietic progenitors for sickle cell anemia, and transplanted to sick mice [44]. This was the first application of these cells to a clinical setting. The iPS cell work has been repeated in human cells [43, 45]. Human iPS cells were derived by introducing 4 genes, Oct4, Nanog, Sox2, and Lin28, to human fibroblasts; cells resembling ES cells were obtained [45]. While these cells avoid the ethical and political implications of ES cells, they currently require genetic reprogramming, and thus encounter the aforementioned obstacles, including the risk of tumor production. There is yet little known about true ES cells, let alone the new iPS cells, and therefore one must take precautions when evaluating the clinical application of these cells.

PROMOTING THE SURVIVAL AND THERAPEUTIC POTENTIAL OF TRANSPLANTED CELLS

The microenvironment in the injured brain is hazardous to transplanted cells. It has been shown that a large number of transplanted cells may die after transplantation [46]. For instance, 70-90% of implanted dopaminergic neurons in the striatum die after transplantation [47, 48]. In our ES cell transplantation investigation, 30% of neural lineage-induced ES cells died 3 days after transplantation into the ischemic rat brain [49]. Several factors may affect cell survival in the acute phase of cerebral infarction, including limited blood supply, hypoxia, trophic factor deficiency, oxidative stress, inflammatory response, and others [50]. The situation is even more severe in the ischemic core region where viable vasculature and direct trophic support are absent. Reperfusion injury, likely caused by accumulation of free radicals and inflammatory mediators, further deteriorates the microenvironment [51]. The death of transplanted cells and consequential immune reactions adds additional burdens to the host tissue that has already been compromised by cellular debris [52, 53]. Thus, anti-death strategies have been explored to promote the survival of transplanted cells and increase the therapeutic potential of transplantation therapy. These methods include continuous infusion of neurotrophic factors, genetic manipulation by overexpressing anti-apoptotic and growth factor genes, and knocking down pro-apoptotic genes [48, 49, 54, 55]. For instance, we have tested the protective effect of over-expressing the anti-apoptotic gene bcl-2 in ES cells and showed increased cell survival of these cells after transplantation into the post-ischemic brain of rats [49]. The bcl-2-overexpressing cells also were differentiated better and improved functional outcome when compared to the control ES cells. Human neural stem cells genetically modified to overexpress VEGF were transplanted into a mouse model of intracerebral hemorrhage, which increased angiogenesis and improved functional recovery [56]. The cells resulted in the proliferation of endogenous microvessels in the ischemic area; the VEGF-overexpressing cells survived better than the control cells [56].

While these studies aid in implicating important factors in promoting stroke survival, genetic modifications add another concern in clinical applications and are generally shunned upon due to the stigma associated with them, including safety issues associated with permanent gene alterations and, in addition to being clinically unfeasible, there are emerging concerns on the efficacy of targeting just one single gene or one signaling pathway. To address this issue our recent investigations have attempted to avoid the obstacles presented by permanent modification of genes. As an initial step, we have tested the potential use of pretreatment of stem cells with sublethal hypoxia and other preconditioning methods prior to transplantation.

Hypoxic/ischemic preconditioning (HP), also known as "hypoxic/ischemic tolerance", is a powerful endogenous phenomenon in which brief episodes of a sub-toxic ischemic/hypoxic insult *in vitro* or *in vivo* induce robust protection against future severe insults [57-60]. HP induces "classical" or "early" protection that lasts 1-2 hrs as well as "late" or "delayed" protection that reappears several hours after preconditioning and lasts up to days or weeks [59, 61]. The early and late effects of HP exist in every species tested and have been successfully induced in many organs and preparations including central neurons [57, 61-63]. Human tissues such as the heart and brain can be preconditioned [60, 64], suggesting clinical implications in human ischemia [62, 63]. Exposure to sublethal hypoxia alters gene expression and activates multiple intracellular signaling pathways that are involved in cell survival and regenerative processes. These changes may contribute to the adaptive responses observed after hypoxia. For example, following HP, expression of hypoxia-inducible factor-1α (HIF-1α) is upregulated, which shows cytoprotective and angiogenic effects. Hypoxia

can prolong the half-life of several mRNAs, including HIF-1α, VEGF and erythropoietin (EPO) amongst others [65, 66]. Besides, chronic hypoxia has been shown to stimulate and maintain an increase of angiogenesis in the postnatal developing brain [37].

Because cell death induced by various insults shares a number of pathways (e.g. caspase activation in apoptosis and [Ca2+]i accumulation in excitotoxicity), one preconditioning inducer often causes tolerance against injuries induced by other insults, a phenomenon described as "cross tolerance" [67]. In addition to the protective effects, some HP triggers and mediators (e.g. EPO) and certain trophic factors (e.g. VEGF) also stimulate cell proliferation, differentiation, angiogenesis, and neurogenesis in the CNS [68-70], which further validates the idea of using preconditioning as a complementary approach in stem cell transplantation. Until very recently, stem cell transplantation and hypoxic preconditioning have been studied as two separate strategies. We propose that pretreatment of stem cells or progenitors with HP can prime these cells with higher tolerance to the harsh post-ischemia environment, increase their chance to survive and their expression of trophic factors that are critically needed for cell differentiation and endogenous regenerative responses.

In vitro experiments and animal studies have shown that HP treatment of mouse or human ES cells and BMSCs prior to transplantation allows for greater survival and engraftment of these cells into the ischemic heart and brain of adult rats [71-76]. In our study on BMSCs, HP increased expression of pro-survival and pro-angiogenic factors including HIF-1α, Ang-1, VEGF and its receptor, Flk-1, EPO, bcl-2, and bcl-xL. Caspase-3 activation and cell death of HP-treated BMSCs were significantly lower compared with that in control cells both *in vitro* and *in vivo*. Transplantation of HP-treated BMSCs after heart ischemia resulted in an increase in angiogenesis, as well as enhanced morphological and functional benefits of stem cell therapy [73]. HP also significantly enhanced the tolerance of ES cell-derived neurally differentiated cells (ES-NPCs) to apoptotic cell death (40-50% reduction in cell death and caspase-3 activation). The HP protective effects on cultured cells lasted for at least 6 days [74]. HP-primed ES-NPCs survived better 3 days after transplantation into the ischemic brain (30-40% reduction in cell death and caspase-3 activation). Finally, transplanted HP-primed ES-NPCs exhibited extensive neuronal differentiation in the ischemic brain, accelerated and enhanced recovery of sensorimotor function when compared to transplantation of non-HP-treated ES-NPCs [74]. The HP cytoprotective effect was diminished by blocking the EPO receptor, while pretreatment of ES-NPCs with recombinant human EPO mimicked the HP effect, enhancing cell survival against apoptotic insults. This observation supports that EPO is an important mediator in the protective effect of HP and provides an attractive possibility of "chemical preconditioning" instead of using hypoxia for the priming process [74].

A recent study reports that BMSC cultured in hypoxia (1-3% O_2) activate the Akt signaling pathway while maintaining their viability and cell cycle rates. BMSC cultured in hypoxia induced expression of c-Met, the major receptor for hepatocyte growth factor (HGF), and enhanced c-Met signaling. BMSC cultured in hypoxic conditions increased their migration rates. In a murine hindlimb ischemia model, the researchers showed that local expression of HGF is increased in ischemic muscle in this model. Intra-arterial injection of BMSC cultured in normoxic or hypoxic conditions 24 hours after surgical induction of hindlimb ischemia both enhanced revascularization, as compared to saline controls. However, restoration of blood flow was observed significantly earlier in mice that had been injected with hypoxic pre-conditioned BMSC [75]. Thus, the preconditioning strategy for graft cells is likely an effective means of promoting cell survival for transplantation therapy. The upregulated HIF-1α-EPO signaling and increased expression/secretion of growth and survival factors can contribute significantly to the autocrine and paracrine effects that promote tissue repair and functional recovery after ischemia [73, 74, 77].

ENDOGENOUS NEUROGENESIS UPON BRAIN INSULTS

Endogenous stem cells have been found in the neonatal and the adult brain in a variety of rodent and primate models. The areas of neurogenesis in the brain are the subventricular zone (SVZ), the subgranular zone (SGZ) and the dentate gyrus (DG) of the hippocampus. Cells in the SVZ include stem cells and progenitor cells that proliferate and migrate through the rostral migratory stream (RMS) to the olfactory bulb (OB) where they terminally differentiate for the remainder of their lifetime. These cells move via chain migration, using each other as a migratory substrate [78]. One of the main markers currently used to identify migrating precursor cells is doublecortin (DCX), a microtuble-associated protein. DCX is expressed within the SVZ, the RMS, and in the OB in precursors and expression is downregulated in postmitotic cells [78]. When knocked down, mice suffer a severe morphological defect in the RMS that results in delayed neuronal migration and lack of the bipolar morphology of cells necessary for migration [78].

Recently, the endogenous stem cells and their regulations have been more aggressively studied following an insult such as an ischemic event. While triggering massive cell death in the ischemic region, cerebral ischemia stimulate regenerative responses in the tissue adjacent and remote to the impaired area [79, 80]. Cerebral ischemia induces the proliferation of endogenous neural stem/progenitor cells in the SVZ [81, 82], and after stroke these SVZ cells migrate

laterally toward the striatal ischemic boundary with distinct migratory behaviors and retained capacity for cell division [83]. These neuroblasts in the striatum form elongated chain-like cell aggregates similar to those in the normal SVZ, and these chains were observed to be closely associated with thin astrocytic processes and blood vessels. The SVZ-derived neuroblasts differentiated into mature neurons in the striatum, expressing neuronal specific nuclear protein and forming synapses with neighboring striatal cells [84]. In neonatal models, hypoxic-ischemic injury has been shown to increase SVZ proliferation from 1-4 weeks after stroke [85]. The SVZ can regenerate a population of neurons after hypoxia-ischemia that is maintained for months [86]. Taken together, these studies indicate the exciting possibility that some degree of tissue repair after stroke may be induced through endogenous neurogenesis [80].

Bromodeoxyuridine (BrdU) is a thymidine analogue that is incorporated into the DNA during S phase and its administration allows for cell proliferation studies. Many studies rely on BrdU to assess the endogenous post-ischemia proliferative response. More recent studies have also utilized techniques such as retroviral GFP injections to label the proliferating SVZ population. At least one of these methods is necessary to identify proliferation changes following ischemia; ideally, both may be used and co-localization of BrdU- and GFP-positive cells can be identified and quantified via immunohistochemical techniques. Another technique, although less popular, is that of monitoring constitutively-labeled-GFP stem cells *in vivo* using magnetic resonance imaging (MRI) [87]. The ES cells were labeled by a lipofection procedure with an MRI contrast agent, and therefore observation of the exogenous cells allowed for monitoring of migration. The transplanted cells migrated from the contralateral side of the brain to the penumbra of the ischemic region. This emphasizes the existence of migratory or other environmental cues that lure the transplanted cells to the site of injury.

Endothelial nitric oxide synthase (eNOS) knockout mice subjected to MCAO exhibited less SVZ proliferation and decreased angiogenesis, which was partly due to a decrease in BDNF expression, a factor previously shown to enhance SVZ neuronal progenitor cell proliferation [88, 89]. This further emphasizes the effects of ischemia-induced SVZ proliferation on regeneration and functional recovery. The data also brings attention to the relationship between neural cells and the vasculature in the CNS. The impaired neurogenesis in the eNOS deficient mice may be a secondary response of the decreased angiogenesis and endothelial cell proliferation.

Interestingly, the existence of de novo neurogenesis has caused some researchers to question whether transplantation of exogenous stem cells are really necessary, the argument being that therapies directed at enhancing endogenous response may suffice in stroke recovery and is in itself devoid of any political or ethical implications [90]. However, there is so far no strong direct evidence that endogenously generated neuronal and non-neuronal cells are sufficient for tissue repair and functional recoveries, especially after a severe brain injury. It appears reasonable that both endogenous regeneration and transplantation of exogenous cells should be explored for the treatment of stroke.

ENDOGENOUS ANGIOGENESIS UPON BRAIN INSULTS

Angiogenesis refers to the formation of new blood vessels from the pre-existing vascular network; it is a process likely involved in tissue repair after stroke. This process of vascular growth is essential in development, reproduction, and wound healing; it requires proliferation, activation and migration of endothelial cells [91-93]. In a vitro study, cortical neural stem cells co-cultured with endothelial cells exhibited increased self-renewal, inhibited differentiation, and a more progenitor cell proliferation resulted compared to co-culture with other cortical control cells [94]. This result demonstrates the important supporting role for endothelial cells to neuronal cells.

Adult blood vessels undergo remodeling as a direct response to tissue demands. Angiogenesis, or proliferation of vascular endothelial cells, provides an enduring mechanism of restoring local blood flow and functional activity after ischemia. In ischemic stroke patients the number of new vessels surrounding injured tissue is correlated with longer survival [95]. We have demonstrated that microvascular proliferation and remodeling occur after cerebral ischemia in the rat barrel cortex, which increased blood flow and stimulated collateral growth [96]. Recent animal studies have moreover linked increased angiogenesis to improved performance in neurological and behavioral tests [38, 61, 97, 98].

Several growth factors and their receptors have been implicated in controlling the highly regulated angiogenic process and are collectively known as angiogenic factors (see below). VEGF and basic fibroblast growth factor (bFGF) are well known angiogenic factors, while Ang-1 and Ang-2 and their receptors (Tie-1 and Tie-2 receptors) are needed for maturation and stabilization of the newly formed vessels [99-102]. VEGF plays a role in promoting angiogenesis and can also protect cells from apoptotic cell death as well as act as a survival factor for newly formed blood vessels [103]. bFGF has been extensively investigated for its role in angiogenesis. Its administration protects against a wide array of ischemic insults [37, 72, 104]. Tie receptors are receptor tyrosine kinases that are expressed exclusively in endothelial cells. Tie-1 is involved in angiogenic capillary growth while Tie-2 is involved in large vessel remodeling and maintenance of vascular structure [72]. It was reported recently (Lee HJ, Kim

KS *et al.*, 2007) reported that, in an animal model of intracerebral hemorrhage stroke, combined administration of human neural stem cells and VEGF results in improved structural and functional outcome from cerebral ischemia [56]. VEGF-expressing ES-NPCs produced an amount of VEGF four times higher than parental F3 cell line *in vitro*. After transplantation, these cells showed improved survival in the lesion site, increased angiogenesis and behavioral recovery in the mouse model.

Angiogenesis is coupled with neurogenesis in the brain, and neurogenesis occurs within an angiogenic niche [105]. The aggregation of neuroblasts around astrocytic processes and blood vessels [106], suggests that the blood vessels may play an important role in neuroblast migration to injured regions. One common thread that connects angiogenesis and neurogenesis is VEGF, which was identified on the basis of its vascular effects, but has since been recognized as an important signaling molecule in neurogenesis as well [22, 72]. Another link between angiogenesis and neurogenesis is that after angiogenic stimulation, endothelial cells secrete brain-derived neurotrophic factor (BDNF), which induces neurogenesis [107].

PROMOTION OF ENDOGENOUS ANGIOGENESIS AND NEUROGENESIS BY STEM CELL TRANSPLANTATION

A combination therapy of cell transplantation plus a supplemental treatment such as growth factor administration may improve the likelihood that the transplanted cells would survive, proliferate, and make connections with the host tissue, thus 'filling' the vacant ischemic cavity with functional cells. Exogenous treatments can protect against delayed cell death and promote regeneration and growth in the penumbra, thus creating a favorable environment for transplanted cell survival and integration in the host. Moreover, transplanted cells may induce therapeutic effects via stimulating endogenous regenerative mechanisms such as angiogenesis and neurogenesis.

Transplanted stem cells demand metabolic and trophic supports to survive in a hostile milieu, which may compromise the survival of endogenous cells at the brink of dying from an ischemic insult. On the other hand, transplanted cells may differentiate into vascular endothelial cells and secret pro-angiogenic factors that promote endogenous angiogenesis. For example, transplanted BMSCs can stimulate angiogenesis after myocardial ischemia by secreting multiple angiogenic cytokines and differentiating into endothelial cells [108]. BMSC transplantation and nitric oxide donor therapy have individually shown promising effects on stroke recovery [109]. Intravenous infusion of human BMSCs with a nitric oxide donor was investigated to enhance the treatment, and immunohistochemistry revealed an increase in angiogenesis and neurogenesis as well as migrating cells, as defined by DCX-positive cells.

The research on endogenous stem cell regulation and transplantation of different types of stem cells and progenitors is still at an early stage yet rapid and encouraging progresses have been made in both areas. It is reasonable to predict that a better understanding of the mechanism of cell differentiation combined with increased cell survival ability and increased endogenous regenerative responses will greatly facilitate the development of a successful stem cell therapy for the treatment of stroke and other degenerative diseases.

REFERENCES

[1]   Lindvall O, Kokaia Z. Stem cells for the treatment of neurological disorders. Nature 2006; 441(7097): 1094-6.

[2]   Einstein O, Ben-Hur T. The changing face of neural stem cell therapy in neurologic diseases. Arch Neurol 2008; 65(4): 452-6.

[3]   Okano H, Sakaguchi M, Ohki K, Suzuki N, Sawamoto K. Regeneration of the central nervous system using endogenous repair mechanisms. J Neurochem 2007; 102(5): 1459-65.

[4]   Tang Y, Yasuhara T, Hara K, et al. Transplantation of bone marrow-derived stem cells: a promising therapy for stroke. Cell Transplant 2007; 16(2): 159-69.

[5]   Bain G, Ray WJ, Yao M, Gottlieb DI. Retinoic acid promotes neural and represses mesodermal gene expression in mouse embryonic stem cells in culture. Biochem Biophys Res Commun 1996; 223(3): 691-4.

[6]   Qu Y, Vadivelu S, Choi L, et al. Neurons derived from embryonic stem (ES) cells resemble normal neurons in their vulnerability to excitotoxic death. Exp Neurol 2003; 184(1): 326-36.

[7]   Theus MH, Wei L, Francis K, Yu SP. Critical roles of Src family tyrosine kinases in neuronal differentiation of embryonic stem cells. Exp Cell Res 2006; 312: 3096-107.

[8]   Li Z, Theus MH, Wei L. Role of ERK 1/2 signaling in neuronal differentiation of cultured embryonic stem cells. Dev Growth Differ 2006; 48(8): 513-23.

[9]   Kurozumi K, Nakamura K, Tamiya T, et al. Mesenchymal stem cells that produce neurotrophic factors reduce ischemic damage in the rat middle cerebral artery occlusion model. Mol Ther 2005; 11(1): 96-104.

[10]   Le Blanc K, Frassoni F, Ball L, et al. Mesenchymal stem cells for treatment of steroid-resistant, severe, acute graft-versus-host disease: a phase II study. Lancet 2008; 371(9624): 1579-86.

[11]   Cobb MH. MAP kinase pathways. Prog Biophys Mol Biol 1999; 71(3-4): 479-500.

[12]   Stariha RL, Kim SU. Mitogen-activated protein kinase signalling in oligodendrocytes: a comparison of primary cultures and CG-4. Int J Dev Neurosci 2001; 19(4): 427-37.

[13]   Vaudry D, Stork PJ, Lazarovici P, Eiden LE. Signaling pathways for PC12 cell differentiation: making the right connections. Science 2002; 296(5573): 1648-9.

[14]   Choi J, Krushel LA, Crossin KL. NF-kappaB activation by N-CAM and cytokines in astrocytes is regulated by multiple protein kinases and redox modulation. Glia 2001; 33(1): 45-56.

[15]   Chen J, Li Y, Wang L, et al. Therapeutic benefit of intravenous administration of bone marrow stromal cells after cerebral ischemia in rats. Stroke 2001; 32(4): 1005-11.

[16]   Phinney DG, Isakova I. Plasticity and therapeutic potential of mesenchymal stem cells in the nervous system. Curr Pharm Des 2005; 11(10): 1255-65.

[17]   Li Y, Chen J, Chen XG, et al. Human marrow stromal cell therapy for stroke in rat: neurotrophins and functional recovery. Neurology 2002; 59(4): 514-23.

[18]   Caplan AI, Dennis JE. Mesenchymal stem cells as trophic mediators. J Cell Biochem 2006; 98(5): 1076-84.

[19]   Nishida M, Li TS, Hirata K, Yano M, Matsuzaki M, Hamano K. Improvement of cardiac function by bone marrow cell implantation in a rat hypoperfusion heart model. Ann Thorac Surg 2003; 75(3): 768-73; discussion 73-4.

[20]   Kobayashi T, Hamano K, Li TS, et al. Enhancement of angiogenesis by the implantation of self bone marrow cells in a rat ischemic heart model. J Surg Res 2000; 89(2): 189-95.

[21]   Kinnaird T, Stabile E, Burnett MS, et al. Marrow-derived stromal cells express genes encoding a broad spectrum of arteriogenic cytokines and promote in vitro and in vivo arteriogenesis through paracrine mechanisms. Circ Res 2004; 94(5): 678-85.

[22]   Jin K, Zhu Y, Sun Y, Mao XO, Xie L, Greenberg DA. Vascular endothelial growth factor (VEGF) stimulates neurogenesis in vitro and in vivo. Proc Natl Acad Sci USA 2002; 99(18): 11946-50.

[23]   Li Y, Chen J, Chopp M. Adult bone marrow transplantation after stroke in adult rats. Cell Transplant 2001; 10(1): 31-40.

[24]   Xin H, Li Y, Chen X, Chopp M. Bone marrow stromal cells induce BMP2/4 production in oxygen-glucose-deprived astrocytes, which promotes an astrocytic phenotype in adult subventricular progenitor cells. J Neurosci Res 2006; 83(8): 1485-93.

[25]   Shen LH, Li Y, Chen J, et al. Intracarotid transplantation of bone marrow stromal cells increases axon-myelin remodeling after stroke. Neuroscience 2006; 137(2): 393-9.

[26]   Lu D, Mahmood A, Qu C, Goussev A, Schallert T, Chopp M. Erythropoietin enhances neurogenesis and restores spatial memory in rats after traumatic brain injury. J Neurotrauma 2005; 22(9): 1011-7.

[27]   Li Y, Chen J, Zhang CL, et al. Gliosis and brain remodeling after treatment of stroke in rats with marrow stromal cells. Glia 2005; 49(3): 407-17.

[28]   Zhang R, Zhang Z, Wang L, et al. Activated neural stem cells contribute to stroke-induced neurogenesis and neuroblast migration toward the infarct boundary in adult rats. J Cereb Blood Flow Metab 2004; 24(4): 441-8.

[29]   Chen J, Zhang ZG, Li Y, et al. Intravenous administration of human bone marrow stromal cells induces angiogenesis in the ischemic boundary zone after stroke in rats. Circ Res 2003; 92(6): 692-9.

[30]   Lu D, Mahmood A, Wang L, Li Y, Lu M, Chopp M. Adult bone marrow stromal cells administered intravenously to rats after traumatic brain injury migrate into brain and improve neurological outcome. Neuroreport. 2001; 12(3): 559-63.

[31]   Lu D, Li Y, Wang L, Chen J, Mahmood A, Chopp M. Intraarterial administration of marrow stromal cells in a rat model of traumatic brain injury. J Neurotrauma 2001; 18(8): 813-9.

[32]   Li Y, Chen J, Wang L, Lu M, Chopp M. Treatment of stroke in rat with intracarotid administration of marrow stromal cells. Neurology 2001; 56(12): 1666-72.

[33]   Chen J, Sanberg PR, Li Y, et al. Intravenous administration of human umbilical cord blood reduces behavioral deficits after stroke in rats. Stroke 2001; 32(11): 2682-8.

[34]   Hess DC, Hill WD, Martin-Studdard A, Carroll J, Brailer J, Carothers J. Bone marrow as a source of endothelial cells

and NeuN-expressing cells After stroke. Stroke 2002; 33(5): 1362-8.

[35] Zhao LR, Duan WM, Reyes M, Keene CD, Verfaillie CM, Low WC. Human bone marrow stem cells exhibit neural phenotypes and ameliorate neurological deficits after grafting into the ischemic brain of rats. Exp Neurol 2002; 174(1): 11-20.

[36] Borlongan CV, Tajima Y, Trojanowski JQ, Lee VM, Sanberg PR. Transplantation of cryopreserved human embryonal carcinoma-derived neurons (NT2N cells) promotes functional recovery in ischemic rats. Exp Neurol 1998; 149(2): 310-21.

[37] Taguchi A, Soma T, Tanaka H, *et al.* Administration of CD34+ cells after stroke enhances neurogenesis via angiogenesis in a mouse model. J Clin Invest 2004; 114(3): 330-8.

[38] Shyu WC, Lin SZ, Yang HI, Tzeng YS, Pang CY, Yen PS, *et al.* Functional recovery of stroke rats induced by granulocyte colony-stimulating factor-stimulated stem cells. Circulation 2004; 110(13): 1847-54.

[39] Lepore AC, Neuhuber B, Connors TM, *et al.* Long-term fate of neural precursor cells following transplantation into developing and adult CNS. Neuroscience 2006; 139(2): 513-30.

[40] Swain RA, Harris AB, Wiener EC, *et al.* Prolonged exercise induces angiogenesis and increases cerebral blood volume in primary motor cortex of the rat. Neuroscience 2003; 117(4): 1037-46.

[41] Philips MF, Mattiasson G, Wieloch T, *et al.* Neuroprotective and behavioral efficacy of nerve growth factor-transfected hippocampal progenitor cell transplants after experimental traumatic brain injury. J Neurosurg 2001; 94(5): 765-74.

[42] Takahashi K, Yamanaka S. Induction of pluripotent stem cells from mouse embryonic and adult fibroblast cultures by defined factors. Cell 2006; 126(4): 663-76.

[43] Nakagawa M, Koyanagi M, Tanabe K, *et al.* Generation of induced pluripotent stem cells without Myc from mouse and human fibroblasts. Nat Biotechnol 2008; 26(1): 101-6.

[44] Mendel DB, Laird AD, Smolich BD, *et al.* Development of SU5416, a selective small molecule inhibitor of VEGF receptor tyrosine kinase activity, as an anti-angiogenesis agent. Anticancer Drug Des 2000; 15(1): 29-41.

[45] Yu J, Vodyanik MA, Smuga-Otto K, *et al.* Induced pluripotent stem cell lines derived from human somatic cells. Science 2007; 318(5858): 1917-20.

[46] Sortwell CE, Pitzer MR, Collier TJ. Time course of apoptotic cell death within mesencephalic cell suspension grafts: implications for improving grafted dopamine neuron survival. Exp Neurol 2000; 165(2): 268-77.

[47] Brundin P, Barbin G, Isacson O, *et al.* Survival of intracerebrally grafted rat dopamine neurons previously cultured *in vitro*. Neurosci Lett 1985; 61(1-2): 79-84.

[48] Zawada WM, Zastrow DJ, Clarkson ED, Adams FS, Bell KP, Freed CR. Growth factors improve immediate survival of embryonic dopamine neurons after transplantation into rats. Brain Res 1998; 786(1-2): 96-103.

[49] Wei L, Cui L, Snider BJ, *et al.* Transplantation of embryonic stem cells overexpressing Bcl-2 promotes functional recovery after transient cerebral ischemia. Neurobiol Dis 2005; 19(1-2): 183-93.

[50] White BC, Sullivan JM, DeGracia DJ, *et al.* Brain ischemia and reperfusion: molecular mechanisms of neuronal injury. J Neurol Sci 2000; 179(S 1-2): 1-33.

[51] Martin LJ, Al-Abdulla NA, Brambrink AM, Kirsch JR, Sieber FE, Portera-Cailliau C. Neurodegeneration in excitotoxicity, global cerebral ischemia, and target deprivation: A perspective on the contributions of apoptosis and necrosis. Brain Res Bull 1998; 46(4): 281-309.

[52] Manoonkitiwongsa PS, Jackson-Friedman C, McMillan PJ, Schultz RL, Lyden PD. Angiogenesis after stroke is correlated with increased numbers of macrophages: the clean-up hypothesis. J Cereb Blood Flow Metab 2001; 21(10): 1223-31.

[53] Modo M, Stroemer RP, Tang E, Patel S, Hodges H. Effects of implantation site of dead stem cells in rats with stroke damage. Neuroreport 2003; 14(1): 39-42.

[54] Chen J, Li Y, Wang L, Lu M, Chopp M. Caspase inhibition by Z-VAD increases the survival of grafted bone marrow cells and improves functional outcome after MCAo in rats. J Neurol Sci 2002; 199(1-2): 17-24.

[55] Park S, Kim EY, Ghil GS, *et al.* Genetically modified human embryonic stem cells relieve symptomatic motor behavior in a rat model of Parkinson's disease. Neurosci Lett 2003; 353(2): 91-4.

[56] Lee HJ, Kim KS, Park IH, Kim SU. Human neural stem cells over-expressing VEGF provide neuroprotection, angiogenesis and functional recovery in mouse stroke model. PLoS ONE 2007; 2(1): e156.

[57] Murry CE, Jennings RB, Reimer KA. Preconditioning with ischemia: a delay of lethal cell injury in ischemic myocardium. Circulation 1986; 74(5): 1124-36.

[58] Bruer U, Weih MK, Isaev NK, *et al.* Induction of tolerance in rat cortical neurons: hypoxic preconditioning. FEBS Lett 1997; 414(1): 117-21.

[59] Bolli R. The late phase of preconditioning. Circ Res 2000; 87(11): 972-83.

[60] Prass K, Scharff A, Ruscher K, *et al.* Hypoxia-induced stroke tolerance in the mouse is mediated by erythropoietin. Stroke 2003; 34(8): 1981-6.

[61] Sugiura S, Kitagawa K, Tanaka S, *et al.* Adenovirus-mediated gene transfer of heparin-binding epidermal growth factor-like growth factor enhances neurogenesis and angiogenesis after focal cerebral ischemia in rats. Stroke 2005; 36(4): 859-64.

[62] Post H, Heusch G. Ischemic preconditioning. Experimental facts and clinical perspective. Minerva Cardioangiol 2002; 50(6): 569-605.

[63] Schaller B, Graf R. Cerebral ischemic preconditioning. An experimental phenomenon or a clinical important entity of stroke prevention? J Neurol 2002; 249(11): 1503-11.

[64] Tomai F, Crea F, Chiariello L, Gioffre PA. Ischemic preconditioning in humans: models, mediators, and clinical relevance. Circulation 1999; 100(5): 559-63.

[65] Jones NM, Bergeron M. Hypoxic preconditioning induces changes in HIF-1 target genes in neonatal rat brain. J Cereb Blood Flow Metab 2001; 21(9): 1105-14.

[66] Paulding WR, Czyzyk-Krzeska MF. Hypoxia-induced regulation of mRNA stability. Adv Exp Med Biol 2000; 475: 111-21.

[67] Kirino T. Ischemic tolerance. J Cereb Blood Flow Metab 2002; 22(11): 1283-96.

[68] Chong ZZ, Kang JQ, Maiese K. Hematopoietic factor erythropoietin fosters neuroprotection through novel signal transduction cascades. J Cereb Blood Flow Metab 2002; 22(5): 503-14.

[69] Buemi M, Cavallaro E, Floccari F, *et al.* The pleiotropic effects of erythropoietin in the central nervous system. J Neuropathol Exp Neurol 2003; 62(3): 228-36.

[70] Studer L, Csete M, Lee SH, *et al.* Enhanced proliferation, survival, and dopaminergic differentiation of CNS precursors in lowered oxygen. J Neurosci 2000; 20(19): 7377-83.

[71] Takahashi M, Li TS, Suzuki R, *et al.* Cytokines produced by bone marrow cells can contribute to functional improvement of the infarcted heart by protecting cardiomyocytes from ischemic injury. Am J Physiol Heart Circ Physiol 2006; 291(?): H886-93.

[72]   Wei L, Keogh CL, Whitaker VR, Theus MH, Yu SP. Angiogenesis and stem cell transplantation as potential treatments of cerebral ischemic stroke. Pathophysiology 2005; 12(1): 47-62.

[73]   Hu X, Yu SP, Fraser JL, *et al.* Transplantation of hypoxia-preconditioned mesenchymal stem cells improves infarcted heart function via enhanced survival of implanted cells and angiogenesis. J Thorac Cardiovasc Surg 2008; 135(4): 799-808.

[74]   Theus MH, Wei L, Cui L, *et al. In vitro* hypoxic preconditioning of embryonic stem cells as a strategy of promoting cell survival and functional benefits after transplantation into the ischemic rat brain. Exp Neurol 2008; 210(2): 656-70.

[75]   Rosova I, Dao M, Capoccia B, Link D, Nolta JA. Hypoxic Preconditioning Results in Increased Motility and Improved Therapeutic Potential of Human Mesenchymal Stem Cells. Stem Cells 2008; 26(8): 2173-82.

[76]   Wang JA, Chen TL, Jiang J, *et al.* Hypoxic preconditioning attenuates hypoxia/reoxygenation-induced apoptosis in mesenchymal stem cells. Acta Pharmacol Sin 2008; 29(1): 74-82.

[77]   Francis K, Wallace G, Li Y, Wei L, Yu SP. Novel use of hypoxic preconditioning to enhance the survival of human embryonic stem cells after transplantation to the ischemic brain. Soc Neurosci Abstr 2007; 113.3.

[78]   Koizumi H, Higginbotham H, Poon T, Tanaka T, Brinkman BC, Gleeson JG. Doublecortin maintains bipolar shape and nuclear translocation during migration in the adult forebrain. Nat Neurosci 2006; 9(6): 779-86.

[79]   Fan Y, Yang GY. Therapeutic angiogenesis for brain ischemia: a brief review. J Neuroimmune Pharmacol 2007; 2(3): 284-9.

[80]   Wei L, Yin K, Lee J-M, *et al.* Restorative Potential of Angiogenesis after Ischemic Stroke In: Maiese K, Ed. Neuronal and Vascular Plasticity: Elucidating Basic Cellular Mechanisms for Future Therapeutic Discovery. Boston, Dordrecht, London: Kluwer Academic Publishers; 2003. pp. 75-95.

[81]   Jin K, Minami M, Lan JQ, *et al.* Neurogenesis in dentate subgranular zone and rostral subventricular zone after focal cerebral ischemia in the rat. Proc Natl Acad Sci USA 2001; 98(8): 4710-5.

[82]   Tonchev AB, Yamashima T, Sawamoto K, Okano H. Enhanced proliferation of progenitor cells in the subventricular zone and limited neuronal production in the striatum and neocortex of adult macaque monkeys after global cerebral ischemia. J Neurosci Res 2005; 81(6): 776-88.

[83]   Zhang RL, LeTourneau Y, Gregg SR, *et al.* Neuroblast division during migration toward the ischemic striatum: a study of dynamic migratory and proliferative characteristics of neuroblasts from the subventricular zone. J Neurosci 2007; 27(12): 3157-62.

[84]   Yamashita T, Ninomiya M, Hernandez AP, *et al.* Subventricular zone-derived neuroblasts migrate and differentiate into mature neurons in the post-stroke adult striatum. J Neurosci 2006; 26(24): 6627-36.

[85]   Ong J, Plane JM, Parent JM, Silverstein FS. Hypoxic-ischemic injury stimulates subventricular zone proliferation and neurogenesis in the neonatal rat. Pediatr Res 2005; 58(3): 600-6.

[86]   Yang Z, Covey MV, Bitel CL, Ni L, Jonakait GM, Levison SW. Sustained neocortical neurogenesis after neonatal hypoxic/ischemic injury. Ann Neurol 2007; 61(3): 199-208.

[87]   Hoehn M, Kustermann E, Blunk J, Wiedermann D, Trapp T, Wecker S, *et al.* Monitoring of implanted stem cell migration *in vivo*: a highly resolved *in vivo* magnetic resonance imaging investigation of experimental stroke in rat. Proc Natl Acad Sci USA 2002; 99(25): 16267-72.

[88]   Chen J, Zhang C, Jiang H, *et al.* Atorvastatin induction of VEGF and BDNF promotes brain plasticity after stroke in mice. J Cereb Blood Flow Metab 2005; 25(2): 281-90.

[89]   Borghesani PR, Peyrin JM, Klein R, *et al.* BDNF stimulates migration of cerebellar granule cells. Development 2002; 129(6): 1435-42.

[90]   Abrahams JM, Gokhan S, Flamm ES, Mehler MF. De novo neurogenesis and acute stroke: are exogenous stem cells really necessary? Neurosurgery 2004; 54(1): 150-5; discussion 5-6.

[91]   Arsic N, Zentilin L, Zacchigna S, *et al.* Induction of functional neovascularization by combined VEGF and angiopoietin-1 gene transfer using AAV vectors. Mol Ther 2003; 7(4): 450-9.

[92]   Folkman J, Shing Y. Angiogenesis. J Biol Chem 1992; 267(16): 10931-4.

[93]   Ellsworth JL, Garcia R, Yu J, Kindy MS. Fibroblast growth factor-18 reduced infarct volumes and behavioral deficits after transient occlusion of the middle cerebral artery in rats. Stroke 2003; 34(6): 1507-12.

[94]   Shen Q, Goderie SK, Jin L, *et al.* Endothelial cells stimulate self-renewal and expand neurogenesis of neural stem cells. Science 2004; 304(5675): 1338-40.

[95]   Krupinski J, Kaluza J, Kumar P, Kumar S, Wang JM. Role of angiogenesis in patients with cerebral ischemic stroke. Stroke 1994; 25(9): 1794-8.

[96]   Wei L, Erinjeri JP, Rovainen CM, Woolsey TA. Collateral growth and angiogenesis around cortical stroke. Stroke 2001; 32(9): 2179-84.

[97]   Kaya D, Gursoy-Ozdemir Y, Yemisci M, Tuncer N, Aktan S, Dalkara T. VEGF protects brain against focal ischemia without increasing blood-brain permeability when administered intracerebroventricularly. J Cereb Blood Flow Metab 2005; 25(9): 1111-8.

[98]   Zhang L, Zhang RL, Wang Y, *et al.* Functional recovery in aged and young rats after embolic stroke: treatment with a phosphodiesterase type 5 inhibitor. Stroke 2005; 36(4): 847-52.

[99]   Eliceiri BP, Cheresh DA. Adhesion events in angiogenesis. Curr Opin Cell Biol 2001; 13(5): 563-8.

[100]   Zhang ZG, Zhang L, Tsang W, *et al.* Correlation of VEGF and angiopoietin expression with disruption of blood-brain barrier and angiogenesis after focal cerebral ischemia. J Cereb Blood Flow Metab 2002; 22(4): 379-92.

[101]   Scott BB, Zaratin PF, Gilmartin AG, *et al.* TNF-alpha modulates angiopoietin-1 expression in rheumatoid synovial fibroblasts via the NF-kappa B signalling pathway. Biochem Biophys Res Commun 2005; 328(2): 409-14.

[102]   North S, Moenner M, Bikfalvi A. Recent developments in the regulation of the angiogenic switch by cellular stress factors in tumors. Cancer Lett 2005; 218(1): 1-14.

[103]   Gerber HP, Dixit V, Ferrara N. Vascular endothelial growth factor induces expression of the antiapoptotic proteins Bcl-2 and A1 in vascular endothelial cells. J Biol Chem 1998; 273(21): 13313-6.

[104]   Kawamata T, Alexis NE, Dietrich WD, Finklestein SP. Intracisternal basic fibroblast growth factor (bFGF) enhances behavioral recovery following focal cerebral infarction in the rat. J Cereb Blood Flow Metab 1996; 16(4): 542-7.

[105]   Palmer TD, Willhoite AR, Gage FH. Vascular niche for adult hippocampal neurogenesis. J Comp Neurol 2000; 425(4): 479-94.

[106]   Fasolo A, Peretto P, Bonfanti L. Cell migration in the rostral migratory stream. Chem Senses. 2002; 27(6): 581-2.

[107]   Greenberg DA, Jin K. From angiogenesis to neuropathology. Nature 2005; 438(7070): 954-9.

[108]   Hamano K, Li TS, Kobayashi T, Kobayashi S, Matsuzaki M, Esato K. Angiogenesis induced by the implantation of

self-bone marrow cells: a new material for therapeutic angiogenesis. Cell Transplant 2000; 9(3): 439-43.

[109] Wang J, Li W, Min J, Ou Q, Chen J, Song E. Intrasplenic transplantation of allogeneic hepatocytes modified by

BCL-2 gene protects rats from acute liver failure. Transplant Proc 2004; 36(10): 2924-6.

74 *Experimental Stroke, 2008, 1, 74-82*

Post-ischemic Neurogenesis and Brain Repair: Growth Factors and Cytokines

Yi-Ping Yan[1],*, Raghu Vemuganti[1,2,3] and Robert J. Dempsey[1,3]

Department of Neurological Surgery[1], Neuroscience Training Program[2] and Cardiovascular Research Center[3], University of Wisconsin-Madison, WI 53792, USA; E-mail: yan@neurosurg.wisc.edu

Abstract: Stroke is the major cause of neurologic death and disability in the adult population. The persistence of neurogenesis in the adult mammalian brain has brought hope that endogenous neural progenitors may be a potential source to repair the damaged brain after cerebral ischemia. In the adult mammalian brain, neurogenesis takes place in specific regions, including the sub-ventricular zone (SVZ) of the lateral ventricle, the sub-granular zone (SGZ) of the dentate gyrus (DG) in the hippocampus and the posterior peri-ventricle (PPV) dorsal to the hippocampus. Accumulating evidence indicates that cerebral ischemia stimulates neurogenesis in adult brain. Numerous attempts in the past to better understand the complicated mechanisms of ischemia-induced neurogenesis have revealed several crucial processes such as proliferation of neural progenitors, migration and differentiation of newly-generated cells, as well as functional incorporation of these cells in the injured brain. However, the molecular mechanisms regulating these steps are far from clearly understood. This review summarizes the role of growth factors and cytokines in the regulation of neurogenesis following cerebral ischemia. The functional significance of post-ischemic neurogenesis, as well as the future research directions to achieve improved functional recovery after stroke by enhancing this endogenous process of brain repair are also discussed.

Keywords: Cerebral ischemia, neural progenitor, growth factors, cytokines, sub-ventricular zone, dentate gyrus.

1. INTRODUCTION

Cerebral ischemia remains the major cause of neurologic death and disability in the adult population. Considerable work has been done to define the brain's initial response to ischemia, which is often an unsuccessful attempt to ameliorate the effects of ischemia and repair the damage. Neurogenesis, the process of generating functional neurons, was traditionally believed to take place in the mammalian central nervous system (CNS) only during embryonic stages. However, the pioneering work by Altman & Das almost four decades ago suggested continuing neurogenesis in the adult brain of rodents [1, 2]. Since the early 1990s, a large body of work has demonstrated that new neurons are indeed born in restricted regions in the adult mammalian CNS, especially the sub-ventricular zone (SVZ) of the lateral ventricle and the sub-granular zone (SGZ) of the dentate gyrus (DG) in the hippocampus [3, 4]. The discovery of neurogenesis in the adult mammalian brain has brought hope that this endogenous mechanism of cell replacement might be further enhanced to repair the damaged brain after cerebral ischemia. Hence, many studies have been performed in animal models of ischemia to elucidate how neurogenesis is affected in the adult brain after cerebral ischemia. Understanding the mechanisms of ischemia-induced neurogenesis would allow us to facilitate this endogenous process of brain repair to improve the functional recovery of stroke victims. Ischemia-induced neurogenesis involves several steps:

proliferation of neural progenitors, and migration, survival, maturation and functional incorporation of these newly-generated cells. To date, the information regarding the molecular mechanisms regulating these steps following ischemia is still fragmentary. As ischemia induces very complicated environmental changes in the brain, it is reasonable to believe that no one factor will affect all steps and some factors will affect just one step of post-ischemic neurogenesis. In this article, we will summarize the role of growth factors and cytokines in the regulation of post-ischemic neurogenesis.

2. NEUROGESIS FOLLOWING GLOBAL CEREBRAL ISCHEMIA

The animal models of global cerebral ischemia replicate the consequences of cardiac arrest which causes a short-term complete interruption of cerebral blood flow. Global ischemia induces selective neuronal death in vulnerable populations of cells such as hippocampal CA1 pyramidal neurons. Therefore, many studies use this model to investigate the effect of global ischemia on neurogenesis in the DG of the hippocampus.

2.1. Global ischemia induced neural progenitor proliferation

To examine the level of neural progenitor proliferation in the brain, the common used method is injection of 5-bromo-2'-deoxyuridine (BrdU), a thymidine analog that incorporates into newly synthesized DNA during the S-phase of mitosis, thus labeling the dividing cells. The BrdU labeled cells can then be detected with immunohistochemistry. By using this technique, an enhanced proliferation of neural progenitors in the SGZ of the DG was observed in gerbil [5-7], rat [8-10], mouse [11] and monkey [12] following global ischemia. The temporal profile of neural progenitor proliferation in the SGZ varies among studies, which may be due to the differences in the duration of ischemia and the animal species used. Generally, the increased cell proliferation was observed to start at 3-4 days, peak at 7-10 days, and gradually decline to control level by 3-5 weeks after global ischemia [5, 6, 8, 9, 11]. The level of progenitor proliferation in SGZ is affected by the duration of ischemia, but not by the intensity of CA1 cell death [5]. Compared with the sham-operated animals, the proliferation of neural progenitors does not increase in the SGZ after 2 min of ischemia in gerbil. Elongation of ischemia to 4 min induces a marked increase in the neural progenitor proliferation similar to the level induced by 10 min ischemia [5].

Following global ischemia, an increased proliferation of neural progenitors was also observed in other neurogenic regions such as the SVZ [13-15] and the posterior peri-ventricle (PPV), a part of the lateral ventricle wall [16]. The increase in number of BrdU labeled cells in the SVZ was observed at 7-14 days after global ischemia in gerbil [13], rat [16] and monkey [14, 15].

2.2. Differentiation and maturation of newly-generated cells following global ischemia

The newly-generated cells in the SGZ were shown to express doublecortin (DCX) and highly polysialylated neural cell adhesion molecule (PSA-NCAM) several days after ischemia, indicating they have become immature migrating neuroblasts [17, 18]. These neuroblasts migrate to the granule cell layer (GCL) of DG and differentiate into neurons that express mature neuronal markers such as neuronal nuclear antigen (NeuN), calbindin, and microtubule-associated protein-2 (MAP-2) [5, 8, 9, 17, 18]. The glial differentiation of newborn cells is very rare in GCL [5, 8, 9, 17], but some proliferating cells in the hilus of the DG differentiate into astrocytes [5]. The survival of the newly-generated neurons in the GCL was shown to decrease in the aged animals compared to the young animals [8]. This indicates that aged brain may lack some factors that support the survival of newly-generated neurons.

As mentioned above, global ischemia induces intense neuronal death in the hippocampal CA1 region. The fundamental question is whether the newly-generated neurons in the hippocampus can substitute neurons lost after global ischemia. The first evidence to this comes from Nakatomi and colleagues. They found that new neurons were generated in the hippocampal CA1 region 28 days after global ischemia in rats [16].

This phenomenon was also observed in a gerbil global ischemic model [7]. The neural progenitors located in the PPV adjacent to the hippocampus proliferated in response to an ischemic insult. Infusion of FGF-2 and EGF into the lateral ventricle during day 12-15 after ischemia further increased the proliferation of neural progenitors in the PPV. The proliferating progenitors were shown to migrate from the PPV into the CA1 region and differentiate into hippocampal pyramidal neurons which integrate into the existing brain circuitry and contribute to the functional recovery after global ischemia [16].

3. NEUROGESIS FOLLOWING FOCAL CEREBRAL ISCHEMIA

3.1. Focal ischemia induced neural progenitor proliferation

In contrast to global ischemia, focal ischemia is induced by occlusion of a cerebral artery, which produces irreversible brain damage in the core region of ischemia and a partially reversible injury in the surrounding penumbral area. By using animal models of focal ischemia, an enhanced neural progenitor proliferation has been observed in both the SVZ [19-22] and the DG [19, 22-26] in rodents. Due to the differences in the animal species and the variations in the duration of middle cerebral artery occlusion (MCAO) among studies, slightly different temporal courses of neural progenitor proliferation in the ipsilateral SVZ were reported. The enhanced proliferation in the ipsilateral SVZ starts as early as 2 days after focal ischemia [20]. The rate of proliferation reaches its peak at 1-2 weeks, gradually returns to the level of sham control by 3-4 weeks after focal ischemia [19, 20, 22]. The tendency of neural progenitor proliferation in the ipsilateral SGZ of the DG is similar to that in the ipsilateral SVZ with a peak proliferation at about 5-7 days after ischemia [19, 22, 23, 25]. Focal ischemia can also induce an increase in neural progenitor proliferation in remote areas such as the contralateral SVZ [19] and the contralateral DG [22-24]. Compared to the level of neural progenitor proliferation in the ipsilateral DG following a 2 h MCAO, less proliferation was observed in the ipsilateral DG after a 30 min MCAO [23]. This suggests that the magnitude of neural progenitor proliferation in the DG is affected by the duration of MCAO. Currently, it is unclear if the duration of MCAO also affects the proliferation of neural progenitors in the SVZ.

3.2. Migration and differentiation of newly-generated cells after focal ischemia

The BrdU positive cells in the SGZ of the DG express DCX, Musashi-1 or proliferating cell nuclear antigen (PCNA) in the first week after focal ischemia, indicating they are neuroblasts [19, 22, 24]. The number of BrdU positive cells in the DG dramatically decreased at 4 weeks after BrdU administration. This suggests that the majority of the newly-generated cells in the DG die during the maturation. The surviving newborn cells migrate into the GCL of the DG, and differentiate into NeuN or calbindin positive neurons by 3-4 week after ischemia [22, 25, 27]. A small portion of the surviving BrdU positive cells in the hilus of the DG express glial fibrillary acidic protein (GFAP), an astroglial marker [24, 25, 27]. However, it is not clear whether the newly-generated cells migrate from the SGZ into the hilus and differentiate into astrocytes or whether it is a indication of glial genesis in the hilus after ischemia.

Under normal conditions, the neuroblasts originating from the neural progenitors in the SVZ migrate via the rostral migratory stream (RMS) and differentiate into interneurons in the olfactory bulb [4]. Following focal ischemia, a large number of neuroblasts from the ipsilateral SVZ divert from the RMS and redirect towards the damaged striatum and cortex [21, 28-33]. This lateral migration of neuroblasts from the ipsilateral SVZ into the ischemic striatum lasts for several months following focal ischemia [34]. However, only a small fraction of these newly-generated cells actually differentiate into mature neurons in the ischemic brain [21, 28, 32, 35]. This suggests that the injured brain does not have a suitable environment for the survival of newly-generated cells.

Ischemia-induced neurogenesis was also observed in the ipsilateral cortex in photochemically-induced cortical microvascular occlusion and transient MCAO rat models [36, 37]. However, the origin of these newborn neurons is unclear. Multipotent precursors have been isolated from the adult rat cortex, which generate only glia *in vivo* but can differentiate into neurons after exposure to high concentration of FGF-2 *in vitro* [38]. Cortical neurogenesis has been reported in the adult rats [39] and primates [40-42] under physiological conditions, but this result was not confirmed by other studies [43-47]. Therefore, it may be possible that precursors which reside in the cortex alter their potential to generate neurons under pathological conditions [48, 49].

4. THE ROLE OF GROWTH FACTORS AND CYTOKINES IN THE REGULATION OF POST-ISCHEMIC NEUROGENESIS

4.1. Fibroblast growth factor 2 (FGF-2) and factors of epidermal growth factor (EGF) family

FGF-2 and EGF have been identified as stimulators of neural stem cell proliferation, and are routinely used for the maintenance of neural stem cells *in vitro*. Following focal or global ischemia, the expression of FGF2 [50-55] and heparin-binding EGF (HB-EGF) [56], a protein of EGF family, was reported to be increased in the brain, indicating their potential role as stimulators of post-ischemic neural progenitor proliferation. The direct evidence comes from FGF-2 deficient mice. Compared with wild-type littermates, the proliferation of neural progenitors in the SGZ of

the DG was reported to be attenuated in the FGF-2 knockout mice following a 20 min MCAO [57]. Furthermore, intraventricular delivery of the virus expressing FGF-2 into the FGF-2 deficient and wild type mice enhances the proliferation of neural progenitors in the DG following focal ischemia [57]. Several other studies have shown that administration of exogenous EGF [58, 59], FGF-2 [60], EGF and FGF-2 [16, 61, 62] or HB-EGF [63] further enhances the proliferation of neural progenitors in the ischemic brain following focal or global ischemia. Over-expression of FGF-2 [64, 65] or HB-EGF [66] in the ischemic brain by viral delivery also induces a short-term as well as long-term stimulation of post-ischemic neural progenitor proliferation. These results suggest that FGF-2 and proteins in the EGF family are stimulators for proliferation of neural progenitors in the ischemic brain.

4.2. Insulin-like growth factor-1 (IGF-1)

IGF-1 is a growth-promoting peptide hormone with neurotrophic properties. It is also a potent endogenous mitogen both in the developmental and adult brain. Transgenic mice overexpressing IGF-1 have an increased density of neurons and larger brain size [67], while IGF-1 hemizygous knockout mice have a 10% smaller brain size than wild type littermates [68]. Peripheral or intraventricular infusion of IGF-1 has been shown to increase the proliferation of neural progenitors in the DG in normal adult rats [69] and prevent an aging-associated decrease of neurogenesis in the DG [70]. *In vitro*, the neural progenitors isolated from the DG express the IGF-1 receptor (IGF-1R), and after addition of IGF-1 to the culture medium, they proliferate in the absence of FGF-2, the most commonly used mitogen for the adult neural progenitor expansion [71]. Our studies have shown that infusion of IGF-1 into the lateral ventricle further enhances focal ischemia-induced neural progenitor proliferation in the DG [22]. After focal ischemia, an up-regulated expression of IGF-1 was observed in activated astrocytes in the penumbral cortex and striatum [72]. Blockade of IGF-1 activity by infusing IGF-1 neutralizing antibody into the lateral ventricle decreases post-ischemic neural progenitor proliferation in the DG and SVZ [72], whereas over-expression of IGF-1 in the ischemic brain further increases the proliferation of neural progenitors in the ipsilateral SVZ [73]. Therefore, IGF-1 is an endogenous factor responsible for focal ischemia-induced neural progenitor proliferation.

4.3. Vascular endothelial growth factor (VEGF) and glial cell derived neurotrophic factor (GDNF)

VEGF is an angiogenic protein with neurotrophic and neuroprotective characteristics. Early studies have shown that adult neural progenitors express VEGF and its receptors [74-76]. VEGF stimulates the proliferation of cultured neural stem cells obtained from the embryonic cortex [74, 77] as well as neural progenitors isolated from the adult rat brain [76]. Intraventricular infusion of VEGF enhances the proliferation of neural progenitors in the DG and SVZ [74], and increases the survival of newly-generated cells in the DG and olfactory bulb in normal rats [76]. VEGF's effect on neurogenesis was also observed in ischemic conditions. Infusion of VEGF into the lateral ventricle increases the survival of newly-generated cells in both the ipsilateral DG and SVZ after focal ischemia [78]. Blocking the VEGF receptor attenuates the proliferation of neural progenitors and the survival of the newly-generated cells in the DG following global ischemia [79]. Both increased proliferation of neural progenitors and survival of newborn cells were also observed in VEGF over-expressing ischemic animals [80, 81]. These results suggest that VEGF is a proliferative factor for neural progenitors and/or a survival factor for the newborn cells.

GDNF, a neurotrophic factor, has been shown to increase adult neurogenesis in normal animals [82]. After focal and global ischemia, the expression of GDNF in the brain was shown to be up-regulated [83-85]. In our previous studies, we have shown that intraventricular infusion of GDNF into ischemic animals induced by transient MCAO further enhances the proliferation of neural progenitors and the survival of the newly-generated cells in the ipsilateral DG [22]. Similar results were reported by a recent study, which showed that infusion of GDNF into the ipsilateral striatum further increased the neural progenitor proliferation in the ipsilateral SVZ and the survival of newborn cells in the ischemic striatum [86]. These studies suggest that GDNF is a proliferative and survival factor in the post-ischemic brain.

4.4. Erythropoietin (EPO)

EPO, a 34 kDa glycoprotein, is a crucial growth factor that promotes the proliferation, survival, and differentiation of mammalian erythroid progenitor cells [87]. In the adult CNS, the expression of EPO and its receptors have been observed in multiple regions including the hippocampus and the SVZ [88-91]. EPO promotes neuronal differentiation of cultured adult neural progenitors from the SVZ [91] and increases the proliferation of neural stem cells from the embryonic hippocampus [92]. Systemically delivered EPO enhances the proliferation of neural progenitors in the hippocampus of adult mouse [93], whereas brain-specific deletion of EPO receptor by generation of a conditional knockout showed a decreased proliferation of neural progenitors in the SVZ [94] and the hippocampus [92]. This indicates that EPO is a regulator of adult neurogenesis by promoting the proliferation and neuronal differentiation of neural progenitors.

EPO also plays a role in ischemia-induced neurogenesis. In a focal ischemic model, EPO treatment further increases the proliferation of neural progenitors in the ipsilateral SVZ and the lateral migration of neuroblasts from the SVZ to the ischemic

boundary of the cortex and striatum [95]. This ischemia-induced lateral migration of neuroblasts is reduced in conditional EPO receptor knockout mice [94]. Currently, it is not clear whether EPO directly or indirectly stimulates the migration of neural progenitors. Neuroblasts migrate into the ischemic areas after stroke in close association with blood vessels and astrocytic processes [32, 33, 35, 96]. EPO stimulates not only neurogeneisis but also angiogenesis after cerebral ischemia [95]. Therefore, it is possible that EPO's effect on post-ischemic neuroblast migration may be through its effect on post-ischemic angiogenesis.

4.5. Stem cell factor (SCF) and granulocyte colony-stimulating factor (G-CSF)

SCF and G-CSF are two hematopoietic cytokines that play an important role in regulating hematopoiesis. Several studies have shown that SCF and G-CSF also play a role in adult neurogenesis in both non-ischemic [97] and ischemic conditions [98-103]. In the brain of adult rodents, the SCF receptor cKit and G-CSF receptor are expressed in the neurogenic regions including the SVZ and the DG [98, 103]. *In vitro*, SCF stimulates the proliferation of neural stem cells from the embryonic brain [98], while G-CSF drives neuronal differentiation of adult neural progenitors [100]. *In vivo*, administration of SCF [103], G-CSF [99, 100, 102] or both [101, 103] further stimulate the proliferation of neural progenitors in the ipsilateral SVZ and enhance neuronal differentiation of newborn cells in the ischemic brain after focal ischemia. These results indicate that SCF and G-CSF are factors that promote the proliferation and neuronal differentiation of neural progenitors.

4.6. Brain-derived neurotrophic factor (BDNF)

BDNF is a neurotrophic factor, which plays an important role in neuronal survival and differentiation. In normal animals, infusion of BDNF has been shown to increase adult neurogenesis [104-107]. After focal and global ischemia, the expression of BDNF in the brain was observed to be up-regulated [108-110]. Therefore, it is conceivable that BDNF might be a factor that regulates post-ischemic neurogenesis.

Following global ischemia, an increased expression of BDNF has been observed in the DG [111]. Over-expression of BDNF by adenovirus in the hippocampus did not alter the number of BrdU positive cells, but suppressed the number of newly-generated neurons in the DG following global ischemia [112]. To explore whether the post-ischemic increase in endogenous BDNF affects ischemia-induced neurogenesis in the DG, TrkB-Fc, a fusion protein combining the extracellular binding domain of BDNF to its high-affinity receptor TrkB, was infused into the lateral ventricle of ischemic rats to block the activity of endogenous BDNF. Consistent with the prior results [112], infusion of TrkB-Fc does not affect the total number of BrdU positive cells, but increases the number of newly-generated neurons in the DG following global ischemia [113]. These results suggest that BDNF may not affect the proliferation of neural progenitors and the survival of newly-generated cells, but counteracts neuronal differentiation of newly-generated cells in the DG following global ischemia.

BDNF also plays a role in the migration of neuroblasts after focal ischemia. Compared with wild-type mice, the number of neuroblasts in the ipsilateral striatum was reported to be increased in the BDNF heterozygous mice after focal ischemia [114]. However, other studies showed that over-expression of BDNF by adeno-associated virus in the ipsilateral striatum [115] or BDNF treatment through intravenous injection [116] also increased the number of focal ischemia-induced migratory neuroblasts in the ipsilateral striatum. The mechanism behind these contradictory results is not clear, but may be caused by differences in ischemic models and animal species. Moreover, whether BDNF attracts the migration of neuroblasts directly or alters the expression of other factors to affect neuroblast migration indirectly needs to be elucidated.

4.7. Stromal cell derived factor-1 (SDF-1)

As discussed before, the neuroblasts derived from the ipsilateral SVZ divert from the RMS and redirect toward the damaged striatum and cortex following focal ischemia. This suggests that factors produced in the ischemic areas of the brain attract the redirected migration of neuroblasts. SDF-1, a CXC chemokine, plays an important role in mediating recruitment of hematopoietic stem cells [117] as well as in regulating the migration of neural cells in the developing brain [118, 119]. After focal ischemia, an up-regulated expression of SDF-1 has been observed in the ischemic brain [34, 35, 120-122]. Neural progenitors isolated from the SVZ of adult rodents express the SDF-1 receptor CXCR4 [34, 121, 123]. CXCR4 is also expressed in neural progenitors in the SVZ [124] and in migrating neuroblasts in the ischemic brain [35]. SDF-1 induces a directed migration of neural progenitors *in vitro* [34, 121, 123] and further promotes focal ischemia-induced lateral migration of neuroblasts [34]. Blockade of the SDF-1 receptor CXCR4 decreases the migration of neuroblasts from the ipsilateral SVZ towards the ischemic boundary following focal ischemia [34, 35], indicating that SDF-1 is an attractant for neuroblast migration into the ischemic brain.

4.8. Monocyte chemoattractant protein-1 (MCP-1)

MCP-1, a CC chemokine, is a chemoattractant for monocytes/macrophages, T lymphocytes, basophils, and NK cells [125]. Previous studies showed that MCP-1 induced the migration of cultured neural progenitors across a chemotaxis chamber *in vitro* [126]. Neural progenitors isolated from the SVZ express MCP-1 receptor CCR2 [127]. CCR2 is also expressed in neural progenitors in the SVZ *in vivo*

[124]. We and others have shown that the expression of MCP-1 is up-regulated in the ischemic brain [33, 128, 129]. When MCP-1 is infused into the striatum of a normal rat brain, it induces the migration of neuroblasts from the SVZ to the infusion site [33]. Compared with the wild-type littermates, the number of migrating neuroblasts in the ipsilateral striatum is significantly decreased after focal ischemia in knockout mice that lack either MCP-1 or its receptor CCR2 [33]. Therefore, MCP-1 is one of the factors that attract newly-formed neuroblasts to migrate from neurogenic regions to the damaged regions following focal ischemia.

4.9. Tumor necrosis factor-α (TNF-α) and other factors

TNF-α, a pro-inflammatory cytokine, exerts its biological effects through activation of two distinct receptor subtypes, TNF-R1 and TNF-R2 [130]. TNF-α inhibits the neuronal differentiation and induces neuronal cell death of cultured embryonic neural progenitors [131]. However, inhibition of TNF-α by infusion of an antibody into the lateral ventricle has been shown to impair the survival of the newly-generated neuroblasts in the ipsilateral striatum and the DG after focal ischemia [132]. It has been demonstrated that TNF-R1 and TNF-R2 have differential actions in neurogenesis. TNF-R1 acts as a suppressor of progenitor proliferation, whereas TNF-R2 can improve survival of the newly formed neurons [133]. Therefore, the different effect of TNF-α on adult neurogenesis may depend on the activation of its receptor subtype. Recently, other factors such as bone morphogenetic protein-7 (BMP-7) and galectin-1 are identified to be stimulators of post-ischemic neural progenitor proliferation [134, 135].

5. THE FUNCTIONAL SIGNIFICANCE OF POST-ISCHEMIC NEUROGENESIS

After cerebral ischemia, enhanced neurogenesis is not only observed in animal models, but also in human stroke patients [136, 137]. The newly-generated cells have the potential to differentiate into neurons, astrocytes and oligodentrocytes to replace brain cells lost after ischemia. They may also produce growth factors that play a role in stabilizing synaptically dysfunctional neurons or sustaining injured neuronal circuits. As the hippocampus is a key structure in learning and memory processes, post-ischemic neurogenesis in the hippocampus may be involved in the recovery of cognitive deficits. Enhancement of post-ischemic neurogenesis in the hippocampus has been shown to facilitate the recovery of cognitive functions [16], while animals with impaired hippocampal neurogenesis show a poor performance in the Morris water maze task after global ischemia [138]. In focal ischemic animals, treatments with EPO [95], BDNF [116] galectin-1 [135], or SCF and G-CSF [101, 103] further stimulate post-ischemic neurogenesis in the SVZ and improve the recovery of motor functions. However, whether post-ischemic neurogenesis contributes to functional recovery after ischemia is uncertain because these studies do not account for the effects of other processes such as the recovery of cellular dysfunction, angiogenesis, and synaptogenesis on functional recovery. In order to elucidate the role of post-ischemic neurogenesis in functional recovery, we need to develop techniques to specifically eliminate neurogenesis in the adult brain. In spite of this, it is reasonable to believe that neurogenesis is a normal healing process of the brain to repair itself after an ischemic insult. Future investigations may target how to promote the survival of the newly-generated cells and induce them to functionally incorporate into the existing circuits, which may lead to novel therapies for stroke victims.

REFERENCES

[1] Altman J, Das GD. Autoradiographic and histological evidence of post-natal hippocampal neurogenesis in rats. J Comp Neurol 1965; 124: 319-35.

[2] Altman J. Autoradiographic and histological studies of postnatal neurogenesis. IV. Cell proliferation and migration in the anterior forebrain, with special reference to persisting neurogenesis in the olfactory bulb. J Comp Neurol 1969; 137: 433-57.

[3] Gage FH. Mammalian neural stem cells. Science 2000; 287: 1433-8.

[4] Alvarez-Buylla A, Garcia-Verdugo JM. Neurogenesis in adult subventricular zone. J Neurosci 2002; 22: 629-34.

[5] Liu J, Solway K, Messing RO, Sharp FR. Increased neurogenesis in the dentate gyrus after transient global ischemia in gerbils. J Neurosci 1998; 18: 7768-78.

[6] Iwai M, Hayashi T, Zhang WR, Sato K, Manabe Y, Abe K. Induction of highly polysialylated neural cell adhesion molecule (PSA-NCAM) in postischemic gerbil hippocampus mainly dissociated with neural stem cell proliferation. Brain Res 2001; 902: 288-93.

[7] Schmidt W, Reymann KG. Proliferating cells differentiate into neurons in the hippocampal CA1 region of gerbils after global cerebral ischemia. Neurosci Lett 2002; 334: 153-6.

[8] Yagita Y, Kitagawa K, Ohtsuki T, et al. Neurogenesis by progenitor cells in the ischemic adult rat hippocampus. Stroke 2001; 32: 1890-6.

[9] Kee NJ, Preston E, Wojtowicz JM. Enhanced neurogenesis after transient global ischemia in the dentate gyrus of the rat. Exp Brain Res 2001; 136: 313-20.

[10] Kawai T, Takagi N, Miyake-Takagi K, Okuyama N, Mochizuki N, Takeo S. Characterization of BrdU-positive neurons induced by transient global ischemia in adult hippocampus. J Cereb Blood Flow Metab 2004; 24: 548-55.

[11] Takagi Y, Nozaki K, Takahashi J, Yodoi J, Ishikawa M, Hashimoto N. Proliferation of neuronal precursor cells in the dentate gyrus is accelerated after transient forebrain ischemia in mice. Brain Res 1999; 831: 283-7.

[12] Tonchev AB, Yamashima T, Zhao L, Okano HJ, Okano H. Proliferation of neural and neuronal progenitors after global brain ischemia in young adult macaque monkeys. Mol Cell Neurosci 2003; 23: 292-301.

[13] Iwai M, Sato K, Kamada H, et al. Temporal profile of stem cell division, migration, and differentiation from subventricular zone to olfactory bulb after transient forebrain ischemia in gerbils. J Cereb Blood Flow Metab 2003: 23: 331-41.

[14] Tonchev AB, Yamashima T, Sawamoto K, Okano H. Enhanced proliferation of progenitor cells in the subventricular zone and limited neuronal production in the

[15] striatum and neocortex of adult macaque monkeys after global cerebral ischemia. J Neurosci Res 2005; 81: 776-88.
Tonchev AB, Yamashima T, Chaldakov GN. Distribution and phenotype of proliferating cells in the forebrain of adult macaque monkeys after transient global cerebral ischemia. Adv Anat Embryol Cell Biol 2007; 191: 1-106.

[16] Nakatomi H, Kuriu T, Okabe S, et al. Regeneration of hippocampal pyramidal neurons after ischemic brain injury by recruitment of endogenous neural progenitors. Cell 2002; 110: 429-41.

[17] Iwai M, Sato K, Omori N, et al. Three steps of neural stem cells development in gerbil dentate gyrus after transient ischemia. J Cereb Blood Flow Metab 2002; 22: 411-9.

[18] Tanaka R, Yamashiro K, Mochizuki H, et al. Neurogenesis after transient global ischemia in the adult hippocampus visualized by improved retroviral vector. Stroke 2004; 35: 1454-9.

[19] Jin K, Minami M, Lan JQ, et al. Neurogenesis in dentate subgranular zone and rostral subventricular zone after focal cerebral ischemia in the rat. Proc Natl Acad Sci USA 2001; 98: 4710-15.

[20] Zhang RL, Zhang ZG, Zhang L, Chopp M. Proliferation and differentiation of progenitor cells in the cortex and the subventricular zone in the adult rat after focal cerebral ischemia. Neuroscience 2001; 105: 33-41.

[21] Parent JM, Vexler ZS, Gong C, Derugin N, Ferriero DM. Rat forebrain neurogenesis and striatal neuron replacement after focal stroke. Ann Neurol 2002; 52: 802-13.

[22] Dempsey RJ, Sailor KA, Bowen KK, Tureyen K, Vemuganti R. Stroke-induced progenitor cell proliferation in adult spontaneously hypertensive rat brain: effect of exogenous IGF-1 and GDNF. J Neurochem 2003; 87: 586-97.

[23] Arvidsson A, Kokaia Z, Lindvall O. N-methyl-D-aspartate receptor-mediated increase of neurogenesis in adult rat dentate gyrus following stroke. Eur J Neurosci 2001; 14: 10-8.

[24] Takasawa K, Kitagawa K, Yagita Y, et al. Increased proliferation of neural progenitor cells but reduced survival of newborn cells in the contralateral hippocampus after focal cerebral ischemia in rats. J Cereb Blood Flow Metab 2002; 22: 299-307.

[25] Zhu DY, Liu SH, Sun HS, Lu YM. Expression of inducible nitric oxide synthase after focal cerebral ischemia stimulates neurogenesis in the adult rodent dentate gyrus. J Neurosci 2003; 23: 223-9.

[26] Türeyen K, Vemuganti R, Sailor KA, Bowen KK, Dempsey RJ. Transient focal cerebral ischemia-induced neurogenesis in the dentate gyrus of the adult mouse. J Neurosurg 2004; 101: 799-805.

[27] Komitova M, Perfilieva E, Mattsson B, Eriksson PS, Johansson BB. Effects of cortical ischemia and postischemic environmental rnrichment on hippocampal cell genesis and differentiation in the adult rat. J Cereb Blood Flow Metab 2002; 22: 852-60.

[28] Arvidsson A, Collin T, Kirik D, Kokaia Z, Lindvall O. Neuronal replacement from endogenous precursors in the adult brain after stroke. Nat Med 2002; 8: 963-70.

[29] Jin K, Sun Y, Xie L, et al. Directed migration of neuronal precursors into the ischemic cerebral cortex and striatum. Mol Cell Neurosci 2003; 24: 171-89.

[30] Zhang R, Zhang Z, Wang L, et al. Activated neural stem cells contribute to stroke-induced neurogenesis and neuroblast migration toward the infarct boundary in adult rats. J Cereb Blood Flow Metab 2004; 24: 441-8.

[31] Gotts JE, Chesselet MF. Migration and fate of newly born cells after focal cortical ischemia in adult rats. J Neurosci Res 2005; 80: 160-71.

[32] Yamashita T, Ninomiya M, Hernández Acosta P, et al. Subventricular zone-derived neuroblasts migrate and differentiate into mature neurons in the post-stroke adult striatum J Neurosci 2006; 26: 6627-36.

[33] Yan YP, Sailor KA, Lang BT, Park SW, Vemuganti R, Dempsey RJ. Monocyte chemoattractant protein-1 plays a

critical role in neuroblast migration after focal cerebral ischemia. J Cereb Blood Flow Metab 2007; 27: 1213-24.

[34]   Thored P, Arvidsson A, Cacci E, et al. Persistent production of neurons from adult brain stem cells during recovery after stroke. Stem Cells 2006; 24: 739-47.

[35]   Ohab JJ, Fleming S, Blesch A, Garmichael ST. A neurovascular niche for neurogenesis after stroke. J Neurosci 2006; 26: 13007-16.

[36]   Gu W, Brännström T, Wester P. Cortical neurogenesis in adult rats after reversible photothrombotic stroke. J Cereb Blood Flow Metab 2000; 20: 1166-73.

[37]   Jiang W, Gu W, Brännström T, Rosqvist R, Wester P. Cortical neurogenesis in adult rats after transient middle cerebral artery occlusion. Stroke 2001; 32: 1201-7.

[38]   Palmer TD, Markakis EA, Willhoite AR, Safar F, Gage FH. Fibroblast growth factor-2 activates a latent neurogenic program in neural stem cells from diverse regions of the adult CNS. J Neurosci 1999; 19: 8487-97.

[39]   Dayer AG, Cleaver KM, Abouantoun T, Cameron HA. New GABAergic interneurons in the adult neocortex and striatum are generated from different precursors. Cell Biol 2005; 168: 415-27.

[40]   Gould E, Reeves AJ, Graziano MS, Gross CG. Neurogenesis in the neocortex of adult primates. Science 1999; 286: 548-52.

[41]   Gould E, Vail N, Wagers M, Gross CG. Adult-generated hippocampal and neocortical neurons in macaques have a transient existence. Proc Natl Acad Sci USA 2001; 98: 10910-7.

[42]   Bernier PJ, Bedard A, Vinet J, Levesque M, Parent A. Newly generated neurons in the amygdala and adjoining cortex of adult primates. Proc Natl Acad Sci USA 2002; 99: 11464-9.

[43]   Kornack DR, Rakic P. Cell proliferation without neurogenesis in adult primate neocortex. Science 2001; 294: 2127-30.

[44]   Ehninger D, Kempermann G. Regional effects of wheel running and environmental enrichment on cell genesis and microglia proliferation in the adult murine neocortex. Cereb Cortex 2003; 13: 845-51.

[45]   Koketsu D, Mikami A, Miyamoto Y, Hisatsune T. Nonrenewal of neurons in the cerebral neocortex of adult macaque monkeys. J Neurosci 2003; 23: 937-42.

[46]   Spalding KL, Bhardwaj RD, Buchholz BA, Druid H, Frisén J. Retrospective birth dating of cells in humans. Cell 2005; 122: 133-43.

[47]   Bhardwaj RD, Curtis MA, Spalding KL, et al. Neocortical neurogenesis in humans is restricted to development. Proc Natl Acad Sci USA 2006; 103: 12564-8.

[48]   Magavi SS, Leavitt BR, Macklis JD. Induction of neurogenesis in the neocortex of adult mice. Nature 2000; 405: 951-5.

[49]   Chen J, Magavi SS, Macklis JD. Neurogenesis of corticospinal motor neurons extending spinal projections in adult mice. Proc Natl Acad Sci USA 2004; 101: 16357-62.

[50]   Kiyota Y, Takami K, Iwane M, et al. Increase in basic fibroblast growth factor-like immunoreactivity in rat brain after forebrain ischemia. Brain Res 1991; 545: 322-8.

[51]   Takami K, Iwane M, Kiyota Y, Miyamoto M, Tsukuda R, Shiosaka S. Increase of basic fibroblast growth factor immunoreactivity and its mRNA level in rat brain following transient forebrain ischemia. Exp Brain Res 1992; 90: 1-10.

[52]   Kumon Y, Sakaki S, Kadota O, et al. Transient increase in endogenous basic fibroblast growth factor in neurons of ischemic rat brains. Brain Res 1993; 605: 169-74.

[53]   Endoh M, Pulsinelli WA, Wagner JA. Transient global ischemia induces dynamic changes in the expression of bFGF and the FGF receptor. Brain Res Mol Brain Res 1994; 22: 76-88.

[54]   Speliotes EK, Caday CG, Do T, Weise J, Kowall NW, Finklestein SP. Increased expression of basic fibroblast growth factor (bFGF) following focal cerebral infarction in the rat. Brain Res Mol Brain Res 1996; 39: 31-42.

[55]   Lin TN, Te J, Lee M, Sun GY, Hsu CY. Induction of basic fibroblast growth factor (bFGF) expression following focal cerebral ischemia. Brain Res Mol Brain Res 1997; 49: 255-65.

[56]   Kawahara N, Mishima K, Higashiyama S, Taniguchi N, Tamura A, Kirino T. The gene for heparin-binding epidermal growth factor-like growth factor is stress-inducible: its role in cerebral ischemia. J Cereb Blood Flow Metab 1999; 19: 307-20.

[57]   Yoshimura S, Takagi Y, Harada J, et al. FGF-2 regulation of neurogenesis in adult hippocampus after brain injury. Proc Natl Acad Sci USA 2001; 98: 5874-9.

[58]   Teramoto T, Qiu J, Plumier JC, Moskowitz MA. EGF amplifies the replacement of parvalbumin-expressing striatal interneurons after ischemia. J Clin Invest 2003; 111: 1125-32.

[59]   Ninomiya M, Yamashita T, Araki N, Okano H, Sawamoto K. Enhanced neurogenesis in the ischemic striatum following EGF-induced expansion of transit-amplifying cells in the subventricular zone. Neurosci Lett 2006; 403: 63-7.

[60]   Wada K, Sugimori H, Bhide PG, Moskowitz MA, Finklestein SP. Effect of basic fibroblast growth factor treatment on brain progenitor cells after permanent focal ischemia in rats. Stroke 2003; 34: 2722-8.

[61]   Türeyen K, Vemuganti R, Bowen KK, Sailor KA, Dempsey RJ. EGF and FGF-2 infusion increases post-ischemic neural progenitor cell proliferation in the adult rat brain. Neurosurgery 2005; 57: 1254-63.

[62]   Baldauf K, Reymann KG. Influence of EGF/bFGF treatment on proliferation, early neurogenesis and infarct volume after transient focal ischemia. Brain Res 2005; 1056: 158-67.

[63]   Jin K, Sun Y, Xie L, Childs J, Mao XO, Greenberg DA. Post-ischemic administration of heparin-binding epidermal growth factor-like growth factor (HB-EGF) reduces infarct size and modifies neurogenesis after focal cerebral ischemia in the rat. J Cereb Blood Flow Metab 2004; 24: 399-408.

[64]   Matsuoka N, Nozaki K, Takagi Y, et al. Adenovirus-mediated gene transfer of fibroblast growth factor-2 increases BrdU-positive cells after forebrain ischemia in gerbils. Stroke 2003; 34: 1519-25.

[65]   Leker RR, Soldner F, Velasco I, Gavin DK, Androutsellis-Theotokis A, McKay RD. Long-lasting regeneration after ischemia in the cerebral cortex. Stroke 2007; 38: 153-61.

[66]   Sugiura S, Kitagawa K, Tanaka S, et al. Adenovirus-mediated gene transfer of heparin-binding epidermal growth factor-like growth factor enhances neurogenesis and angiogenesis after focal cerebral ischemia in rats. Stroke 2005; 36: 859-64.

[67]   O'Kusky JR, Ye P, D'Ercole AJ. Insulin-like growth factor-I promotes neurogenesis and synaptogenesis in the hippocampal dentate gyrus during postnatal development. J Neurosci 2000; 20: 8435-42.

[68]   Beck KD, Powell-Braxton L, Widmer HR, Valverde J, Hefti F. Igf1 gene disruption results in reduced brain size, CNS hypomyelination, and loss of hippocampal granule and striatal parvalbumin-containing neurons. Neuron 1995; 14: 717-30.

[69]   Aberg MA, Aberg ND, Hedbacker H, Oscarsson J, Eriksson PS. Peripheral infusion of IGF-I selectively induces neurogenesis in the adult rat hippocampus. J Neurosci 2000; 20: 2896-903.

[70]   Lichtenwalner RJ, Forbes ME, Bennett SA, Lynch CD, Sonntag WE, Riddle DR. Intracerebroventricular infusion of insulin-like growth factor-I ameliorates the age-related decline in hippocampal neurogenesis. Neuroscience 2001; 107: 603-13.

[71]   Aberg MA, Aberg ND, Palmer TD, et al. IGF-I has a direct proliferative effect in adult hippocampal progenitor cells. Mol Cell Neurosci 2003; 24: 23-40.

[72]   Yan YP, Sailor KA, Vemuganti R, Dempsey RJ. Insulin-like growth factor-1 is an endogenous mediator of focal

ischemia-induced neural progenitor proliferation. Eur J Neurosci 2006; 24: 45-54.

[73] Zhu W, Fan Y, Frenzel T, *et al.* Insulin Growth Factor-1 Gene Transfer Enhances Neurovascular Remodeling and Improves Long-Term Stroke Outcome in Mice. Stroke 2008; 39: 1254-61.

[74] Jin K, Zhu Y, Sun Y, Mao XO, Xie L, Greenberg DA. Vascular endothelial growth factor (VEGF) stimulates neurogenesis in vitro and in vivo. Proc Natl Acad Sci USA 2002; 99: 11946-50.

[75] Maurer MH, Tripps WK, Feldmann RE, Kuschinsky W. Expression of vascular endothelial growth factor and its receptors in rat neural stem cells. Neurosci Lett 2003; 344: 165-8.

[76] Schänzer A, Wachs FP, Wilhelm D, *et al.* Direct stimulation of adult neural stem cells in vitro and neurogenesis in vivo by vascular endothelial growth factor. Brain Pathol 2004; 14: 237-48.

[77] Zhu Y, Jin K, Mao XO, Greenberg DA. Vascular endothelial growth factor promotes proliferation of cortical neuron precursors by regulating E2F expression. FASEB J 2003; 17: 186-93.

[78] Sun Y, Jin K, Xie L, *et al.* VEGF-induced neuroprotection, neurogenesis, and angiogenesis after focal cerebral ischemia. J Clin Invest 2003; 111: 1843-51.

[79] Kawai, T, Takagi N, Mochizuki N, *et al.* Inhibitor of vascular endothelial growth factor receptor tyrosine kinase attenuates cellular proliferation and differentiation to mature neurons in the hippocampal dentate gyrus after transient forebrain ischemia in the adult rat. Neuroscience 2006; 141: 1209-16.

[80] Wang YQ, Guo X, Qiu MH, Feng XY, Sun FY. VEGF overexpression enhances striatal neurogenesis in brain of adult rat after a transient middle cerebral artery occlusion. J Neurosci Res 2007; 85: 73-82.

[81] Wang Y, Jin K, Mao XO, *et al.* VEGF-overexpressing transgenic mice show enhanced post-ischemic neurogenesis and neuromigration. J Neurosci Res 2007; 85: 740-7.

[82] Chen Y, Ai Y, Slevin JR, Maley BE, Gash DM. Progenitor proliferation in the adult hippocampus and substantia nigra induced by glial cell line-derived neurotrophic factor. Exp Neurol 2005; 196: 87-95.

[83] Abe K, Hayashi T. Expression of the glial cell line-derived neurotrophic factor gene in rat brain after transient MCA occlusion. Brain Res 1997; 776: 230-4.

[84] Wei G, Wu G, Cao X. Dynamic expression of glial cell line-derived neurotrophic factor after cerebral ischemia. Neuroreport 2000; 11: 1177-83.

[85] Miyazaki H, Nagashima K, Okuma Y, Nomura Y. Expression of glial cell line-derived neurotrophic factor induced by transient forebrain ischemia in rats. Brain Res 2001; 922: 165-72.

[86] Kobayashi T, Ahlenius H, Thored P, Kobayashi R, Kokaia Z, Lindvall O. Intracerebral infusion of glial cell line-derived neurotrophic factor promotes striatal neurogenesis after stroke in adult rats. Stroke 2006; 37: 2361-7.

[87] Krantz SB. Erythropoietin. Blood 1991; 77: 419-34.

[88] Digicaylioglu M, Bichet S, Marti HH, *et al.* Localization of specific erythropoietin binding sites in defined areas of the mouse brain. Proc Natl Acad Sci USA 1995; 92: 3717-20.

[89] Marti HH, Wenger RH, Rivas LA, *et al.* Erythropoietin gene expression in human, monkey and murine brain. Eur J Neurosci 1996; 8: 666-76.

[90] Morishita E, Masuda S, Nagao M, Yasuda Y, Sasaki R. Erythropoietin receptor is expressed in rat hippocampal and cerebral cortical neurons, and erythropoietin prevents in vitro glutamate-induced neuronal death. Neuroscience 1997; 76: 105-16.

[91] Shingo T, Sorokan ST, Shimazaki T, Weiss S. Erythropoietin regulates the *in vitro* and *in vivo* production of neuronal progenitors by mammalian forebrain neural stem cells. J Neurosci 2001; 21: 9733-43.

[92] Chen ZY, Asavaritikrai P, Prchal JT, Noguchi CT. Endogenous erythropoietin signaling is required for normal neural progenitor cell proliferation. Biol Chem 2007; 282: 25875-83.

[93] Ransome MI, Turnley AM. Systemically delivered Erythropoietin transiently enhances adult hippocampal neurogenesis. J Neurochem 2007; 102: 1953-65.

[94] Tsai PT, Ohab JJ, Kertesz N, *et al.* A critical role of erythropoietin receptor in neurogenesis and post-stroke recovery. J Neurosci 2006; 26: 1269-74.

[95] Wang L, Zhang Z, Wang Y, Zhang R, Chopp M. Treatment of stroke with erythropoietin enhances neurogenesis and angiogenesis and improves neurological function in rats. Stroke 2004; 35: 1732-7.

[96] Thored P, Wood J, Arvidsson A, Cammenga J, Kokaia Z, Lindvall O. Long-term neuroblast migration along blood vessels in an area with transient angiogenesis and increased vascularization after stroke. Stroke 2007; 38: 3032-9.

[97] Jung KH, Chu K, Lee ST, *et al.* Granulocyte colony-stimulating factor stimulates neurogenesis via vascular endothelial growth factor with STAT activation. Brain Res 2006; 1073-1074: 190-201.

[98] Jin K, Mao XO, Sun Y, Xie L, Greenberg DA. Stem cell factor stimulates neurogenesis *in vitro* and *in vivo*. J Clin Invest 2002; 110: 311-9.

[99] Shyu WC, Lin SZ, Yang HI, *et al.* Functional recovery of stroke rats induced by granulocyte colony-stimulating factor-stimulated stem cells. Circulation 2004; 110: 1847-54.

[100] Schneider A, Krüger C, Steigleder T, *et al.* The hematopoietic factor G-CSF is a neuronal ligand that counteracts programmed cell death and drives neurogenesis. J Clin Invest 2005; 115: 2083-98.

[101] Kawada H, Takizawa S, Takanashi T, *et al.* Administration of hematopoietic cytokines in the subacute phase after cerebral infarction is effective for functional recovery facilitating proliferation of intrinsic neural stem/progenitor cells and transition of bone marrow-derived neuronal cells. Circulation 2006; 113: 701-10.

[102] Sehara Y, Hayashi T, Deguchi K, *et al.* Potentiation of neurogenesis and angiogenesis by G-CSF after focal cerebral ischemia in rats. Brain Res 2007; 1151: 142-9.

[103] Zhao LR, Singhal S, Duan WM, Mehta J, Kessler JA. Brain repair by hematopoietic growth factors in a rat model of stroke. Stroke 2007; 38: 2584-91.

[104] Zigova T, Pencea V, Wiegand SJ, Luskin MB. Intraventricular administration of BDNF increases the number of newly generated neurons in the adult olfactory bulb. Mol Cell Neurosci 1998; 11: 234-45.

[105] Pencea V, Bingaman KD, Wiegand SJ, Luskin MB. Infusion of brain-derived neurotrophic factor into the lateral ventricle of the adult rat leads to new neurons in the parenchyma of the striatum, septum, thalamus, and hypothalamus. J Neurosci 2001; 21: 6706-17.

[106] Benraiss A, Chmielnicki E, Lerner K, Roh D, Goldman SA. Adenoviral brain-derived neurotrophic factor induces both neostriatal and olfactory neuronal recruitment from endogenous progenitor cells in the adult forebrain. J Neurosci 2001; 21: 6718-31.

[107] Scharfman H, Goodman J, Macleod A, Phani S, Antonelli C, Croll S. Increased neurogenesis and the ectopic granule cells after intrahippocampal BDNF infusion in adult rats. Exp Neurol 2005; 192: 348-56.

[108] Lindvall O, Ernfors P, Bengzon J, *et al.* Differential regulation of mRNAs for nerve growth factor, brain-derived neurotrophic factor, and neurotrophin 3 in the adult rat brain following cerebral ischemia and hypoglycemic coma. Proc Natl Acad Sci USA 1992; 89: 648-52.

[109] Takeda A, Onodera H, Sugimoto A, Kogure K, Obinata M, Shibahara S. Coordinated expression of messenger RNAs for nerve growth factor, brain-derived neurotrophic factor and neurotrophin-3 in the rat hippocampus following transient forebrain ischemia. Neuroscience 1993; 55: 23-31.

[110]   Kokaia Z, Zhao Q, Kokaia M, *et al*. Regulation of brain-derived neurotrophic factor gene expression after transient middle cerebral artery occlusion with and without brain damage. Exp Neurol 1995; 136: 73-88.

[111]   Kokaia Z, Nawa H, Uchino H, *et al*. Regional brain-derived neurotrophic factor mRNA and protein levels following transient forebrain ischemia in the rat. Mol Brain Res 1996; 38: 139-44.

[112]   Larsson E, Mandel RJ, Klein RL, Muzyczka N, Lindvall O, Kokaia Z. Suppression of insult-induced neurogenesis in adult rat brain by brain-derived neurotrophic factor. Exp Neurol 2002; 177: 1-8.

[113]   Gustafsson E, Lindvall O, Kokaia Z. Intraventricular infusion of TrkB-Fc fusion protein promotes ischemia-induced neurogenesis in adult rat dentate gyrus. Stroke 2003; 34: 2710-5.

[114]   Nygren J, Kokaia M, Wieloch T. Decreased expression of brain-derived neurotrophic factor in BDNF(+/-) mice is associated with enhanced recovery of motor performance and increased neuroblast number following experimental stroke. J Neurosci Res 2006; 84: 626-31.

[115]   Gustafsson E, Andsberg G, Darsalia V, *et al*. Anterograde delivery of brain-derived neurotrophic factor to striatum via nigral transduction of recombinant adeno-associated virus increases neuronal death but promotes neurogenic response following stroke. Eur J Neurosci 2003; 17: 2667-78.

[116]   Schäbitz WR, Steigleder T, Cooper-Kuhn CM, *et al*. Intravenous brain-derived neurotrophic factor enhances poststroke sensorimotor recovery and stimulates neurogenesis. Stroke 2007; 38: 2165-72.

[117]   Broxmeyer HE. Chemokines in hematopoiesis. Curr Opin Hematol 2008; 15: 49-58.

[118]   Stumm RK, Zhou C, Ara T, *et al*. CXCR4 regulates interneuron migration in the developing neocortex. J Neurosci 2003; 23: 5123-30.

[119]   López-Bendito G, Sánchez-Alcañiz JA, Pla R, *et al*. Chemokine signaling controls intracortical migration and final distribution of GABAergic interneurons. J Neurosci 2008; 28: 1613-24.

[120]   Stumm RK, Rummel J, Junker V, *et al*. A dual role for the SDF-1/CXCR4 chemokine receptor system in adult brain: isoform-selective regulation of SDF-1 expression modulates CXCR4-dependent neuronal plasticity and cerebral leukocyte recruitment after focal ischemia. J Neurosci 2002; 22: 5865-78.

[121]   Imitola J, Raddassi K, Park KI, *et al*. Directed migration of neural stem cells to sites of CNS injury by the stromal cell-derived factor 1alpha/CXC chemokine receptor 4 pathway. Proc Natl Acad Sci USA 2004; 101: 18117-22.

[122]   Hill W, Hess DC, Martin-Studdard A, *et al*. SDF-1 (CXCL12) is upregulated in the ischemic penumbra following stroke: association with bone marrow cell homing to injury. J Neuropathol Exp Neurol 2004; 63: 84-96.

[123]   Robin AM, Zhang ZG, Wang L, *et al*. Stromal cell-derived factor 1alpha mediates neural progenitor cell motility after focal cerebral ischemia. J Cereb Blood Flow Metab 2006; 26: 125-34.

[124]   Tran PB, Banisadr G, Ren D, Chenn A, Miller RJ. Chemokine receptor expression by neural progenitor cells in neurogenic regions of mouse brain. J Comp Neurol 2007; 500: 1007-33.

[125]   Rossi D, Zlotnik A. The biology of chemokines and their receptors. Ann Rev Immunol 2000; 18: 217-42.

[126]   Widera D, Holtkamp W, Entschladen F, *et al*. MCP-1 induces migration of adult neural stem cells. Eur J Cell Biol 2004; 83: 381-7.

[127]   Ji JF, He BP, Dheen ST, Tay SS. Expression of chemokine receptor CXCR4, CCR2, CCR5 and CX3CR1 in neural progenitor cells isolated from the subventricular zone of the adult rat brain. Neurosci Lett 2004; 355: 236-40.

[128]   Wang X, Yue TL, Barone FC, Feuerstein GZ. Monocyte chemoattractant protein-1 messenger RNA expression in rat ischemic cortex. Stroke 1995; 26: 661-5.

[129]   Che X, Ye W, Panga L, Wu DC, Yang GY. Monocyte chemoattractant protein-1 expressed in neurons and astrocytes during focal ischemia in mice. Brain Res 2001; 902: 171-7.

[130]   Wajant H, Pfizenmaier K, Scheurich P. Tumor necrosis factor signaling. Cell Death Differ 2003; 10: 45-65.

[131]   Liu YP, Lin HI, Tzeng SF. Tumor necrosis factor-alpha and interleukin-18 modulate neuronal cell fate in embryonic neural progenitor culture. Brain Res 2005; 1054: 152-8.

[132]   Heldmann U, Thored P, Claasen JH, Arvidsson A, Kokaia Z, Lindvall O. TNF-alpha antibody infusion impairs survival of stroke-generated neuroblasts in adult rat brain. Exp Neurol 2005; 196: 204-8.

[133]   Iosif RE, Ekdahl CT, Ahlenius H, *et al*. Tumor necrosis factor receptor 1 is a negative regulator of progenitor proliferation in adult hippocampal neurogenesis. J Neurosci 2006; 26: 9703-12.

[134]   Chou J, Harvey BK, Chang CF, Shen H, Morales M, Wang Y. Neuroregenerative effects of BMP7 after stroke in rats. J Neurol Sci 2006; 240: 21-9.

[135]   Ishibashi S, Kuroiwa T, Sakaguchi M, *et al*. Galectin-1 regulates neurogenesis in the subventricular zone and promotes functional recovery after stroke. Exp Neurol 2007; 207: 302-13.

[136]   Jin K, Wang X, Xie L, *et al*. Evidence for stroke-induced neurogenesis in the human brain. Proc Natl Acad Sci USA 2006; 103: 13198-202.

[137]   Macas J, Nern C, Plate KH, Momma S. Increased generation of neuronal progenitors after ischemic injury in the aged adult human forebrain. J Neurosci 2006; 26: 13114-19.

[138]   Raber J, Fan Y, Matsumori Y, *et al*. Irradiation attenuates neurogenesis and exacerbates ischemia-induced deficits. Ann Neurol 2004; 55: 381-9.

Experimental Stroke, 2008, 1, 83-89

Brain Aging, Neurogenesis and Experimental Stroke

Kunlin Jin

Buck Institute for Age Research, California, CA 94945, USA; E-mail: kjin@buckinstitute.org

Abstract: Aging is associated with a striking increase in the incidence of stroke and neurodegenerative diseases, both of which are major causes of disability among those aged 70 years and older in the United States. Despite progress in understanding the molecular mechanisms of neuronal cell death in these diseases, widely effective treatments remain elusive. Adult endogenous neural stem cells hold great promise for brain repair because of their unique location within the central nervous system, their potential to proliferate and to differentiate into all major neural lineages, and their ability to incorporate functionally into existing neuronal circuitry after stroke. Nevertheless, the ability to exploit these cells for therapeutic purposes is hampered by the lack of knowledge about the biological behaviors of neural stem cells in the adult brain, and the cellular and molecular signals that control the generation of a functional neuron from adult neural stem cells after stroke, particularly in the aged brain. Therefore, it is essential to better understand the biological behaviors of neural stem cells and how neural stem cells are regulated after stroke in the aged brain, since stroke affects mainly the aged population. In this regard, brain aging and neurogenesis after focal cerebral ischemia are reviewed in this chapter.

INTRODUCTION

Stroke is a major cause of death and disability in the elderly [1, 2]. However, *in vivo* experimental stroke studies, including the evaluation of neuroprotective and cell replacement strategies, have relied almost universally on models of stroke in young adult animals due to their availability, lower cost and fewer health problems [3]. Compared to mature young adults, the elderly show substantial declines of baseline functions and adaptive capacities in their tissues and organs, including brain. Old populations are thus more severely impaired by stroke than are young populations, and show poorer functional recovery [4]. The persistent failure of human trials targeted at neuroprotective agents, effective in animal model of stroke, further indicates that the discrepancy between animal models and human diseases could have important clinical application [5]. Therefore, a better understanding of how age affects the response to therapeutic interventions after stroke is crucially important for rational development of effective treatment. Neural stem cells are the self-renewing, multipotent cells that generate the main phenotypes of the nervous system. The existence of neural stem cells in the adult brain has been postulated. Damaged cells or tisssue may be replaced by endogenous neural stem cells, thus opening a new avenue for the treatment of stroke. This review seeks to integrate what is known about the responses of endogenous neural stem cells resided in the neurogenic regions of aged brain to experimental stroke.

BRAIN AGING AND AGE-RELATED CHANGES IN THE BRAIN

Aging is a complex natural process that occurs from birth to death, and encompasses physical, social, psychological, and spiritual changes that potentially involves every molecule, cell, and organ in the body. Aging can also be defined as an increasing probability of death with the passage of time, and is characterized by functional decline due to histological and biochemical changes in tissues and organ systems. In its broadest sense, aging merely refers to changes that occur during a lifespan. Many tissues, organs and organ systems show decrements in function with age or exhibit some age-related increase in disease incidence. These decrements in function disadvantage the aging population, leading to decreases in health and activity and subsequent decreases in the ability of individuals to take care of themselves and in overall quality of life.

Brain aging is of great concern since **i)** brain aging greatly increases the risk of aged-related neurological diseases such as Alzheimer's disease (AD), Parkinson's disease (PD) and stroke, which remain major causes of disabilities and mortality in the elderly [6]. Current interventional approaches often fail to treat the underlying cause of pathogenesis; **ii)** brain aging is a cause of impairments in cognitive, motor, sensory and other behaviors in the elderly [7], accompanied with altered morphology and neural circuitry. Although these changes generally do not themselves result in neurodegeneration, the functional decline in aged brain worsens in the presence of neurodegenerative disease. Therefore, therapy, which alleviates aging and age-related disorders, is a primary goal in aging research; **iii)** brain may play a key role in control of lifespan. An example of such is that mice with mutations resulting in abnormally small pituitary glands or decreased levels of growth hormone experience a longer lifespan than normal mice [8]. In addition, *Caenorhabditis elegans* with mutations in insulin-like signaling pathways have an expanded lifespan when the mutant proteins are expressed in neurons, but not in other cells [9].

Although cognitive abilities often decline during normal brain aging, the structural and functional changes that underline such deficits and the mechanisms that regulate

Kunlin Jin / Guo-Yuan Yang (Eds.)

them are poorly understood. The number of neurons and connections in most regions of the aging brain remain essentially stable, but aging-related cognitive deficits could arise from changes in neuronal communication and from dysregulation of the dynamic replacement of neurons, glia and synapse. Functional magnetic resonance imaging (MRI) and positron emission tomography studies suggest that age-related memory changes may relate to altered functional activation of the prefrontal cortex and hippocampus [10]. Anatomical and electrophysiological studies indicate that the hippocampus of the aged rat sustains a loss of synapses in the dentate gyrus, a loss of functional synapses in CA1 region, a decrease in the NMDA (N-methyl-D-aspartic acid)-receptor-mediated response at perforant path synapses onto dentate gyrus granule cells, and an alteration of Ca(2+) regulation in CA1 region [7]. These changes may contribute to the observed age-related impairments of synaptic plasticity, which include deficits in the induction and maintenance of long-term potentiation (LTP), lower thresholds for depotentiation and long-term depression (LTD). This shift in the balance of LTP and LTD could, in turn, impair the encoding and enhance the erasure of memories, and therefore contribute to cognitive deficits [11]. Altered synaptic plasticity may also change the dynamic interactions among cells in hippocampal networks, causing deficits in the storage and retrieval of information about the spatial organization of the environment [11]. Successful memory formation requires a coordinated pattern of activation and deactivation in a distributed memory network that is altered by the process of aging. A recent study suggests that a failure in the ability to deactivate specific regions in the default mode network and consequent disruption of reciprocal neural activity between medial temporal lobe (MTL) and parietal memory systems may underlie age-associated memory impairment [12].

RESPONSE OF THE AGED BRAIN TO STROKE

Stroke is the rapidly developing loss of brain functions due to a disturbance in the blood vessels supplying blood to the brain, which can result from ischemia (lack of blood supply) caused by thrombosis or embolism, or due to a hemorrhage. Almost 90% are ischemic in origin. Ischemia stroke can be classified into global and focal cerebral ischemia. The focal cerebral ischemia model used most often in rodents involves occlusion of the middle cerebral artery (MCAO), and typically gives rise to localized brain infarction [13], which recapitulates many of the pathophysiological and histopathological features of patients with stroke. Studies of stroke in experimental animals have demonstrated the neuroprotective efficacy of a variety of interventions, but upon clinical testing, the strategies often failed to show benefit for aged human. One possible explanation for this discrepancy may be that although stroke in humans usually afflicts the elderly [1, 2], most experimental studies of cerebral ischemia have employed young-adult

animals, due to their greater availability, lower cost and fewer health problems, which thus may not fully reproduce the effects of ischemia on neural tissue in aged subjects [4]. In agreement with that, several anti-excitotoxic candidates including antagonists to the NMDA receptor such as MK801 and to the AMPA receptor such as NBQX were found to be less effective neuroprotectants in aged animal than young animals after experimental stroke [14]. We found that aged rats (24-month-old) given basic fibroblast growth factor (FGF-2) pre-ischemia showed better symmetry of movement and forepaw outstretching, and reduced infarct volumes, compared to rats treated with vehicle, but no significant improvement was found in aged rats given FGF-2 after focal ischemia. In contrast, young adult (3-month-old) rats treated with FGF-2 for 3 days beginning 24 hr post-ischemia showed significant neurobehavioral improvement and better histological outcome [15]. Abnormalities in glycolytic flux, lactate production, oxidation and energy production are more pronounced with advancing age, indicating a reduced ability of the brain to adapt to stress [16]. Consistent with these observations, ischemic changes are more pronounced with advancing age in models of both global and focal cerebral ischemia, as are post-ischemic behavioral abno-rmallities [15, 17-20], along with molecular and cytolo-gical responses listed in Table 1 (modified from [4]).

Table 1. Response of the Young Adult and Aged Brain to Stroke [4]

Cellular event/function	Change after stroke		References
	Young adult	Aged	
Mortality rate	lower	increased	[13, 19, 20]
Infarct size	similar	similar	[13, 22]
Cell death	delayed	early, increased	[17, 22]
Inflammation	delayed	precipitous	[21, 23]
Scar formation	delayed	precipitous	[24]
Functional recovery	rapid	delayed, incomplete	[25]
DNA damage	delayed	increased	[26]
Protein damage	delayed	increased	[27]
Neurogenesis	increased	increased	[25, 28, 29]
Oxidative stress	delayed	increased	[26]

In this light, the aged post-acute animal model that have been developed using aged rats and mice [15, 17, 21], is more relevant to human stroke and are helpful for evaluating the effect of aging on cerebral ischemic injury, as well as potential neural stem/progenitor cells (NSC)-based therapies.

NEUROGENESIS IN AGED BRAIN

Neurogenesis, a process by which neurons are created, continues throughout adulthood in the rostral subventricular zone (SVZ) lining the lateral ventricles and the subgranular zone (SGZ) of the hippocampal dentate gyrus (DG) in mice [30], rats [28], non-human primates [31] and humans [32]. However the rate of neurogenesis in the dentate SGZ declines with age [33-

35]. Similarly, other and our studies show that neurogenesis in the SVZ also decrease by greater than 50% compared to that seen in a young-adult brain [36, 37], though both SVZ astrocytes and adjacent ependymal cells remain relatively constant. Neurogenesis persists in the DG in elderly rodents [35] and humans [32, 38, 39] to maintain an equilibrium between production of newborn cells and neuronal loss. By electrophysiological analysis, newly generated hippocampal granule cells in aged and young mice were found to share identical physiological properties. Hence, although the rate of neurogenesis tapers with aging, a population of highly excitable young neurons indistinguishable from those found in younger animals is continuously generated. Newborn cells that exhibit appropriate migration and prolonged survival, and newly generated cells that differentiate into neurons, remain stable during aging. However, in newly formed neurons of the middle-aged and aged DG, the expression of mature neuronal markers such as NeuN is delayed and early dendritic growth is retarded. Therefore, the presence of far fewer new granule cells in the aged DG is not due to alterations in the long-term survival and phenotypic differentiation of newly generated cells but solely to diminished production of new cells. The results support neuronal fate choice, migration and enduring surviva of newly born cells remains stable even during aging but its ability to promote rapid neuronal maturation and dendritic growth is diminished as early as middle age [40]. Maintenance of the fundamental properties of NSCs even at advanced age suggests that stimulation of neurogenesis may constitute a valid strategy to counteract age-related neuronal loss and cognitive declines [41].

In theory, the age-related decline in neurogenesis could result from reduced proliferation or increased death rate of NSCs. Surprisingly, intraventricular administration of a caspase-3 inhibitor failed to restore the number of BrdU-positive cells in the aged SGZ, suggesting that the age-related decline in neurogenesis may be attributable primarily to reduced proliferation of NSCs [42]. The mechanism involved in decreased neurogenesis is unclear, but appears to be influenced in part by a reduction in epidermal growth factor receptor (EGFR) signaling, which results in associated deficits in fine olfactory discrimination [43]. Levels of both EGFR and transforming growth factor-α (TGF-α) are reduced in aged mice and the TGF-hypomorphic mutant mouse, *waved-1*, phenocopies aged mice with reduced levels of SVZ neurogenesis and loss of refined olfaction [43]. Significant declines of other neurogenic factors such as FGF-2, insulin-like growth factor-1 (IGF-1) and vascular endothelial growth factor (VEGF) [44] are also found in the aging hippocampus, and may contribute to reduced neurogenesis [45]. In apparent support of multiple growth factor involvement, we find that infusion of FGF-2 or heparin-binding-EGF (HB-EGF) into the aged brain is able to restore SVZ neurogenesis to levels found in young adult [36]. Restoration of IGF-1 levels also significantly restored neurogenesis in aged brain [46]. In addition, hippocampal neurogenesis is greater in aged mice that live in an enriched environment or receive

NMDA receptor antagonists [47], show a reduction in corticosteroid levels [34], or exercise by running [48]. The changes are associated with significant improvements in learning parameters, exploratory behavior, and locomotor activity [49]. On the other hand, there is no direct evidence to indicate that the aged brain retains the ability to react to functional challenges is due to a neurogenic response.

Neural stem cells only reside in certain regions of the adult brain, suggesting the microenvironments within an organism where stem cells reside - the neural stem cell niches that controls their renewal and maturation [50-52], which is further highlighted by the limitations on differentiation of adult-derived neural stem cells following engraftment back to non-neurogenic regions [53]. Stem cell niche may include cells, extracellular-matrix components in the stem-cell niche and the three-dimensional spaces they form [54]. Decline in neurogenesis could also result from age-related changes in the local niche and in the systemic milieu of the organism that influences all cells. Studies of the importance of such changes in the stem cell niche have been described in the germline stem cell niche in *Drosophila* [55]. Thus, even in the absence of significant aging of stem cells themselves, neural stem cell functionality could show a marked age-related decline due to decrements in the signals within the local and systemic environment that modulate the function of stem cells or their progeny [56].

ROLE OF NEUROGENESIS IN NORMAL ADULT BRAIN

Whether neurogenesis is required for maintenance of normal brain functions remains a matter of debate. Understanding these roles will be important in determining if newly generated cells can replace neurons that are lost as a result of neurodegenerative disease and brain injuries such as stroke. Several lines of evidence suggest that cells derived from the adult SVZ or SGZ play an important role in leaning and memory of normal brain: **(1)** there is a link between neurogenesis and cognition. For example, voluntary running increases SGZ cell proliferation, along with improvement of water maze performance (spatial learning) and selectively enhances dentate gyrus long-term potentiation (LTP) [57]. Aged runners show faster acquisition and better retention of the maze than age-matched controls, and the decline in neurogenesis in aged brain is reversed to 50% of young control levels by running [48]. Moreover, fine morphology of new neurons do not differ between young and aged runners, suggesting that voluntary exercise ameliorates some of the deleterious morphological and behavioral consequences of aging [48]. In addition to physical exercise, environment has also a major impact on SGZ neurogenesis. For example, exposure to an enriched environment between 3 to 13 wk of age was found to increase survival of newly born cells [58], and also led to better recognition memory [59]. Training in a hippocampus-dependent learning task (i.e., Morris water maze) induces immediate early gene protein expression in newborn dentate granule cells [60]; **(2)** New neurons are integrated into memory networks. SGZ-derived cells develop dendritic projections, and extend their axons along the expected trajectory, reaching the dendrites of CA3 pyramidal cells [61]. These cells receive synaptic inputs [62], and develop synaptic responsiveness and other electrophysiological properties similar to those of existing granule cells [63, 64]. Newborn neurons can incorporate into neuronal networks, as demonstrated by functional synaptic transmission [63] and synaptic integration [65], and can form axons that can be backfilled [66]. More importantly, these new neurons are incorporated into dentate gyrus circuits, supporting spatial memory in an age-dependent manner [67] and also suggesting that new neurons make a unique contribution to memory processing in the dentate gyrus; **(3)** Production of newly generated cells in adult SVZ, SGZ and olfactory bulb (OB) is tightly regulated by physiological processes such as exercise [57] and stress [68], as well as by pathological conditions such as stroke [28] and epilepsy [30]. Antidepressants also increase neurogenesis [64]; **(4)** Blocking adult neurogenesis by treatment with the antimitotic agents such as methylazo-methanol acetate (MAM) [60] or low-dose irradiation of either whole brain or restricted brain regions [69, 70] or using genetically engineered mice to specifically eliminate neural progenitors, such as the GFAP-TK mice in which the proliferating GFAP+ progenitors are susceptible to ganciclovir (GCV) treatment [71], disturbs performance on a hippocampus-dependent learning task, whereas a hippocampus-independent version of the same task is spared. The findings suggest that newly generated neurons in the hippocampus play a role in the formation of hippocampal-dependent memory. Notably, learning contextual fear conditioning tasks are impaired in irradiated rats or mice, ganciclovir-treated GFAP-TK mice [71] and Tlx conditional knockout [72], but not in mice treated with MAM [60]. The cause of such a discrepancy may originate from differences in behavioral testing protocols, the animal species, or genetic backgrounds. For example, only very young cells are targeted by the MAM treatment, whereas both young cells and mature newborn neurons are affected in irradiated animals and GFAP-TK mice. Therefore, it is possible that immature and mature newborn neurons play different roles in learning [64]; **(5)** aging is associated with functional deficits on hippocampus-dependent memory tasks, accompanied by structural alterations. Neurogenesis seems to be related to both performance deficits on hippocampus-dependent tasks and hippocampal volume reduction [73]. In addition, the integration of newly generated neurons into hippocampal circuitry decreases with aging [74]. These findings suggest that the decline in neurogenesis in aged brain may associate with deficit of learning and memory.

NEUROGENESIS IN AGED BRAIN AFTER STROKE

Substantial evidence documents that proliferation of NSCs in the adult brain increases after brain injuries. In the young-adult animal, stroke induces the proliferation of endogenous NSCs located in the SVZ (focal ischemia) [28] and in the dentate SGZ (global ischemia) [75]. Despite an age-related reduction in basal SVZ proliferation, NSCs in the SVZ of aged rats [29] and human [76] retain the capacity for proliferation and lesion-directed migration in response to cerebral ischemia, although the response is less robust than in younger animals. Interestingly, the absolute number of stroke-generated new striatal neurons is similar in young and aged rats [77]. Stroke-induced compensatory neurogenesis may also occur in the human brain. A recent study shows that cells expressing the polysialylated neural cell adhesion molecule (PSA-NCAM) are generated in the SVZ in human stroke brain, in relation to brains of comparable age without obvious neuropathologic changes. In addition, the number of Ki67-positive cells in the ipsilateral SVZ without concomitant apoptotic cell death is increased. Newborn cells migrate along the olfactory tracts, but it is unclear whether they also migrate into the damaged regions [78]. In a study of aged patients with ischemic stroke, we found that a number of cells expressing cell proliferative protein markers such as Ki67, minichromosome maintenance deficient 2 (MCM2) and proliferating cell nuclear antigen (PCNA), were observed in the ischemic penumbra surrounding cerebral cortical infarct [76]. Double and triple immunostaining showed that these dividing cells co-expressed several NSC protein markers including doublecortin (DCX), TUC-4, βIII tubulin and PSA-NCAM, but not cell death marker such as the activated form of caspase-3, suggesting that the aged human brain retains a capacity to respond to ischemic injuries [76].

Migration of newly generated cells into ischemic regions is one of the most striking features of ischemia-induced neurogenesis. Newborn cells migrate in chains from the SVZ to the penumbra regions (peri-infarct) of ischemic striatum near the SVZ that typically degenerate in most rodent models of focal cerebral ischemia [44]. Some of these cells express phenotypic markers of mature neurons, including neuronal-specific nuclear protein (NeuN), and region-specific mature neuronal markers, such as calbindin and dopamine and cAMP-regulated phosphoprotein-32 [79, 80], and form synapses [81], which are preferentially vulnerable to ischemia, consistent with differentiation towards a phenotype appropriate for cell replacement [79, 82]. Newly generated cells can also migrate from the ipsilateral SVZ and the rostral migratory stream (RMS) to the penumbra region of cortex cross tissue boundaries of striatum and white matter [83-85]. However, in the contralateral hemisphere, newborn neurons were restricted to the SVZ and a small chain of emigrating cells [79, 85]. After transient global forebrain ischemia, newborn cells can also migrate to the hippocampus and replace CA1 pyramidal neurons damaged by ischemia [86]. These findings suggest that endogenous mechanisms exist to guide such cells toward ischemic brain lesions.

Molecular and cellular mechanisms of cell migration after focal ischemia may be more complex, which may include extracellular signposts provided by the extracellular matrix (ECM) and by other cell types to direct migrating cells in transit, such as the chemotactic factor, stromal cell-derived factor 1α (SDF-1α) [87] and matrix metalloproteinases (MMPs) [88]. The studies on ischemia-induced migration of newborn cells point to some general principles of ischemia-induced cell migration. For example, newborn neurons can migrate long distances to reach ischemic brain lesions. In doing so, they appear to rely more or less on stereotypical pathways, which include not only routes observed normally in adult neurogenesis, like the RMS, but also pathways associated with developmental neuromigration. Alternative routes for migration from the adult SVZ include the lateral cortical stream [89] and ventral migratory mass [84] in the brain after stroke. Recent studies show that the neuroblast migration may associate with peri-infarct blood vessels in a region of active vascular remodeling. Blood vessels in cortical penumbra express SDF1 and angiopoietin 1 (Ang1), and their neighboring neuroblasts express their receptors CXC-chemokine receptor-4 (CXCR4) and Tie2. Gain- and loss-of-function experiments within the SDF1 and Ang1 systems demonstrate distinct roles in promoting post-stroke neuroblast migration and localization within peri-infarct cortex. Systemic administration of SDF1ß and Ang1 promote behavioral recovery during the period of neuroblast migration but do not affect the long-term survival of regenerated neurons in peri-infarct cortex. These findings suggest that a unique neurovascular niche is present in cortical penumbra, in which angiogenesis and neurogenesis are linked through specific vascular growth factors and chemokines in a process that is associated with behavioral recovery [90, 91]. Our study showed that although bran injury was able to increase neurogenesis in aged brain as young adult animals does; the migration of newly generated cells dramatically reduced in the aged brain compared to young adult brain [15]. Therefore, the capability of endogenous neural stem cells for brain repair is largely limited in aged brain, suggesting that such differences need to be considered in developing cell therapeutic agents for stroke. Elucidating the molecular basis for this phenomenon in the aging brain could yield novel approaches to neurorestoration by neurogenesis after stroke.

FUNCTIONAL CONTRIBUTION OF NEUROGENESIS AFTER STROKE

Whether the stroke-induced new neurons contribute to functional recovery remain largely unknown. Evidence for functional neuronal replacement in the damaged regions has been reported from rat after global cerebral ischemia. Intraventricular administration of growth factors including FGF-2 and EGF generated hippocampal CA1 neurons derived from the DG. The newly generated cells could integrate into the existing local neuronal circuitry, which may play a role in ameliorating neurological deficits [86]. There is no direct evidence to show that neurogenesis contributes to functional recovery after stroke.

CONCLUSION

Stroke remains the third leading cause of death. Even among those who survive stroke, disability due to hemiparesis, gait disorders, aphasia and other deficits is common, and ~20% of stroke survivors require institutional care at 6 months post-stroke. This long-term disability contributes to the average lifetime cost for stroke care of ~$140,000 and an annual national cost of ~$54 billion [1]. The most recent major advance in treatment, the use of thrombolytic agents to dissolve clots in the acute aftermath of stroke, appears to be effective only within about the first 3 hours after onset of symptoms [92]; therefore, widely effective treatment for stroke remains elusive, emphasizing the need for new therapeutic developments. The potential therapeutic impact of neural stem cells in replacing cells and tissues damaged due to stroke opens enormous possibilities based on the facts that neural stem cells can differentiate into different neural lineages *in vivo* [93, 94], and transplantation of these cells have already been shown to hold exciting potential for replacing damaged brain tissue for the treatment of many neurological diseases [95-98]. The demonstration of neurogenesis in the regions in adult brains and of the presence of proliferating cells with the ability to give rise to neurons in the ischemic regions of brains after cerebral ischemia have reinvigorated our hopes of rebuilding damaged tissues by endogenous neural cell replacement. However, little is known about whether aged brain will affect the biological behaviors of neural stem cells to the same extent that it does in younger brain; whether these differentiated neuronal cells can integrate into the local neural circuits and actually contribute the functional recovery of aged brain; and whether newly generated neural cells functionally contribute to the outcome recovery, and whether manipulation of adult neurogenesis will significantly improve the outcome after experimental stroke, if the amount of neuron replacement from endogenous NSCs is minimal in aged brain.

ACKNOWLEDGES

This work is supported by National Institute of Health (NIH) grant AG21980 (K.J.).

REFERENCES

[1]   Ramirez-Lassepas M. Stroke and the aging of the brain and the arteries. Geriatrics 1998; 53: S44-48.

[2]   Arnold KG. Cerebral blood flow in geriatrics--a review. Age Ageing 1981; 10: 5-9.

[3]   Harris NR, Rumbaut RE. Age-related responses of the microcirculation to ischemia-reperfusion and inflammation. Pathophysiology 2001; 8: 1-10.

[4]   Popa-Wagner A, Carmichael ST, Kokaia Z, Kessler C, Walker LC. The response of the aged brain to stroke: too much, too soon? Curr Neurovasc Res 2007; 4: 216-227.

[5]   Kidwell CS, Liebeskind DS, Starkman S, Saver JL. Trends in acute ischemic stroke trials through the 20th century. Stroke 2001; 32: 1349-1359.

[6]   Trojanowski JQ. Alzheimer's disease centers and the dementias of aging program of the national institute on aging: a brief overview. J Alzheimers Dis 2001; 3: 249-251.

[7]   Yankner BA, Lu T, Loerch P. The aging brain. Annu Rev Pathol 2008; 3: 41-66.

[8]   Holzenberger M. The GH/IGF-I axis and longevity. Eur J Endocrinol 2004; 151 (Suppl 1): S23-27.

[9]   Lin K, Hsin H, Libina N, Kenyon C. Regulation of the Caenorhabditis elegans longevity protein DAF-16 by insulin/IGF-1 and germline signaling. Nat Genet 2001; 28: 139-145.

[10]   Persson J, Sylvester CY, Nelson JK, Welsh KM, Jonides J, Reuter-Lorenz PA. Selection requirements during verb generation: differential recruitment in older and younger adults. Neuroimage 2004; 23: 1382-1390.

[11]   Rosenzweig ES, Barnes CA. Impact of aging on hippocampal function: plasticity, network dynamics, and cognition. Prog Neurobiol 2003; 69: 143-179.

[12]   Miller SL, Celone K, DePeau K, et al. Age-related memory impairment associated with loss of parietal deactivation but preserved hippocampal activation. Proc Natl Acad Sci USA 2008; 105: 2181-2186.

[13]   Ginsberg MD, Busto R. Rodent models of cerebral ischemia. Stroke 1989; 20: 1627-1642.

[14]   Suzuki Y, Takagi Y, Nakamura R, Hashimoto K, Umemura K. Ability of NMDA and non-NMDA receptor antagonists to inhibit cerebral ischemic damage in aged rats. Brain Res 2003; 964: 116-120.

[15]   Won SJ, Xie L, Kim SH, et al. Influence of age on the response to fibroblast growth factor-2 treatment in a rat model of stroke. Brain Res 2006; 1123: 237-244.

[16]   Hoyer S. Ischemia in aged brain. Gerontology 1987; 33: 203-206.

[17]   Popa-Wagner A, Dinca I, Yalikun S, Walker L, Kroemer H, Kessler C. Accelerated delimitation of the infarct zone by capillary-derived nestin-positive cells in aged rats. Curr Neurovasc Res 2006; 3: 3-13.

[18]   Yao H, Sadoshima S, Ooboshi H, Sato Y, Uchimura H, Fujishima M. Age-related vulnerability to cerebral ischemia in spontaneously hypertensive rats. Stroke 1991; 22: 1414-1418.

[19]   Cada A, de la Torre JC, Gonzalez-Lima F. Chronic cerebrovascular ischemia in aged rats: effects on brain metabolic capacity and behavior. Neurobiol Aging 2000; 21: 225-233.

[20]   Lindner MD, Gribkoff VK, Donlan NA, Jones TA. Long-lasting functional disabilities in middle-aged rats with small cerebral infarcts. J Neurosci 2003; 23: 10913-10922.

[21]   Wang LC, Futrell N, Wang DZ, Chen FJ, Zhai QH, Schultz LR. A reproducible model of middle cerebral artery occlusion, compatible with long-term survival, in aged rats. Stroke 1995; 26: 2087-2090.

[22]   Brown AW, Marlowe KJ, Bjelke B. Age effect on motor recovery in a post-acute animal stroke model. Neurobiol Aging 2003; 24: 607-614.

[23]   Zhang L, Zhang RL, Wang Y, et al. Functional recovery in aged and young rats after embolic stroke: treatment with a phosphodiesterase type 5 inhibitor. Stroke 2005; 36: 847-852.

[24]   Badan I, Buchhold B, Hamm A, et al. Accelerated glial reactivity to stroke in aged rats correlates with reduced functional recovery. J Cereb Blood Flow Metab 2003; 23: 845-854.

[25]   Badan I, Platt D, Kessler C, Popa-Wagner A. Temporal dynamics of degenerative and regenerative events associated with cerebral ischemia in aged rats. Gerontology 2003; 49: 356-365.

[26]   Li Y, Chen J, Chopp M. Adult bone marrow transplantation after stroke in adult rats. Cell Transplant 2001; 10: 31-40.

[27]   Roberts EL, Jr., Chih CP, Rosenthal M. Age-related changes in brain metabolism and vulnerability to anoxia. Adv Exp Med Biol 1997; 411: 83-89.

[28]   Jin K, Minami M, Lan JQ, et al. Neurogenesis in dentate subgranular zone and rostral subventricular zone after focal cerebral ischemia in the rat. Proc Natl Acad Sci USA 2001; 98: 4710-4715.

[29]   Jin K, Minami M, Xie L, et al. Ischemia-induced neurogenesis is preserved but reduced in the aged rodent brain. Aging Cell 2004; 3: 373-377.

[30]   Yoshimura S, Takagi Y, Harada J, et al. FGF-2 regulation of neurogenesis in adult hippocampus after brain injury. Proc Natl Acad Sci USA 2001; 98: 5874-5879.

[31]   McDermott KW, Lantos PL. Distribution and fine structural analysis of undifferentiated cells in the primate subependymal layer. J Anat 1991; 178: 45-63.

[32]   Eriksson PS, Perfilieva E, Bjork-Eriksson T, et al. Neurogenesis in the adult human hippocampus. Nat Med 1998; 4: 1313-1317.

[33]   Kuhn HG, Dickinson-Anson H, Gage FH. Neurogenesis in the dentate gyrus of the adult rat: age-related decrease of neuronal progenitor proliferation. J Neurosci 1996; 16: 2027-2033.

[34]   Cameron HA, McKay RD. Restoring production of hippocampal neurons in old age. Nat Neurosci 1999; 2: 894-897.

[35]   Gould E, Reeves AJ, Fallah M, Tanapat P, Gross CG, Fuchs E. Hippocampal neurogenesis in adult Old World primates. Proc Natl Acad Sci USA 1999; 96: 5263-5267.

[36]   Jin K, Sun Y, Xie L, et al. Neurogenesis and aging: FGF-2 and HB-EGF restore neurogenesis in hippocampus and subventricular zone of aged mice. Aging Cell 2003; 2: 175-183.

[37]   Luo J, Daniels SB, Lennington JB, Notti RQ, Conover JC. The aging neurogenic subventricular zone. Aging Cell 2006; 5: 139-152.

[38]   Sanai N, Tramontin AD, Quinones-Hinojosa A, et al. Unique astrocyte ribbon in adult human brain contains neural stem cells but lacks chain migration. Nature 2004; 427: 740-744.

[39]   Curtis MA, Kam M, Nannmark U, et al. Human neuroblasts migrate to the olfactory bulb via a lateral ventricular extension. Science 2007; 315: 1243-1249.

[40]   Rao MS, Hattiangady B, Abdel-Rahman A, Stanley DP, Shetty AK. Newly born cells in the ageing dentate gyrus display normal migration, survival and neuronal fate choice but endure retarded early maturation. Eur J Neurosci 2005; 21: 464-476.

[41]   Couillard-Despres S, Winner B, Karl C, et al. Targeted transgene expression in neuronal precursors: watching young neurons in the old brain. Eur J Neurosci 2006; 24: 1535-1545.

[42]   Tang H, Wang Y, Xie L, et al. Effect of neural precursor proliferation level on neurogenesis in rat brain during aging and after focal ischemia. Neurobiol Aging 2009; 30: 299-308.

[43]   Enwere E, Shingo T, Gregg C, Fujikawa H, Ohta S, Weiss S. Aging Results in reduced epidermal growth factor receptor signaling, diminished olfactory neurogenesis, and deficits in fine olfactory discrimination. J Neurosci 2004; 24: 8354-8365.

[44]   Greenberg DA, Jin K. Growth factors and stroke. NeuroRx 2006; 3: 458-465.

[45]   Shetty AK, Hattiangady B, Shetty GA. Stem/progenitor cell proliferation factors FGF-2, IGF-1, and VEGF exhibit early decline during the course of aging in the hippocampus: role of astrocytes. Glia 2005; 51: 173-186.

[46]   Li Y, Huang TT, Carlson EJ, et al. Dilated cardiomyopathy and neonatal lethality in mutant mice lacking manganese superoxide dismutase. Nat Genet 1995; 11: 376-381.

[47]   Nacher J, Alonso-Llosa G, Rosell DR, McEwen BS. NMDA receptor antagonist treatment increases the production of new neurons in the aged rat hippocampus. Neurobiol Aging 2003; 24: 273-284.

[48]   van Praag H, Shubert T, Zhao C, Gage FH. Exercise Enhances Learning and Hippocampal Neurogenesis in Aged Mice. J. Neurosci. 2005; 25: 8680-8685.

[49]   Kempermann G, Gast D, Gage FH. Neuroplasticity in old age: Sustained fivefold induction of hippocampal neurogenesis by long-term environmental enrichment. Ann Neurol 2002; 52: 135-43.

[50]   Goetz AK, Scheffler B, Chen H-X, et al. Temporally restricted substrate interactions direct fate and specification of neural precursors derived from embryonic stem cells. Proc Natl Acad Sci USA 2006; 103: 11063-11068.

[51]   Lemischka IR, Moore KA. Stem cells: interactive niches. Nature 2003; 425: 778-779.

[52]   Ahn S, Joyner AL. In vivo analysis of quiescent adult neural stem cells responding to Sonic hedgehog. Nature 2005; 437: 894-897.

[53]   Suhonen JO, Peterson DA, Ray J, Gage FH. Differentiation of adult hippocampus-derived progenitors into olfactory neurons in vivo. Nature 1996; 383: 624-627.

[54]   Kearns SM, Laywell ED, Kukekov VK, Steindler DA. Extracellular matrix effects on neurosphere cell motility. Exp Neurol 2003; 182: 240-244.

[55]   Xie T, Spradling AC. A niche maintaining germ line stem cells in the Drosophila ovary. Science 2000; 290: 328-330.

[56]   Rando TA. Stem cells, ageing and the quest for immortality. Nature 2006; 441: 1080-1086.

[57]   van Praag H, Christie BR, Sejnowski TJ, Gage FH. Running enhances neurogenesis, learning, and long-term potentiation in mice. Proc Natl Acad Sci USA 1999; 96: 13427-13431.

[58]   Kempermann G, Kuhn HG, Gage FH. Experience-induced neurogenesis in the senescent dentate gyrus. J Neurosci 1998; 18: 3206-3212.

[59]   Bruel-Jungerman E, Laroche S, Rampon C. New neurons in the dentate gyrus are involved in the expression of enhanced long-term memory following environmental enrichment. Eur J Neurosci 2005; 21: 513-521.

[60]   Shors TJ, Miesegaes G, Beylin A, Zhao M, Rydel T, Gould E. Neurogenesis in the adult is involved in the formation of trace memories. Nature 2001; 410: 372-376.

[61]   Hastings NB, Gould E. Rapid extension of axons into the CA3 region by adult-generated granule cells. J Comp Neurol 1999; 413: 146-154.

[62]   Bayer SA. Neuron production in the hippocampus and olfactory bulb of the adult rat brain: addition or replacement? Ann N Y Acad Sci 1985; 457: 163-172.

[63]   Song HJ, Stevens CF, Gage FH. Neural stem cells from adult hippocampus develop essential properties of functional CNS neurons. Nat Neurosci 2002; 5: 438-445.

[64]   Zhao C, Deng W, Gage FH. Mechanisms and functional implications of adult neurogenesis. Cell 2008; 132: 645-660.

[65]   Ramirez-Amaya V, Marrone DF, Gage FH, Worley PF, Barnes CA. Integration of New Neurons into Functional Neural Networks. J Neurosci 2006; 26: 12237-12241.

[66] Cameron HA, Woolley CS, McEwen BS, Gould E. Differentiation of newly born neurons and glia in the dentate gyrus of the adult rat. Neuroscience 1993; 56: 337-344.

[67] Kee N, Teixeira CM, Wang AH, Frankland PW. Preferential incorporation of adult-generated granule cells into spatial memory networks in the dentate gyrus. Nat Neurosci 2007; 10: 355-362.

[68] Gould E, Tanapat P, McEwen BS, Flugge G, Fuchs E. Proliferation of granule cell precursors in the dentate gyrus of adult monkeys is diminished by stress. Proc Natl Acad Sci USA 1998; 95: 3168-3171.

[69] Santarelli L, Saxe M, Gross C, *et al.* Requirement of Hippocampal Neurogenesis for the Behavioral Effects of Antidepressants. Science 2003; 301: 805-809.

[70] Snyder JS, Hong NS, McDonald RJ, Wojtowicz JM. A role for adult neurogenesis in spatial long-term memory. Neuroscience 2005; 130: 843-852.

[71] Saxe MD, Battaglia F, Wang J-W, *et al.* Sofroniew MV, Kandel ER, Santarelli L, Hen R, Drew MR. Ablation of hippocampal neurogenesis impairs contextual fear conditioning and synaptic plasticity in the dentate gyrus. Proc Natl Acad Sci USA 2006; 103: 17501-17506.

[72] Zhang CL, Zou Y, He W, Gage FH, Evans RM. A role for adult TLX-positive neural stem cells in learning and behaviour. Nature 2008; 451: 1004-1007.

[73] Driscoll I, Howard SR, Stone JC, *et al.* The aging hippocampus: a multi-level analysis in the rat. Neuroscience 2006; 139: 1173-1185.

[74] Wati H, Kudo K, Qiao C, Kuroki T, Kanba S. A decreased survival of proliferated cells in the hippocampus is associated with a decline in spatial memory in aged rats. Neurosci Lett 2006; 399: 171-174.

[75] Liu J, Solway K, Messing RO, Sharp FR. Increased neurogenesis in the dentate gyrus after transient global ischemia in gerbils. J Neurosci 1998; 18: 7768-7778.

[76] Jin K, Wang X, Xie L, *et al.* Evidence for stroke-induced neurogenesis in the human brain. Proc Natl Acad Sci USA 2006; 103: 13198-13202.

[77] Darsalia V, Heldmann U, Lindvall O, Kokaia Z. Stroke-induced neurogenesis in aged brain. Stroke 2005; 36: 1790-1795.

[78] Macas J, Nern C, Plate KH, Momma S. Increased generation of neuronal progenitors after ischemic injury in the aged adult human forebrain. J Neurosci 2006; 26: 13114-13119.

[79] Arvidsson A, Collin T, Kirik D, Kokaia Z, Lindvall O. Neuronal replacement from endogenous precursors in the adult brain after stroke. Nat Med 2002; 8: 963-970.

[80] Parent JM, Vexler ZS, Gong C, Derugin N, Ferriero DM. Rat forebrain neurogenesis and striatal neuron replacement after focal stroke. Ann Neurol 2002; 52: 802-813.

[81] Yamashita T, Ninomiya M, Hernandez AP. Subventricular zone-derived neuroblasts migrate and differentiate into mature neurons in the post-stroke adult striatum. J Neurosci 2006; 26: 6627-6636.

[82] Teramoto T, Qiu J, Plumier J-C, Moskowitz MA. EGF amplifies the replacement of parvalbumin-expressing striatal interneurons after ischemia. J Clin Invest 2003; 111: 1125-1132.

[83] Tsai PT, Ohab JJ, Kertesz N, *et al.* A critical role of erythropoietin receptor in neurogenesis and post-stroke recovery. J Neurosci 2006; 26: 1269-1274.

[84] De Marchis S, Fasolo A, Puche AC. Subventricular zone-derived neuronal progenitors migrate into the subcortical forebrain of postnatal mice. J Comp Neurol 2004; 476: 290-300.

[85] Jin K, Sun Y, Xie L, *et al.* Directed migration of neuronal precursors into the ischemic cerebral cortex and striatum. Mol Cell Neurosci 2003; 24: 171-189.

[86] Nakatomi H, Kuriu T, Okabe S, *et al.* Regeneration of hippocampal pyramidal neurons after ischemic brain injury. Cell 2002; 110: 429-441.

[87] Imitola J, Raddassi K, Park KI, *et al.* Directed migration of neural stem cells to sites of CNS injury by the stromal cell-derived factor 1{alpha}/CXC chemokine receptor 4 pathway. Proc Natl Acad Sci USA 2004; 101: 18117-18122.

[88] Lee SR, Kim HY, Rogowska J, *et al.* Involvement of matrix metalloproteinase in neuroblast cell migration from the subventricular zone after stroke. J Neurosci 2006; 26: 3491-3495.

[89] Nguyen-Ba-Charvet KT, Picard-Riera N, Tessier-Lavigne M, *et al.* Multiple roles for slits in the control of cell migration in the rostral migratory stream. J Neurosci 2004; 24: 1497-1506.

[90] Ohab JJ, Fleming S, Blesch A, Carmichael ST. A neurovascular niche for neurogenesis after stroke. J Neurosci 2006; 26: 13007-13016.

[91] Thored P, Wood J, Arvidsson A, Cammenga J, Kokaia Z, Lindvall O. Long-term neuroblast migration along blood vessels in an area with transient angiogenesis and increased vascularization after stroke. Stroke 2007; 38: 3032-3039.

[92] Brott T, Bogousslavsky J. Treatment of acute ischemic stroke. N Engl J Med 2000; 343: 710-722.

[93] Brivanlou AH, Gage FH, Jaenisch R, Jessell T, Melton D, Rossant J. Stem cells. Setting standards for human embryonic stem cells. Science 2003; 300: 913-916.

[94] Fricker RA, Carpenter MK, Winkler C, Greco C, Gates MA, Bjorklund A. Site-specific migration and neuronal differentiation of human neural progenitor cells after transplantation in the adult rat brain. J Neurosci 1999; 19: 5990-6005.

[95] Lindvall O, Kokaia Z. Stem cells for the treatment of neurological disorders. Nature 2006; 441: 1094-1096.

[96] Emsley JG, Mitchell BD, Magavi SS, Arlotta P, Macklis JD. The repair of complex neuronal circuitry by transplanted and endogenous precursors. NeuroRx 2004; 1: 452-471.

[97] Kerr DA, Llado J, Shamblott MJ, *et al.* Human embryonic germ cell derivatives facilitate motor recovery of rats with diffuse motor neuron injury. J Neurosci 2003; 23: 5131-5140.

[98] Klein S, Svendsen CN. Stem cells in the injured spinal cord: reducing the pain and increasing the gain. Nat Neurosci 2005; 8: 259-260.

Erythropoietin and Ischemic Brain Remodeling

Zheng Gang Zhang[1,*]**, Michael Chopp**[1,2]

[1]*Department of Neurology, Henry Ford Health Sciences Center, 2799 W. Grand Boulevard, Detroit, Michigan 48202;* [2]*Department of Physics, Oakland University, Rochester, Michigan 48309, USA;*

Address correspondence to: Dr. Zheng Gang Zhang, Department of Neurology, Henry Ford Hospital, 2799 West Grand Boulevard, Detroit, MI 48202, USA; Tel: 313-916-5456; Fax: 313-916-1318; Email: zhazh@neuro.hfh.edu

Abstract: Erythropoietin (EPO) is a hematopoietic cytokine and has the neuroprotective effect for treatment of acute ischemic stroke. Emerging data indicate that EPO also plays an important role in brain remodeling after stroke. This chapter reviews the effect of EPO on neurogenesis and angiogenesis and signaling pathways that mediate EPO-enhanced coupling of neurovascular niche in the ischemic brain.

1. INTRODUCTION

Erythropoietin (EPO) is a naturally occurring cytokine most widely recognized for its role in stimulating the maturation, differentiation and survival of hematopoietic progenitor cells [1,2]. However, EPO also plays a role in neuroprotection [3-5]. EPO mediates its biological effects through binding to its receptor, EPOR [1,5-8]. In the brain, neurons, glia and endothelial cells express EPO and EPOR [3,4]. Exogenous EPO penetrates the blood brain barrier (BBB) after systemic administration of recombinant human EPO (rhEPO) [4,9-13]. The neuroprotective effect of EPO for treatment of acute ischemic stroke has been extensively studied in experimental stroke [3-5].

Carbamylated EPO (CEPO) has been observed in patients suffering from end-stage renal disease [14,15]. CEPO does not show any binding to the classical EPOR *in vitro* or stimulate a hematopoietic response *in vivo*, but nevertheless has been shown to exert neuroprotective effects when administered following cerebral ischemia or other types of neuronal injury [12]. Although the specific cellular mechanisms responsible for the neuroprotective effect of CEPO, and the relationships between signaling pathways that mediate the beneficial effects of rhEPO and CEPO remain to be fully elucidated, the protective effects of CEPO may involve signaling through the common β receptor (CD 131) [16].

In addition to their neuroprotective effect, recent experimental studies show that EPO and CEPO regulate neurogenesis and angiogenesis in adult rodent brain during stroke recovery. This article reviews data on the effect of EPO and CEPO on neurogenesis and angiogenesis in ischemic brain. The reader is referred to excellent reviews of the neuroprotective effect of EPO on acute stroke [1,2,8].

2. NEUROGENESIS

In the adult rodent brain, neurogenesis occurs primarily in the subventricular zone (SVZ) of the lateral ventricle and in the subgranular zone (SGZ) of the dentate gyrus [17-20]. The SVZ contains migratory neuroblasts, actively proliferating progenitor cells and quiescent neural stem cells, which last for the life-time of the animal [21-25]. Neuroblasts in the SVZ travel the rostral migratory stream (RMS) to the olfactory bulb (OB) where they differentiate into interneurons [26-28]. Transient and permanent occlusion of the middle cerebral artery (MCA) results in increased neurogenesis in the ipsilateral SVZ, and neuroblasts in the SVZ migrate towards the ischemic boundary regions of the striatum and cortex, where they exhibit phenotypes of mature neurons [29-44]. Thus, ischemic brain generates new neurons to replenish damaged neurons [34,36,45]. Stroke-induced neurogenesis has also recently been demonstrated in the adult human brain, even in advanced age patients [46]. However, neurogenesis in response to stroke is limited and many newborn neurons die [34].

EPO/EPOR mediates neurogenesis in developing and adult brains [47-51]. During embryonic development, EPO and EPOR are highly expressed in the brain and EPOR knockout mice exhibit decreases of neuronal progenitor cells (50). In the adult brain, EPOR is expressed in the SVZ [47,48,51]. Incubation of neural progenitor cells isolated from the SVZ of the adult rodent with rhEPO substantially increases neuronal population [47]. Intraventricular infusion of rhEPO enhances neurogenesis in the SVZ, while blocking EPO by an EPO neutralizing antibody abolishes EPO-enhanced neurogenesis in the adult mouse [48]. Using different genetical manipulations, two groups independently demonstrate that knockout of brain *EPOR* substantially reduces neural progenitor cell proliferation in the SVZ of the adult mouse [51,52]. EPO/EPOR also regulates ischemia-increased neurogenesis [47,51,52]. Neural progenitor cells derived from the ischemic SVZ upregulate EPO gene expression and produce more neurons than the cells from the normal SVZ [47]. Application of an EPO neutralizing antibody suppress ischemia-increased neurons [47]. Conditional knockout of brain *EPOR* results in reduction of ischemia-increased neurogenesis in a model of cortical ischemia [51]. Intraperitoneal administration of rhEPO augments neurogenesis in the ischemic SVZ and striatal ischemic boundary of the adult rat when the treatment is initiated 24h after embolic MCA occlusion [47]. In postnatal rats, treatment of transient focal cerebral ischemia and hypoxia/ischemia with rhEPO also substantially increases neurogenesis [53,54]. Exogenous EPO increases the number of proliferating neuroblasts, identified by BrdU (a marker of proliferating cells), and doublecortin (DCX, a marker of neuroblasts) in the SVZ, but does not alter the number of apoptotic cells in the SVZ [47,53,54]. These data suggest that exogenous EPO further enhances neurogenesis in the ischemic brain.

In vitro study shows that CEPO, a well-characterized EPO derivative, enhances neurogenesis [55]. Incubation of SVZ neural progenitor cells derived from the adult mouse substantially increases neurons but not astrocytes [55]. In contrast to EPO, knockout of EPOR in neural progenitor cells does not abolish CEPO-increased neurogenesis [55]. These data suggest that EPOR is not required for the effect of CEPO on adult neural progenitor cells, although CEPO mediates neuroprotection in the CNS by binding to a heteroreceptor, consisting of the classical EPOR and the common β receptor (CD131) [16]. Studies on whether other receptors regulate the biological function of CEPO in neural progenitor cells are warranted.

3. COUPLING OF ANGIOGENESIS AND NEUROGENESIS

Angiogenesis is a multi step process involving endothelial cell proliferation, migration, tube formation, branching and anastomosis [56,57]. Vascular endothelial growth factor (VEGF) is a potent angiogenic factor and it reacts with the VEGF receptor 2 (VEGFR2) [58,59]. EPO stimulates migration and proliferation of endothelial cells derived from various organs including the brain [5,60]. Systemic administration of rhEPO substantially increases angiogenesis in the ischemic brain [47,53,61]. VEGF appears to regulate EPO-induced angiogenesis. Administration of rhEPO elevates brain VEGF levels, which are associated with angiogenesis in the ischemic brain [47]. Blocking VEGF by a specific VEGFR 2 antagonist suppresses EPO-induced capillary tube formation *in vitro* [47]. Knockout of *EPOR* results in reduction of VEGF and impairment of angiogenesis in response to hindlimb ischemia [62].

The vascular niche affects the neurogenic behavior of neural stem and progenitor cells [63-65]. Neurogenesis in the dentate gyrus is anatomically colocalized to endothelial precursors in the adult rat [64]. Endothelial cells promote the survival and differentiation of neuronal

precursors isolated from the rat SVZ *in vitro* [63,66]. Stroke-induced angiogenesis and neurogenesis are coupled [67,68]. Endothelial cells activated by ischemia promote neural progenitor cell differentiation into neurons, whereas blockage of angiogenesis reduces migration of neuroblasts in the SVZ to the ischemic boundary [67,68]. EPO-enhanced angiogenesis is coupled with neurogenesis in the ischemic brain [69,70]. Cerebral endothelial cells activated by rhEPO secrete active forms of matrix metalloproteinase 2 and 9 (MMP2 and MMP9), which promote neuroblast migration [69]. Application of MMP inhibitors abolishes the endothelial enhanced neuroblast migration [69]. On the other hand, EPO elevates VEGF levels in neural progenitor cells, which augments *in vitro* angiogenesis [69]. Blockage of VEGFR2 with a VEGFR2 antagonist or siRNA against VEGFR2 suppresses neural progenitor cell increased angiogenesis [69]. These data indicate that MMPs and VEGF likely mediate coupling of EPO-enhanced angiogenesis and neurogenesis.

4. THE PI3K/AKT AND ERk1/2 PATHWAYS

EPO interacts with its receptor, EPOR, and activates Janus tyrosine kinase 2 (JAK2), which initiates multiple signal transduction pathways including phosphatidylinositol 3-kinase/Akt (PI3K/Akt) and extracellular signal-regulated kinase (ERK1/2) pathways [2,7]. In neural progenitor cells, EPO first activates Akt and its substrate, GSK3α/ß and then activates ERK1/2 [70,71]. Blockage of the PI3K/Akt and ERK1/2 with pharmacological inhibitors suppresses EPO-phosphorylated Akt, GSK3α/ß and ERK1/2 and abrogates EPO-augmented neuronal population [70,71]. In addition, EPO activates the signal transducer and transcriptional activator STAT5 and induces NF-κB translocation in neural progenitor cells [48]. Blockage of NF-κB translocation abolishes the EPO-increased neuronal production [48]. The effect of NF-κB on neural progenitor cells does not involve the regulation of neural progenitor survival because the blockage of NF-κB translocation does not affect the number of apoptotic cells [48]. These data indicate that the PI3K/Akt, ERK1/2, and STAT5 pathways and NF-κB mediate EPO-induced neurogenesis. In cerebral endothelial cells, EPO also activates Akt and ERK1/2, while blockage of the PI3K/Akt or ERK1/2 pathways by pharmacological inhibitors abolished EPO-induced angiogenesis [47,69]. Thus, activation of the PI3K/Akt, ERK1/2, and STAT5 pathways could be signaling mechanisms underlying EPO-enhanced angiogenesis and neurogenesis.

5. PRO-NEURONAL BHLH TRANSCRIP-TION FACTORS, MASH1 AND NGN1

Mammalian achaete-scute homolog 1 (Mash1) and Neurogenin 1 (Ngn1) are pro-neuronal basic helix-loop-helix (bHLH) transcription factors and regulate neurogenesis [72-75]. EPO and CEPO upregulate Mash1 and Ngn1 expression in adult SVZ neural progenitor cells [48,55,71]. Attenuation of endogenous Mash1 and Ngn1 in neural progenitor cells with siRNA reduces CEPO- and EPO-increased neuronal population, respectively [55,71]. In addition, EPO upregulates suppressor of cytokine signaling (SOCS) 2, which induces neural progenitor cells to differentiate into neurons but not astrocytes [76]. Collectively, these data provide indication why administration of rhEPO and CEPO selectively increases the neuronal population but does not augment astrocytes [47,53-55,71,77].

6. THE SONIC HEDGEHOG (SHH) PATHWAY

Shh is a member of the hedgehog family proteins known to exert important regulatory functions in patterning and growth in a large number of tissues during embryogenesis [78-80]. In the mammalian brain, Shh has been shown to regulate progenitor cell proliferation and differentiation [80]. Shh binds to the transmembrane receptor protein, patched (Ptc) which, in the absence of Shh, exerts an inhibitory effect on the seven transmembrane receptor smoothened (Smo) [80]. Binding of Shh to Ptc blocks the inhibitory effect of Ptc on Smo. Once activated, Smo induces a complex series of intracellular reactions that targets the Gli family of transcription factors [80]. Gli1 is the principal effector of Shh signaling in neural progenitor cells [80]. Neural progenitor cells isolated from the SVZ of neonatal mice secrete Shh [81]. In the adult brain, Shh acts as a mitogen in cooperation with epidermal growth factor (EGF) to regulate proliferation of the neural stem cells in adult SVZ and the SGZ of the dentate gyrus [82]. Shh upregulates Mash1 expression in the adult neural progenitor cells [55]. The Shh pathway activated by CEPO mediates CEPO-induced neurogenesis [55]. Blockage of the Shh pathway with cyclopamine, a specific inhibitor of Smo, or siRNA against Gli1 suppresses CEPO-upregulated Mash1 expression and CEPO-increased neurogenesis [55]. Thus, the Shh pathway appears via Mash1 to promote neural progenitor cell differentiation into neurons [55].

7. CONCLUSIONS

EPO-enhanced angiogenesis and neurogenesis contribute to improvement of functional recovery [83-86]. Studies of signaling pathways provide insight into mechanisms of EPO- and CEPO-induced angiogenesis and neurogenesis.

8. ACKNOWLEDGMENTS

This work was supported by NIH grants RO1 NS38292, P50 NS23392, and PO1 NS42345.

9. REFERENCES

[1]   Maiese K, Li F, Chong ZZ. Erythropoietin in the brain: can the promise to protect be fulfilled? Trends Pharmacol Sci 2004; 25(11): 577-583.

[2]   Tonges L, Schlachetzki JC, Weishaupt JH, Bahr M. Hematopoietic cytokines--on the verge of conquering neurology. Curr Mol Med 2007; 7(2): 157-170.

[3]   Marti HH. Erythropoietin and the hypoxic brain. J Exp Biol 2004; 207(Pt 18): 3233-3242.

[4]   Grasso G, Sfacteria A, Cerami A, Brines M. Erythropoietin as a tissue-protective cytokine in brain injury: what do we know and where do we go? Neuroscientist 2004; 10(2): 93-98.

[5]   Ghezzi P, Brines M. Erythropoietin as an antiapoptotic, tissue-protective cytokine. Cell Death Differ 2004; 11 (Suppl 1): S37-44.

[6]   Wojchowski DM, Gregory RC, Miller CP, Pandit AK, Pircher TJ. Signal transduction in the erythropoietin receptor system. Exp Cell Res 1999; 253(1): 143-156.

[7]   Watowich SS. Activation of erythropoietin signaling by receptor dimerization. Int J Biochem Cell Biol 1999; 31(10): 1075-1088.

[8]   Maiese K, Li F, Chong ZZ. New avenues of exploration for erythropoietin. JAMA 2005; 293(1): 90-95.

[9]   Juul S. Erythropoietin in the central nervous system, and its use to prevent hypoxic-ischemic brain damage. Acta Paediatr Suppl 2002; 91(438): 36-42.

[10]   Brines ML, Ghezzi P, Keenan S, et al. Erythropoietin crosses the blood-brain barrier to protect against experimental brain injury. Proc Natl Acad Sci USA 2000; 97(19): 10526-10531.

[11]   Juul SE, McPherson RJ, Farrell FX, Jolliffe L, Ness DJ, Gleason CA. Erytropoietin concentrations in cerebrospinal fluid of nonhuman primates and fetal sheep following high-dose recombinant erythropoietin. Biol Neonate 2004; 85(2): 138-144.

[12]   Leist M, Ghezzi P, Grasso G, et al. Derivatives of erythropoietin that are tissue protective but not erythropoietic. Science 2004; 305(5681): 239-242.

[13]   Wang Y, Zhang ZG, Rhodes K, et al. Post-ischemic treatment with erythropoietin or carbamylated erythropoietin reduces infarction and improves neurological outcome in a rat model of focal cerebral ischemia. Br J Pharmacol 2007; 151(8): 1377-1384.

[14]   Park KD, Mun KC, Chang EJ, Park SB, Kim HC. Inhibition of erythropoietin activity by cyanate. Scand J Urol Nephrol 2004; 38(1): 69-72.

[15]   Mun KC, Golper TA. Impaired biological activity of erythropoietin by cyanate carbamylation. Blood Purif 2000; 18(1): 13-17.

[16]   Brines M, Grasso G, Fiordaliso F, et al. Erythropoietin mediates tissue protection through an erythropoietin and common beta-subunit heteroreceptor. Proc Natl Acad Sci U S A 2004; 101(41): 14907-14912.

[17]   Alvarez-Buylla A, Herrera DG, Wichterle H. The subventricular zone: source of neuronal precursors for brain repair. Prog Brain Res 2000; 127: 1-11.

[18]   Luskin MB, Zigova T, Soteres BJ, Stewart RR. Neuronal progenitor cells derived from the anterior subventricular zone of the neonatal rat forebrain continue to proliferate in vitro and express a neuronal phenotype. Mol Cell Neurosci 1997; 8(5): 351-366.

[19]   Gage FH, Ray J, Fisher LJ. Isolation, characterization, and use of stem cells from the CNS. Annu Rev Neurosci 1995; 18: 159-192.

[20]   Kirschenbaum B, Doetsch F, Lois C, Alvarez-Buylla A. Adult subventricular zone neuronal precursors continue to proliferate and migrate in the absence of the olfactory bulb. J Neurosci 1999; 19(6): 2171-2180.

[21]   Luskin MB. Restricted proliferation and migration of postnatally generated neurons derived from the forebrain subventricular zone. Neuron 1993; 11(1): 173-189.

[22]   Lois C, Alvarez-Buylla A. Long-distance neuronal migration in the adult mammalian brain. Science 1994; 264(5162): 1145-1148.

[23]   Morshead CM, Craig CG, van der Kooy D. In vivo clonal analyses reveal the properties of endogenous neural stem cell proliferation in the adult mammalian forebrain. Development 1998; 125(12): 2251-2261.

[24]   van der Kooy D, Weiss S. Why stem cells? Science 2000; 287(5457): 1439-1441.

[25]   Lois C, Alvarez-Buylla A. Proliferating subventricular zone cells in the adult mammalian forebrain can differentiate into neurons and glia. Proc Natl Acad Sci USA 1993; 90(5): 2074-2077.

[26]   Morshead CM, Reynolds BA, Craig CG, et al. Neural stem cells in the adult mammalian forebrain: a relatively quiescent subpopulation of subependymal cells. Neuron 1994; 13(5): 1071-1082.

[27]   Luskin MB. Neuroblasts of the postnatal mammalian forebrain: their phenotype and fate. J Neurobiol 1998; 36(2): 221-233.

[28]   Garcia-Verdugo JM, Doetsch F, Wichterle H, Lim DA, Alvarez-Buylla A. Architecture and cell types of the adult subventricular zone: in search of the stem cells. J Neurobiol 1998; 36(2): 234-248.

[29]   Zhang RL, Zhang ZG, Zhang L, Chopp M. Proliferation and differentiation of progenitor cells in the cortex and the subventricular zone in the adult rat after focal cerebral ischemia. Neuroscience 2001; 105(1): 33-41.

[30] Jin K, Minami M, Lan JQ, *et al.* Neurogenesis in dentate subgranular zone and rostral subventricular zone after focal cerebral ischemia in the rat. Proc Natl Acad Sci USA 2001; 98(8): 4710-4715.

[31] Yoshimura S, Takagi Y, Harada J, *et al.* FGF-2 regulation of neurogenesis in adult hippocampus after brain injury. Proc Natl Acad Sci USA 2001; 98(10): 5874-5879.

[32] Tonchev AB, Yamashima T, Zhao L, Okano HJ, Okano H. Proliferation of neural and neuronal progenitors after global brain ischemia in young adult macaque monkeys. Mol Cell Neurosci 2003; 23(2): 292-301.

[33] Parent JM, Vexler ZS, Gong C, Derugin N, Ferriero DM. Rat forebrain neurogenesis and striatal neuron replacement after focal stroke. Ann Neurol 2002; 52(6): 802-813.

[34] Arvidsson A, Collin T, Kirik D, Kokaia Z, Lindvall O. Neuronal replacement from endogenous precursors in the adult brain after stroke. Nat Med 2002; 8(9): 963-970.

[35] Liu J, Solway K, Messing RO, Sharp FR. Increased neurogenesis in the dentate gyrus after transient global ischemia in gerbils. J Neurosci 1998; 18(19): 7768-7778.

[36] Zhang R, Zhang Z, Wang L, *et al.* Activated neural stem cells contribute to stroke-induced neurogenesis and neuroblast migration toward the infarct boundary in adult rats. J Cereb Blood Flow Metab 2004; 24(4): 441-448.

[37] Iwai M, Sato K, Omori N, *et al.* Three steps of neural stem cells development in gerbil dentate gyrus after transient ischemia. J Cereb Blood Flow Metab 2002; 22(4): 411-419.

[38] Iwai M, Sato K, Kamada H, *et al.* Temporal profile of stem cell division, migration, and differentiation from subventricular zone to olfactory bulb after transient forebrain ischemia in gerbils. J Cereb Blood Flow Metab 2003; 23(3): 331-341.

[39] Schmidt W, Reymann KG. Proliferating cells differentiate into neurons in the hippocampal CA1 region of gerbils after global cerebral ischemia. Neurosci Lett 2002; 334(3): 153-156.

[40] Tanaka R, Yamashiro K, Mochizuki H, *et al.* Neurogenesis after transient global ischemia in the adult hippocampus visualized by improved retroviral vector. Stroke 2004; 35(6): 1454-1459.

[41] Kee NJ, Preston E, Wojtowicz JM. Enhanced neurogenesis after transient global ischemia in the dentate gyrus of the rat. Exp Brain Res 2001; 136(3): 313-320.

[42] Yagita Y, Kitagawa K, Ohtsuki T, *et al.* Neurogenesis by progenitor cells in the ischemic adult rat hippocampus. Stroke 2001; 32(8): 1890-1896.

[43] Zhu DY, Liu SH, Sun HS, Lu YM. Expression of inducible nitric oxide synthase after focal cerebral ischemia stimulates neurogenesis in the adult rodent dentate gyrus. J Neurosci 2003; 23(1): 223-229.

[44] Thored P, Arvidsson A, Cacci E, *et al.* Persistent production of neurons from adult brain stem cells during recovery after stroke. Stem Cells 2006; 24(3): 739-747.

[45] Jin K, Sun Y, Xie L, *et al.* Directed migration of neuronal precursors into the ischemic cerebral cortex and striatum. Mol Cell Neurosci 2003; 24(1): 171-189.

[46] Macas J, Nern C, Plate KH, Momma S. Increased generation of neuronal progenitors after ischemic injury in the aged adult human forebrain. J Neurosci 2006; 26(50): 13114-13119.

[47] Wang L, Zhang Z, Wang Y, Zhang R, Chopp M. Treatment of stroke with erythropoietin enhances neurogenesis and angiogenesis and improves neurological function in rats. Stroke 2004; 35(7): 1732-1737.

[48] Shingo T, Sorokan ST, Shimazaki T, Weiss S. Erythropoietin regulates the *in vitro* and *in vivo* production of neuronal progenitors by mammalian forebrain neural stem cells. J Neurosci 2001; 21(24): 9733-9743.

[49] Liu C, Shen K, Liu Z, Noguchi CT. Regulated human erythropoietin receptor expression in mouse brain. J Biol Chem 1997; 272(51): 32395-32400.

[50] Yu X, Shacka JJ, Eells JB, *et al.* Erythropoietin receptor signalling is required for normal brain development. Development 2002; 129(2): 505-516.

[51] Tsai PT, Ohab JJ, Kertesz N, *et al.* A critical role of erythropoietin receptor in neurogenesis and post-stroke recovery. J Neurosci 2006; 26(4): 1269-1274.

[52] Chen ZY, Asavaritikrai P, Prchal JT, Noguchi CT. Endogenous erythropoietin signaling is required for normal neural progenitor cell proliferation. J Biol Chem 2007; 282(35): 25875-25883.

[53] Iwai M, Cao G, Yin W, Stetler RA, Liu J, Chen J. Erythropoietin promotes neuronal replacement through revascularization and neurogenesis after neonatal hypoxia/ischemia in rats. Stroke 2007; 38(10): 2795-2803.

[54] Gonzalez FF, McQuillen P, Mu D, *et al.* Erythropoietin enhances long-term neuroprotection and neurogenesis in neonatal stroke. Dev Neurosci 2007; 29(4-5): 321-330.

[55] Wang L, Zhang ZG, Gregg SR, *et al.* The Sonic hedgehog pathway mediates carbamylated erythropoietin-enhanced proliferation and differentiation of adult neural progenitor cells. J Biol Chem 2007; 282(44): 32462-32470.

[56] Risau W. Mechanisms of angiogenesis. Nature 1997; 386(6626): 671-674.

[57] Carmeliet P. Mechanisms of angiogenesis and arteriogenesis. Nat Med 2000; 6(4): 389-395.

[58] Carmeliet P, Collen D. Molecular analysis of blood vessel formation and disease. Am J Physiol 1997; 273(5 Pt 2): H2091-2104.

[59] Risau W, Esser S, Engelhardt B. Differentiation of blood-brain barrier endothelial cells. Pathol Biol (Paris) 1998; 46(3): 171-175.

[60] Jaquet K, Krause K, Tawakol-Khodai M, Geidel S, Kuck KH. Erythropoietin and VEGF exhibit equal angiogenic potential. Microvasc Res 2002; 64(2): 326-333.

[61] Li Y, Lu Z, Keogh CL, Yu SP, Wei L. Erythropoietin-induced neurovascular protection, angiogenesis, and cerebral blood flow restoration after focal ischemia in mice. J Cereb Blood Flow Metab 2007; 27(5): 1043-1054.

[62] Nakano M, Satoh K, Fukumoto Y, *et al.* Important role of erythropoietin receptor to promote VEGF expression and angiogenesis in peripheral ischemia in mice. Circ Res 2007; 100(5): 662-669.

[63] Leventhal C, Rafii S, Rafii D, Shahar A, Goldman SA. Endothelial trophic support of neuronal production and recruitment from the adult mammalian subependyma. Mol Cell Neurosci 1999; 13(6): 450-464.

[64] Palmer TD, Willhoite AR, Gage FH. Vascular niche for adult hippocampal neurogenesis. J Comp Neurol 2000; 425(4): 479-494.

[65] Shen Q, Goderie SK, Jin L, *et al.* Endothelial cells stimulate self-renewal and expand neurogenesis of neural stem cells. Science 2004; 304(5675): 1338-1340.

[66] Louissaint A, Jr., Rao S, Leventhal C, Goldman SA. Coordinated interaction of neurogenesis and angiogenesis in the adult songbird brain. Neuron 2002; 34(6): 945-960.

[67] Teng H, Zhang ZG, Wang L, *et al.* Coupling of angiogenesis and neurogenesis in cultured endothelial cells and neural progenitor cells after stroke. J Cereb Blood Flow Metab 2008; 28(4): 764-771.

[68] Ohab JJ, Fleming S, Blesch A, Carmichael ST. A neurovascular niche for neurogenesis after stroke. J Neurosci 2006; 26(50): 13007-13016.

[69] Wang L, Zhang ZG, Zhang RL, *et al.* Matrix metalloproteinase 2 (MMP2) and MMP9 secreted by erythropoietin-activated endothelial cells promote neural progenitor cell migration. J Neurosci 2006; 26(22): 5996-6003.

[70] Wang L, Chopp M, Gregg SR, *et al.* Neural progenitor cells treated with EPO induce angiogenesis through the production of VEGF. J Cereb Blood Flow Metab 2008; 28(7): 1316-8.

[71] Wang L, Zhang ZG, Zhang RL, *et al.* Neurogenin 1 mediates erythropoietin enhanced differentiation of adult neural progenitor cells. J Cereb Blood Flow Metab 2006; 26(4): 556-564.

[72] Ross SE, Greenberg ME, Stiles CD. Basic helix-loop-helix factors in cortical development. Neuron 2003; 39(1): 13-25.

[73] Kageyama R, Ohtsuka T, Hatakeyama J, Ohsawa R. Roles of bHLH genes in neural stem cell differentiation. Exp Cell Res 2005; 306(2): 343-348.

[74] Parras CM, Galli R, Britz O, *et al.* Mash1 specifies neurons and oligodendrocytes in the postnatal brain. Embo J 2004; 23(22): 4495-4505.

[75] Casarosa S, Fode C, Guillemot F. Mash1 regulates neurogenesis in the ventral telencephalon. Development 1999; 126(3): 525-534.

[76] Turnley AM, Faux CH, Rietze RL, *et al.* Suppressor of cytokine signaling 2 regulates neuronal differentiation by inhibiting growth hormone signaling. Nat Neurosci 2002; 5(11): 1155-1162.

[77] Wang L, Zhang Z, Zhang R, *et al.* Erythropoietin up-regulates SOCS2 in neuronal progenitor cells derived from SVZ of adult rat. Neuroreport 2004; 15(8): 1225-1229.

[78] Cayuso J, Marti E. Morphogens in motion: growth control of the neural tube. J Neurobiol 2005; 64(4): 376-387.

[79] Stecca B, Ruiz i Altaba A. Brain as a paradigm of organ growth: Hedgehog-Gli signaling in neural stem cells and brain tumors. J Neurobiol 2005; 64(4): 476-490.

[80] Ruiz i Altaba A, Palma V, Dahmane N. Hedgehog-Gli signalling and the growth of the brain. Nat Rev Neurosci 2002; 3(1): 24-33.

[81] Rafuse VF, Soundararajan P, Leopold C, Robertson HA. Neuroprotective properties of cultured neural progenitor cells are associated with the production of sonic hedgehog. Neuroscience 2005; 131(4): 899-916.

[82] Palma V, Lim DA, Dahmane N, *et al.* Sonic hedgehog controls stem cell behavior in the postnatal and adult brain. Development 2005; 132(2): 335-344.

[83] Dewar D, Yam P, McCulloch J. Drug development for stroke: importance of protecting cerebral white matter. Eur J Pharmacol 1999; 375(1-3): 41-50.

[84] Kawamata T SE, Finklestein SP. The role of polypeptide growth factors in recovery from stroke. In: Freund HJ SB, and Witte OW, editor. Brain Plasticity. Philadephia: Lippincott-Raven; 1997. pp. 377-382.

[85] Pons TP. Reorganizing the brain [news]. Nat Med 1998; 4(5): 561-562.

[86] Cramer SC, Chopp M. Recovery recapitulates ontogeny. Trends Neurosci 2000; 23(6): 265-271.

94   *Experimental Stroke, 2008, 1,* 94-99

Potential MRI Methodologies and Treatment of Stroke

Quan Jiang

Departments of Neurology, Henry Ford Health Health Systerm, Detroit, Michigan, USA;
E-mail: QJIANG11@hfhs.org

Abstract: Magnetic resonance imaging (MRI) has shown great potential in early detection and characterization of stroke injury. MRI methodologies such as diffusion and perfusion MRI have been successfully applied to both experimental stroke and clinical studies, covering a broad range of questions raised in the early treatment of stroke. However, potential MRI methodologies related to critical issues in the treatment of stroke have not been well reviewed. In the current review, we present an overview of possible MRI methodologies addressing the critical issues related to treatment of stroke, including MRI measurements for predicting and detecting hemorrhagic transformation, as well as staging ischemic tissue.

INTRODUCTION

Stroke refers to a neurological deficit resulting from destruction of brain tissue in a patient with cerebrovascular disease. Following the onset of disease, it evolves markedly over the first few hours -- the so-called therapeutic window -- before entering a prolonged chronic phase [1-5]. To understand the spontaneous evolution and progression of the disease and evaluate the effect of therapeutic interventions, noninvasive imaging is imperative. While computed tomography (CT) is used most often for initial evaluation of stroke, magnetic resonance imaging (MRI) affords greater sensitivity and specificity for detection of an acute ischemic infarct and may help clarify the dynamics of the ongoing pathophysiological processes [1, 2, 6-11]. At the same time, CT scanners are available, lower in cost, more tolerant of patient motion, and superior in allowing access to critically ill patients during scanning. The primary role of CT has been detection of intraparenchymal or extra-axial hematomas that might require acute intervention and exclusion of non-stroke-related processes such as tumor or infection. The promise of early intervention shifts the emphasis toward imaging techniques that provide increased sensitivity and specificity for detection of ischemic injury. Diffusion weighted MRI (DWI) has shown the extreme sensitivity to detect acute cerebral ischemia within minutes after stroke onset [1, 12-15]. Since DWI was first described by Moseley *et al.* [12], it has become a major tool for detection of the ischemic territory and characterization of the acute and subacute development of the stroke process. Perfusion is another MRI technique that has played an important role in studies of stroke. Currently, DWI and perfusion weighted MRI (PWI) are broadly employed for diagnosis and management of stroke. The present review is not meant as an update of stroke diagnosis using MRI, which has been extensively reviewed [16, 17], but rather the application of new MRI methodologies to the critical issues related to treatment of stroke, including their potential for predicting and detecting hemorrhagic transformation as well as staging ischemic tissue.

MRI FOR PREDICTION AND DETECTION OF HEMORRHAGIC TRANSFORMATION

Hemorrhagic transformation (HT) of an ischemic brain is common in stroke patients, occurring in up to 70% of cases [18]. However, it has only been with the advent of sensitive imaging techniques, performed at prescribed times after stroke onset, that the true incidence of HT is becoming clear. Interest in HT after ischemic stroke has been heightened by the introduction of reperfusion strategies designed to remove the occluding clot and re-establish cerebral blood flow. All of the reperfusion strategies proven to be effective in improving functional outcome after ischemic stroke have been associated with an increased risk of HT, which is sometimes fatal [19-21]. Currently, diagnosis of hemorrhage is the domain of computed tomography (CT) rather than MRI, especially in acute stroke [22-24]. The pattern of evolution of hemorrhage described by CT is relatively simple, reflecting the protein content of the tissue at the bleeding site [25, 26], compared with the wealth of information including the stage of development that can be obtained with MRI [8, 27, 28]. HT evolves in several stages which are detectable by MRI, beginning with damage to the blood brain barrier (BBB) as evidenced by leakage of erythrocytes [29]. MRI can predict the site of hemorrhage by measuring the inverse of the apparent forward transfer rate (k_{inv}) for magnetization transfer (MT) and permeability of the BBB [8, 30, 31]. Fig. (1) represents contrast enhanced MRI (CEMRI) (Fig. **1A**), k_{inv} (Fig. **1B**), T_2 (Fig. **1C**), apparent diffusion coefficient of water (ADC_w, Fig. **1D**) and cerebral blood flow (CBF, Fig. **1E**), while the last image in Fig. **1A** is a histological section obtained 48 h after embolization from a rat treated with recombinant tissue plasminogen activator (rt-PA) at 4 h after embolization. The k_{inv} and CEMRI appear to be sensitive to HT soon after embolization.

Kunlin Jin / Guo-Yuan Yang (Eds.)

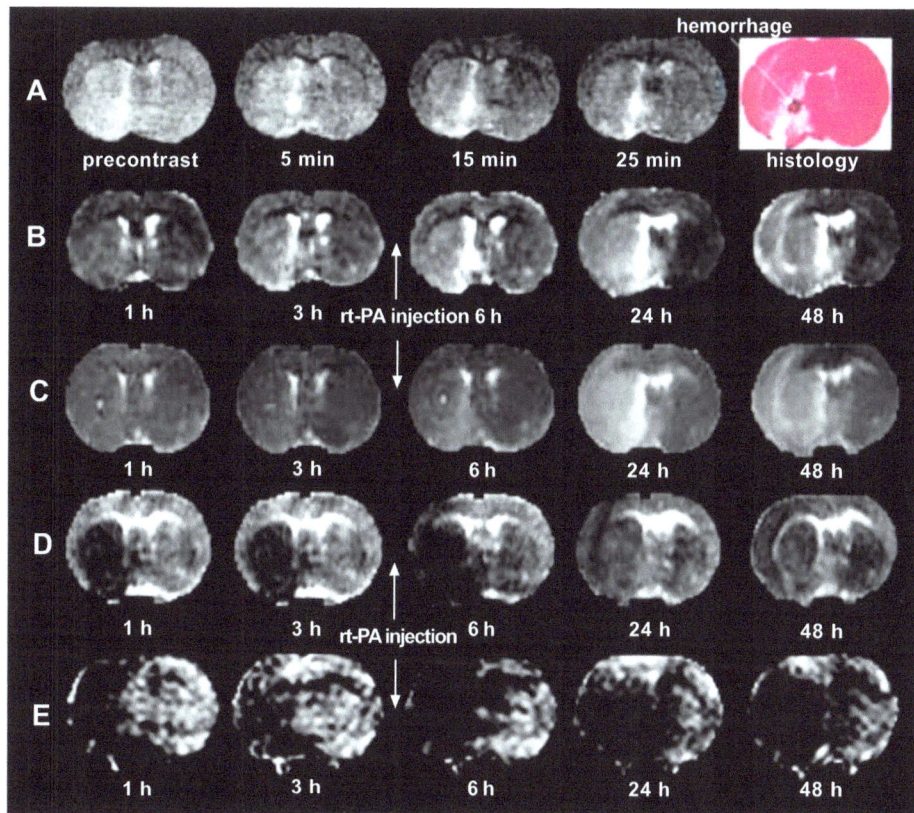

Fig. (1). Typical image set in detecting HT. **A**: Contrast enhanced T_1 weighted MR images, obtained before and after injection of a Gd-DTPA contrast agent at 3 h after rt-PA administration show the increasing contrast in a hyperintense area in the preoptic region. The corresponding histological section obtained at 48 h after embolization demonstrated gross hemorrhage in the left preoptic region. **B**: The temporal evolution of k_{inv} maps obtained at various times from 1 h to 48 h after embolization. k_{inv} maps revealed a small increase in k_{inv} in the area encompassing the territory supplied by the MCA and a large increase in the preoptic region where gross hemorrhage was confirmed by histology. **C**: The T_2 maps revealed a slow increase in T_2 after embolization in the area encompassing the territory supplied by the MCA and a large increase in preoptic region. Compared with the k_{inv} maps, the contrast in T_2 maps between the preoptic region and the rest of the ischemic region was lower and the T_2 maps were difficult to identify the true hemorrhagic region. **D** and **E**: ADC_w and CBF measurements revealed an early decrease both in ADC_w and CBF in the territory supplied by the MCA. However, both measurements do not distinguish the area with HT from the rest of the ischemic region.

Maps of k_{inv} detected HT not only at the delayed time points, but also as early as 3 h after embolization [8]. MT derives from the exchange of nuclear spin magnetization between "free" and "bound" protons and reflects proteolysis [32]. Severe damage to the BBB during the acute ischemic period may involve rapid loss of cellular structure through proteolysis and cause leakage of water and small proteins [8, 32, 33] thereby reducing the weight of the macromolecule pool and increasing k_{inv}.

Early Gd-DTPA enhancement during the acute stage of ischemic stroke appeared to be sensitive to HT. Based on histological analysis, Gd-DTPA enhancement in tissue liable to undergo HT is related to early endothelial cell damage with subsequent severe disruption of the BBB. Thus increases in BBB permeability to small molecules such as Gd-DTPA will pinpoint the regions at risk of HT. Early parenchymal enhancement has also been observed with the suture model of focal ischemia in rats [34], the embolic model in rabbits [35] and the catheter model in baboons [36]. Those studies, similar to ours, found that the enhanced area overestimated the extent of the hemorrhage seen at histology. A similar

overestimation was also observed on the k_{inv} maps and may be related to the disparate parameters measured by CEMRI, MT and histology. Gd-DTPA and water molecules are much smaller than erythrocytes and therefore can cross the BBB earlier and diffuse farther in the hemorrhagic region. Although the enhanced area did not predict the size of the eventual HT, it did distinguish ischemic areas with HT from nonhemorrhagic sites. Smaller molecular indicators may prove to be more efficient markers to predict HT, since it is known to evolve over a period of days or even weeks. Further investigation using indicators of different size is needed in order to adjust the sensitivity and accuracy of HT prediction.

Compared with the k_{inv} maps, the contrast in T_2 maps between the HT region and the rest of the ischemic tissue was lower when contrast infusion was slowly increased. The T_2 maps showed a larger hyperintense region, making it difficult to identify the true bleeding site. ADC_w and CBF could not distinguish HT from the surrounding ischemic region in cases of severe ischemic damage unless thrombolytic treatment was administered early [8].

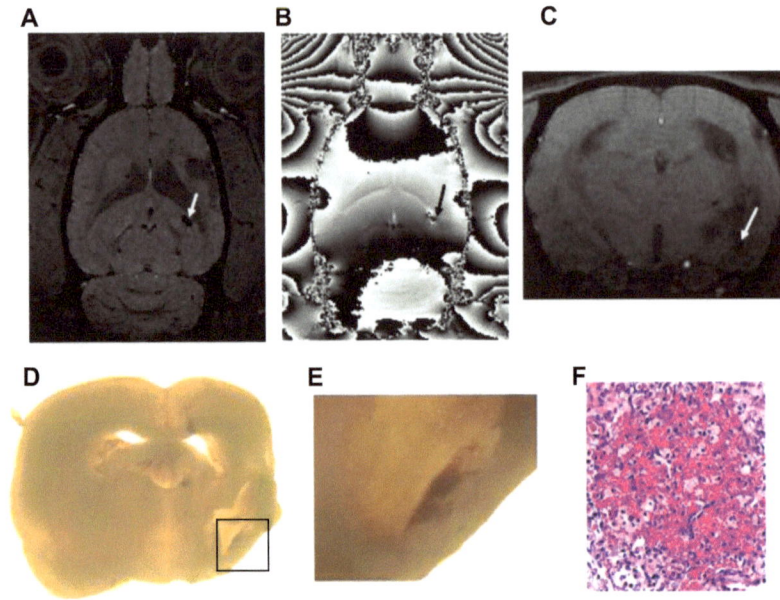

Fig. (2). SWI processed image (**A**), phase image (**B**), and gradient echo image (**C**) detected microhemorrhage (arrows, **A** to **C**). Hemorrhage appeared in the corresponding histological section (**D** and **E**) and confirmed by light microscopy (**F**).

The ability of MRI to sensitively detect and predict hemorrhage using a contrast agent and magnetization transfer may be related to early endothelial damage leading to increased ability of small molecules (*i.e.*, Gd-DTPA contrast agent or small proteins) to traverse the BBB [8]. However, CEMRI only provides indirect, parameter dependent information on increased permeability resulting from damage to the BBB. Quantitative permeability related MRI [30, 31] can provide intrinsic parameters about fibrin leakage after embolic stroke. Two permeability related MRI parameters, the transfer constant (K_i) and the distribution volume (V_p) of the mobile protons, showed greater sensitivity in predicting which areas of cerebral tissue might progress to fibrin leakage [30].

MRI can not only predict HT based on endothelial cell damage and ensuing severe disruption of the BBB but can also identify hemorrhage after it forms. This involves changes in the signal induced by magnetic susceptibility [27, 28]. During hemorrhage, hemoglobin gradually changes from the oxy-, deoxy- (ferrous) and met- (ferric) heme proteins found in erythrocytes to the iron (ferric) storage forms of ferritin and hemosiderin contained within phagocytes, based on the stage of hemorrhage [27]. Traditional MRI images based on T_1, T_2, proton density (PD), and gradient echo sequences exhibit different patterns of hemorrhage at different stages of development [37-40]. However, traditional MRI based on signal intensity is not as sensitive, especially during the hyperacute stage of hemorrhage [23, 24, 27]. The deoxy- and met- heme proteins in erythrocytes and the iron storage forms of ferritin and hemosiderin in phagocytes are paramagnetic molecules that cause signal loss (darkening) in images due to magnetic susceptibility, best seen on susceptibility-weighted $T_2{}^*$ images [27,

41]. Susceptibility weighted $T_2{}^*$ MRI is sensitive enough to detect hemorrhage even in the hyperacute stage [41, 42]. Recently, high resolution susceptibility weighted MRI incorporating phase information (SWI) has proved to be highly sensitive to hemorrhage, even microscopic bleeds [43, 44]. SWI uses fully velocity compensated, radio frequency spoiled, high resolution 3D gradient echo scans [43, 45]. Signals from substances with different susceptibilities (such as hemorrhage) will cause phase differences with adjacent tissues [43, 44]. Hemorrhage can be identified on the processed images, which combine magnitude and phase information to maximize the negative signal intensities of the regions containing degraded hemoglobin [43, 44]. Fig. (**2**) shows a coronal processed SWI image (**A**) with combined magnitude and phase information to maximize the negative signal intensities of the regions containing degraded hemoglobin [45]; phase image (**B**); axial gradient echo (GE) image (**C**); and the corresponding histological section (**D-F**) from a representative rat with 4 h of MCAo, obtained at 3 weeks after MCAo. The small hemorrhage (arrows in **A-C**) was more visible on the processed SWI compared to the traditional GE MRI. The histological section showed bleeding into the left dorsal endopiriform region (**D** and **E**). Light microscopy confirmed HT and microvascular plugging in the right dorsal endopiriform region (**F**).

Prediction and identification of HT before and during the hyperacute stage of hemorrhage is a critical issue related to acute management of stroke. Advances in MRI have improved its reliability for early prediction and identification of HT. Implementing these approaches in patients will provide new opportunities for better manage acute treatment of stroke.

MRI FOR STAGING ISCHEMIC TISSUE

Treatment of stroke is currently restricted to thrombolysis with rt-PA within a three-hour window after ictus [19], so that only a small portion of stroke patients can be treated [46]. This narrow window is derived from statistical data taken from clinical trials [19]. However, the therapeutic window for transformation from reversible to irreversible damage depends on many factors, including the extent of residual perfusion and the specific tissue affected. The treatment window could be greatly extended if reversible tissue damage could be accurately identified and therapy based on the individual patient rather than statistical data. MRI has shown great potential for identifying reversible ischemic damage, and CBF is the most sensitive MRI parameter. The normal range of CBF is 60 to 80 ml/100 g/min, and it could drop to 20-25 ml/100 g/min without loss of function; however, a CBF of 10-20 ml/100 g/min will result in loss of neuronal function although the brain structure is preserved (so-called ischemic penumbra) [47, 48]. The extent of damage also depends on the duration of ischemia, as ischemic damage to the penumbra is reversible if CBF is restored in time. The duration of ischemia and residual CBF are reflected by changes in other MRI measurable biophysical parameters, such as ADC_w, MTC and spin-spin relaxation or T_2. Diffusion weighted imaging (DWI) has shown promise in the early diagnosis of stroke [1, 12, 14, 15, 49-51]. The decline in ADC_w can be detected as soon as 3 min after ischemia [13]. During ischemia, energy depletion, intracellular water accumulation, and changes in cell membrane permeability [12-15, 50] have all been implicated as contributing to the changes in ADC_w. ADC_w is also sensitive to CBF [12, 52]; Busza *et al.* [52] have reported that the decrease in ADC_w is related to the threshold value of CBF. Therefore, in the acute ischemic phase a reduction in ADC_w may be related to a sharp decline in cerebral metabolic energy. Mintorovitch *et al.* [53] demonstrated a significant decline in Na^+, K^+-ATPase activity at 30 and 60 min after MCA occlusion. Threshold values of ADC_w acutely after MCA occlusion may predict which tissues will become reversibly or irreversibly damaged [1, 54, 55]. Hoehn-Berlage *et al.* [54] demonstrated that areas of ATP depletion corresponded to areas with CBF below 18 ± 14 ml/100 g-min. Areas of energy breakdown and tissue acidosis matched areas where ADC_w was reduced to $77 \pm 3\%$ of control 2 h after MCA occlusion in rats. Dardzinski *et al.* [55] showed that infarct area, as measured by TTC staining, correlated highly ($r = 0.89$, $p < 0.0001$) with an ischemic region giving ADC_w values below 0.55 x 10-3 mm^2/s 2 h after MCA occlusion in rats. Although ADC_w predicts cerebral ischemic cell damage, such a prediction is dependent on the time of measurement and duration of ischemia [1]. There is a significant correlation between ADC_w and cell damage 2 h after onset of ischemia and at specific early time points after reperfusion in a transient (2 h) MCA occlusion model in rats [1].

Thus the ability of a single ADC_w measurement to pinpoint the affected tissue and predict biological outcome appears to be linked to a narrow time window requiring precise knowledge of the onset of ischemia. Very early (< 10 minutes) after the onset of stroke, the ischemic damage is reversible, although ADC_w is below the threshold value. Also, using threshold values of ADC_w without including time as a variable will give erroneous information about the status of the tissue, particularly at later time points (such as > 24 h) after onset of ischemia, when ADC_w may appear normal in the ischemic core. Thus it is risky to categorize the process of ischemic changes from reversible to irreversible damage using ADC_w alone, without knowing the precise time of stroke onset.

In clinical practice, patients cannot be studied at the precise moment of stroke onset, nor over time, so that moment-to-moment shifts in ADC_w cannot be observed. Likewise ischemic lesions are highly heterogeneous and exhibit ADC_w values ranging from below to above normal [56]. It needs to establish MRI parameters that are independent of time and give comprehensive information about the histopathological status of the affected tissue at the time of study. Conventional T_2 weighted MRI provides information on vasogenic edema [57]. Elevated T_2 may identify vasogenic tissue and thereby provide complementary information along with ADC_w to distinguish reversible from irreversible tissue damage. T_2 and ADC_w exhibit different temporal profiles in the ischemic brain. ADC_w declines acutely after onset of ischemia, whereas T_2 exhibits a delayed increase compared to ADC_w [1, 58]. By noting that the dynamic shifts in ADC_w and T_2 differ with respect to each other, it may be possible to attribute tissue histopathology to characteristic MR signatures.

Characteristics of ischemic tissue have been evaluated using dual parameter MRI analysis [59, 60] in which ADC_w and T_2 maps were combined into a single image using cluster data. Different MRI signatures based on low, normal and high ADC_w and T_2 values were assigned to tissue histopathology, ranging from normal to pan-necrosis and cavitation [60]. Data from both permanently electrocoagulated and transient suture MCA occlusion models in rats have demonstrated that multimodal integrated MRI parameters can measure the degree of ischemic cell damage [60]. However, the original MRI tissue signature was a supervised model that required an operator to define a rectangular box on a scatter plot of T_2 versus ADC_w using the mean and standard deviation of normal tissue from T_2 and ADC_w maps [2], and the need for supervision to determine cluster centers proved to be a drawback. Fortunately, unsupervised segmentation techniques that minimize the need for human interaction have been developed. To get around the deficiencies of the original model, a novel vector signature methodology using an Iterative Self-Organizing Data Analysis Technique (ISODATA) have been developed for cluster segmentation [61] that is based on the angular separation between normal and abnormal tissue clusters and used this method to accurately classify normal and abnormal cerebral tissue in the experimental stroke [62-67]. The main advantage of the ISODATA method is that it automatically adjusts the number of clusters and thus does not require any initial training. The ISODATA method has proved to be promising for characterization of ischemic cell damage after stroke both in animals and stroke patients [62-67].

Currently, the most popular imaging method for acute stroke therapy is the mismatch concept using DWI and perfusion weighted MRI (PWI) measurements. This is a simplified approach, which assumes that the DWI reflects irreversibly damaged ischemic tissue and PWI reflects the complete area of hypoperfusion. The volume difference between DWI and PWI is also termed DWI/PWI mismatch. The abnormal region on DWI may not be irreversibly damaged totally as discussed above. More precise methods of staging ischemic damage using neuroimaging could provide valuable information in managing acute treatment of stroke.

ACKNOWLEDGMENTS

This work was supported by NIH grants RO1 NS48349, RO1 NS38292, RO1 NS43324, RO1 HL64766, PO1 NS23393, and PO1 NS42345.

REFERENCES

[1]   Jiang Q, Zhang ZG, Chopp M, *et al.* Temporal evolution and spatial distribution of the diffusion constant of water in rat brain after transient middle cerebral artery occlusion. J Neurol Sci 1993; 120(2): 123-30.

[2]   Jiang Q, Chopp M, Zhang ZG, *et al.* The temporal evolution of MRI tissue signatures after transient middle cerebral artery occlusion in rat. J Neurol Sci 1997; 145(1): 15-23.

[3]   Fisher M, Garcia JH. Evolving stroke and the ischemic penumbra. Neurology 1996; 47(4): 884-8.

[4]   Garcia JH, Lassen NA, Weiller C, Sperling B, Nakagawara J. Ischemic stroke and incomplete infarction. Stroke 1996; 27(4): 761-5.

[5]   Back T, Schuler OG. The natural course of lesion development in brain ischemia. Acta Neurochir Suppl 2004; 89: 55-61.

[6]   Jiang Q, Zhang RL, Zhang ZG, *et al.* Magnetic resonance imaging indexes of therapeutic efficacy of recombinant tissue plasminogen activator treatment of rat at 1 and 4 hours after embolic stroke. J Cereb Blood Flow Metab 2000; 20(1): 21-7.

[7]   Jiang Q, Ewing JR, Zhang ZG, *et al.* Magnetization transfer MRI: application to treatment of middle cerebral artery occlusion in rat. J Magn Reson Imaging 2001; 13(2): 178-84.

[8]   Jiang Q, Zhang RL, Zhang ZG, *et al.* Magnetic resonance imaging characterization of hemorrhagic transformation of embolic stroke in the rat. J Cereb Blood Flow Metab 2002; 22(5): 559-68.

[9]   Jiang Q, Zhang RL, Zhang ZG, *et al.* Quantitative Evaluation of BBB Permeability after Embolic Stroke Using MRI. Stroke 2004; 35(1): 333.

[10]   Jiang Q, Zhang ZG, Ding GL, *et al.* Pourabdollah Nejad D S, Athiraman H, Chopp M. Investigation of Neural Progenitor Cell Induced Angiogenesis after Embolic Stroke in Rat using MRI. Neuroimage 2005; 28(3): 698-707.

[11]   Jiang Q, Zhang ZG, Ding GL, *et al.* MRI detects white matter reorganization after neural progenitor cell treatment of stroke. Neuroimage 2006; 32(3): 1080-9.

[12]   Moseley ME, Cohen Y, Mintorovitch J, *et al.* Early detection of regional cerebral ischemia in cats: comparison of diffusion- and T2-weighted MRI and spectroscopy. Magn Reson Med 1990; 14(2): 330-46.

[13]   Davis D, Ulatowski J, Eleff S, *et al.* Rapid monitoring of changes in water diffusion coefficients during reversible ischemia in cat and rat brain. Magn Reson Med 1994; 31(4): 454-60.

[14]   Benveniste H, Hedlund LW, Johnson GA. Mechanism of detection of acute cerebral ischemia in rats by diffusion-weighted magnetic resonance microscopy. Stroke 1992; 23(5): 746-54.

[15]   Helpern J, Ordidge R, Knight R, Jiang Q. Mechanism and Predictive Value of The Decrease in Water Diffusion in Cerebral Ischemia. In: LeBihan D, Ed. Diffusion and Perfusion Magnetic Resonance Imaging Application to Functional MRI. 2nd ed. New York: Raven Press; 1995. p 173-80.

[16]   FIiebach JB, Schellinger PD, Sartor K, Heiland S, Warach S, Hacke W. Stroke MRI. Steinkopff Verlag Darmstadt: Springer; 2003.

[17]   Dijkhuizen RM, Nicolay K. Magnetic resonance imaging in experimental models of brain disorders. J Cereb Blood Flow Metab 2003; 23(12): 1383-1402.

[18]   Lodder J, Krijne-Kubat B, Broekman J. Cerebral hemorrhagic infarction at autopsy: cardiac embolic cause and the relationship to the cause of death. Stroke 1986; 17(4): 626-9.

[19]   NINDS. The National Institute of Neurological Disorders and Stroke rt-PA Stroke Study Group: Tissue plasminogen activator for acute ischemic stroke. N Engl J Med 1995; 333: 1581-7.

[20]   Furlan A, Higashida R, Wechsler L, *et al.* Intra-arterial prourokinase for acute ischemic stroke. The PROACT II study: a randomized controlled trial. Prolyse in Acute Cerebral Thromboembolism. JAMA 1999; 282(21): 2003-11.

[21]   Pessin MS, Teal PA, Caplan LR. Hemorrhagic infarction: guilt by association? AJNR Am J Neuroradiol 1991; 12(6): 1123-6.

[22]   Higashida RT, Furlan AJ. Trial design and reporting standards for intra-arterial cerebral thrombolysis for acute ischemic stroke. Stroke 2003; 34(8): e109-37.

[23]   Higer HP, Pedrosa P, Schaeben W, Bielke G, Meindl S. [Intracranial hemorrhage in MRT]. Radiologe 1989; 29(6): 297-302.

[24]   Jansen O, Heiland S, Schellinger P. [Neuroradiologic diagnosis in acute arterial cerebral infarct. Current status of new methods]. Nervenarzt 1998; 69(6): 465-71.

[25]   Enzmann DR, Britt RH, Lyons BE, Buxton JL, Wilson DA. Natural history of experimental intracerebral hemorrhage: sonography, computed tomography and neuropathology. AJNR Am J Neuroradiol 1981; 2(6): 517-26.

[26]   New P, Scott W. Blood. In: New P, Scott W, Eds. Computed Tomography of Brain and Orbit (EMI Scanning). Baltimore: William & Wilkins; 1975.

[27]   Atlas S, Thulborn K. Intracranial Hemorrhage. In: SW A, editor. Magnetic Resonance Imaging of the Brain and Spine. Volume 1. Philadelphia: Lippincott-Raven Publishers; 2002. pp. 773-832.

[28]   Thulborn K, Brady T. Biochemical basis of the MR appearance of cerebral hemorrhage. 1996; Vol 8; pp. 255-68.

[29]   Hamann GF, Okada Y, del Zoppo GJ. Hemorrhagic transformation and microvascular integrity during focal cerebral ischemia/reperfusion. J Cereb Blood Flow Metab 1996; 16(6): 1373-8.

[30]   Jiang Q, Ewing JR, Ding GL, *et al.* Quantitative evaluation of BBB permeability after embolic stroke in rat using MRI. J Cereb Blood Flow Metab 2005; 25(5): 583-92.

[31] Ewing JR, Knight RA, Nagaraja TN, *et al.* Fenstermacher J. Patlak plots of Gd-DTPA MRI data yield blood-brain transfer constants concordant with those of 14C-sucrose in areas of blood-brain opening. Magn Reson Med 2003; 50(2): 283-92.

[32] Neumar RW, Hagle SM, DeGracia DJ, Krause GS, White BC. Brain m-calpain autolysis during global cerebral ischemia. J Neurochemistry 1996; 66: 421-4.

[33] Ewing JR, Jiang Q, Boska M, *et al.* T1 and magnetization transfer at 7 Tesla in acute ischemic infarct in the rat. Magn Reson Med 1999; 41(4): 696-705.

[34] Knight RA, Barker PB, Fagan SC, Li Y, Jacobs MA, Welch KM. Prediction of impending hemorrhagic transformation in ischemic stroke using magnetic resonance imaging in rats. Stroke 1998; 29(1): 144-51.

[35] Yenari M, de Crespigny A, Palmer J, *et al.* Improved perfusion with rt-PA and hirulog in a rabbit model of embolic stroke. J Cereb Blood Flow Metab 1997; 17(4): 401-11.

[36] Mathews VP, Monsein LH, Pardo CA, Bryan RN. Histologic abnormalities associated with gadolinium enhancement on MR in the initial hours of experimental cerebral infarction. Am J Neuroradiol 1994; 15(3): 3-579.

[37] Hayman LA, Taber KH, Ford JJ, Bryan RN. Mechanisms of MR signal alteration by acute intracerebral blood: old concepts and new theories. AJNR Am J Neuroradiol 1991; 12(5): 899-907.

[38] Hayman LA, Pagani JJ, Kirkpatrick JB, Hinck VC. Pathophysiology of acute intracerebral and subarachnoid hemorrhage: applications to MR imaging. AJR Am J Roentgenol 1989; 153(1): 135-9.

[39] Weingarten K, Zimmerman RD, Cahill PT, Deck MD. Detection of acute intracerebral hemorrhage on MR imaging: ineffectiveness of prolonged interecho interval pulse sequences. AJNR Am J Neuroradiol 1991; 12(3): 475-9.

[40] Bradley WG, Jr. MR appearance of hemorrhage in the brain. Radiology 1993; 189(1): 15-26.

[41] Patel MR, Edelman RR, Warach S. Detection of hyperacute primary intraparenchymal hemorrhage by magnetic resonance imaging. Stroke 1996; 27(12): 2321-4.

[42] Linfante I, Llinas RH, Caplan LR, Warach S. MRI features of intracerebral hemorrhage within 2 hours from symptom onset. Stroke 1999; 30(11): 2263-7.

[43] Ding G, Jiang Q, Li L, *et al.* Angiogenesis detected after embolic stroke in rat brain using magnetic resonance T2*WI. Stroke 2008; 39(5): 1563-8.

[44] Tong KA, Ashwal S, Holshouser BA, *et al.* Hemorrhagic shearing lesions in children and adolescents with posttraumatic diffuse axonal injury: improved detection and initial results. Radiology 2003; 227(2): 332-9.

[45] Sehgal V, Delproposto Z, Haacke EM, *et al.* Clinical applications of neuroimaging with susceptibility-weighted imaging. J Magn Reson Imaging 2005; 22(4): 439-50.

[46] O'Connor RE, McGraw P, Edelsohn L. Thrombolytic therapy for acute ischemic stroke: why the majority of patients remain ineligible for treatment. Ann Emerg Med 1999; 33(1): 9-14.

[47] Ginsberg MD, Pulsinelli WA. The ischemic penumbra, injury thresholds, and the therapeutic window for acute stroke. Ann Neurol 1994; 36(4): 553-4.

[48] Reith W, Hasegawa Y, Latour LL, Dardzinski BJ, Sotak CH, Fisher M. Multislice diffusion mapping for 3-D evolution of cerebral ischemia in a rat stroke model. Neurology 1995; 45(1): 172-7.

[49] Helpern JA, Dereski MO, Knight RA, Ordidge RJ, Chopp M, Qing ZX. Histopathological correlations of nuclear magnetic resonance imaging parameters in experimental cerebral ischemia. Magn Reson Imaging 1993; 11(2): 241-6.

[50] Moonen CT, Pekar J, de Vleeschouwer MH, van Gelderen P, van Zijl PC, DesPres D. Restricted and anisotropic displacement of water in healthy cat brain and in stroke

studied by NMR diffusion imaging. Magn Reson Med 1991; 19(2): 327-32.

[51] Minematsu K, Li L, Sotak CH, Davis MA, Fisher M. Reversible focal ischemic injury demonstrated by diffusion-weighted magnetic resonance imaging in rats. Stroke 1992; 23(9): 1304-1310; discussion 1310-01.

[52] Busza AL, Allen KL, King MD, van Bruggen N, Williams SR, Gadian DG. Diffusion-weighted imaging studies of cerebral ischemia in gerbils. Potential relevance to energy failure. Stroke 1992; 23(11): 1602-12.

[53] Mintorovitch J, Yang GY, Shimizu H, Kucharczyk J, Chan PH, Weinstein PR. Diffusion-weighted magnetic resonance imaging of acute focal cerebral ischemia: comparison of signal intensity with changes in brain water and Na+,K(+)-ATPase activity. J Cereb Blood Flow Metab 1994; 14(2): 332-6.

[54] Hoehn-Berlage M, Eis M, Back T, Kohno K, Yamashita K. Changes of relaxation times (T1, T2) and apparent diffusion coefficient after permanent middle cerebral artery occlusion in the rat: temporal evolution, regional extent, and comparison with histology. Magn Reson Med 1995; 34(6): 824-834.

[55] Dardzinski BJ, Sotak CH, Fisher M, Hasegawa Y, Li L, Minematsu K. Apparent diffusion coefficient mapping of experimental focal cerebral ischemia using diffusion-weighted echo-planar imaging. Magn Reson Med 1993; 30(3): 318-25.

[56] Nagesh V, Welch KM, Windham JP, *et al.* Time course of ADCw changes in ischemic stroke: beyond the human eye. Stroke 1998; 29(9): 1778-82.

[57] Hoehn-Berlage M, Tolxdorff T, Bockhorst K, Okada Y, Ernestus RI. *In vivo* NMR T2 relaxation of experimental brain tumors in the cat: a multiparameter tissue characterization. Magn Reson Imaging 1992; 10(6): 935-47.

[58] Knight RA, Ordidge RJ, Helpern JA, Chopp M, Rodolosi LC, Peck D. Temporal evolution of ischemic damage in rat brain measured by proton nuclear magnetic resonance imaging. Stroke 1991; 22(6): 802-8.

[59] Welch KM, Windham J, Knight RA, *et al.* A model to predict the histopathology of human stroke using diffusion and T2-weighted magnetic resonance imaging [see comments]. Stroke 1995; 26(11): 1983-9.

[60] Jiang Q, Chopp M, Zhang ZG, *et al.* The temporal evolution of MRI tissue signatures after transient middle cerebral artery occlusion in rat. J Neurol Sci 1997; 145(1): 15-23.

[61] Ball GH, Hall DJ. A clustering technique for summarizing multivariate data. Behav Sci 1967; 12(2): 153-5.

[62] Jacobs MA, Knight RA, Soltanian-Zadeh H, *et al.* Unsupervised segmentation of multiparameter MRI in experimental cerebral ischemia with comparison to T2, diffusion, and ADC MRI parameters and histopathological validation. J Magn Reson Imaging 2000; 11(4): 425-37.

[63] Jacobs MA, Mitsias P, Soltanian-Zadeh H, *et al.* Multiparametric MRI tissue characterization in clinical stroke with correlation to clinical outcome: part 2. Stroke 2001; 32(4): 950-7.

[64] Jacobs MA, Zhang ZG, Knight RA, *et al.* A model for multiparametric mri tissue characterization in experimental cerebral ischemia with histological validation in rat: part 1. Stroke 2001; 32(4): 943-9.

[65] Soltanian-Zadeh H, Pasnoor M, Hammoud R, *et al.* MRI tissue characterization of experimental cerebral ischemia in rat. J Magn Reson Imaging 2003; 17(4): 398-409.

[66] Ding G, Jiang Q, Zhang L, *et al.* Multiparametric ISODATA analysis of embolic stroke and rt-PA intervention in rat. J Neurol Sci 2004; 223(2): 135-43.

[67] Li L, Jiang Q, Ding G, *et al.* Map-ISODATA demarcates regional response to combination rt-PA and 7E3 F(ab')2 treatment of embolic stroke in the rat. J Magn Reson Imaging 2005; 21(6): 726-34.

The Use of a Global Statistical Approach for the Design and Data Analysis of Clinical Trials with Multiple Primary Outcomes

Peng Huang[1,*], Robert F. Woolson[2] and Ann-Charlotte Granholm[3]

[1]*Division of Oncology Biostatistics, The Sidney Kimmel Comprehensive Cancer Center, School of Medicine, Johns Hopkins University, 550 North Broadway, Suite 1103, Baltimore, Maryland 21205-2013, USA; E-mail: phuang12@jhmi.edu*

[2]*Department of Biostatistics, Bioinformatics, and Epidemiology, Medical University of South Carolina, USA*

[3]*Department of Neurosciences and the Center on Aging, Medical University of South Carolina, USA*

Abstract: Determining whether one treatment is preferred over others is a major goal of many clinical studies but can be complicated by the situation when no single outcome is sufficient to make the judgment. We present a useful global statistical test technique and the corresponding global treatment effect (GTE) measure for assessing treatment's global preference when multiple outcomes are evaluated together. Applications of these techniques in clinical trial design and data analysis are illustrated.

INTRODUCTION

Many clinical studies seek to determine whether a treatment is beneficial and preferable to other options. Establishing the relative benefit of a treatment involves, in some cases, the easy task of identifying a single most important primary outcome. For many other diseases, however, a single outcome is not sufficient to determine whether a treatment is beneficial, or the single most relevant clinical outcome is difficult, if not impossible, to measure. In this case, several outcomes are used jointly to evaluate a treatment's global benefit. In the TOAST acute ischemic stroke trial [1, 2], for example, subjects' post-treatment functional and neurological conditions were measured via NIH Stroke Scale, Glasgow Outcome Scale, Barthel Index, and motor examination score to evaluate whether subjects receiving a heparinoid had better global clinical outcomes than subjects receiving placebo. Reflecting similar complexity, a trial assessing the safety and efficacy of minocycline in the treatment of rheumatoid arthritis [3] included multiple scale evaluations of 60 diarthrodial joints for tenderness and 58 joints for swelling. When comparing the long-term ability of treatments to retard Parkinson's disease (PD) progression, a single outcome is not sufficient to determine whether a treatment is beneficial. While the Unified Parkinson's Disease Rating Scale (UPDRS) has been widely used in clinical trials, it does not capture all dimensions of disease progression. In addition to the UPDRS, PD clinical trials have incorporated a battery of other outcome measures to assess functional and non-motor aspects of PD decline. These measures have included ratings of global clinical impression, quality of life, motor fluctuations, dyskinesias, depression, cognition, and hallucinations.

In these examples, the use of multiple primary outcomes in clinical trial design and data analysis imposes some significant statistical challenges. First, it is generally unrealistic to specify the joint distribution of multiple outcomes. Second, since different outcomes may be measured in different scales, e.g. continuous, ordered categorical, and it can be difficult to summarize a treatment's global effect across all outcomes. Third, conventional statistical models and software are typically readily available only to compare mean outcome differences. These approaches lack robustness in statistical inference when data have skewed distributions: results observed in one trial may not be repeatable in another trial. Fourth, restrictive assumptions are often added to statistical models for mathematical or computational convenience instead of considering whether they are appropriate to the scientific question under investigation. As pointed out by O'Brien and Geller [4], although many multivariate statistical techniques have been proposed to analyze several outcomes simultaneously, many of them were proposed with a focus on the complex theoretical properties themselves. Insufficient attention has been devoted to careful specification of the medical questions that the proposed and theoretical statistical analysis is intended to address. As a result, analytic procedures are often inappropriately matched to medical questions.

In response to this challenge, O'Brien [5] first introduced a novel and effective *global statistical test* (GST) technique for treatment comparisons to answer a clinical question as "Should we give this treatment to patients?" when no single outcome is sufficient to answer this question. Because a GST is a single multivariate test, it does not require multiple univariate tests to determine a treatment's global benefit. Therefore, there is no penalty vis-a-vis type I error inflation. The major feature of a GST is that it often has a higher power than univariate tests when a treatment shows a consistent and persuasive improvement across all outcomes [6]. For example, in a NINDS t-PA stroke trial [7], t-PA improved all 4 primary outcomes (the Barthel Index, Modified Rankin Scale, Glasgow Outcome Scale, and National Institutes of Health Stroke Scale) with unadjusted univariate p-values of 0.026, 0.019, 0.025, and 0.033 respectively. None of these outcomes was considered significant at alpha=0.05 level after Bonferroni adjustment. However, a GST [8] gives a p-value of 0.008, demonstrating a strong evidence of global treatment benefit. On the other hand, if a treatment shows both strong beneficial and strong harmful effects on different outcomes, the GST will have limited power to identify a treatment benefit. Clinicians are less enthusiastic to recommend such treatment to patients in this circumstance.

This paper is an exposition of how one can apply GST in statistical design and data analysis when multiple primary outcomes are assessed simultaneously to determine whether one treatment should be recommended for use. More specifically, we give detailed step-by-step procedures addressing how to define a treatment's global effect; how to test this global effect at the end of data collection; and how to compute sample size when the GST is to be used to test this global effect. One clinical trial example is used to illustrate how to compute sample size, and two other clinical trial examples are used to illustrate the differences between the GST and commonly used Bonferroni adjustment and Hotelling's T^2 test for multiple outcomes. A summary of various multivariate techniques is given in the discussion section. We focus throughout on the two-sample problem of comparing a single treatment group to a control (or placebo).

Measurement of global treatment effect – the GTE

In many clinical studies, treatment difference on a single outcome is often measured through the standardized mean difference, i.e., the effect size, defined as the ratio, $\Delta\mu/\sigma$, of mean treatment difference ($\Delta\mu$) and the common (or pooled) standard deviation of the two treatment groups. While it is a common sense that the use of effect size requires that mean difference is a meaningful measure of change, this fundamental assumption is often ignored in applications, particularly when data have a skewed distribution. A mean is easily influenced by outlying observations, and, in fact, one outlying observation is enough to completely change conclusions. Acion *et al.* [9] gave an example of comparing the change in global function score from baseline to 6 months between a cognitive behavior therapy group and a standard therapy group. Although all patients in cognitive behavior therapy group had improved their global functional score while all patients except one in

standard therapy group became much worse, the new therapy was not considered beneficial by the effect size based t-test approach due to the measure from one patient in the standard therapy group whose measure has substantially reduced the estimate of treatment effect size. Besides, confusions can arise when outcomes are not measured on a continuous or linear scale. For example, Glasgow Outcome Scale is measured in the following ordinal scale:

> 1=dead, 2=vegetative state, 3=severe disability, 4=moderate disability, 5=good recovery.

Suppose a study reports that a new treatment can increase the mean Glasgow Outcome Scale from 3.9 in placebo to 3.6 with common standard deviation 0.2. This gives effect size of 1.5. Such information would be difficult for a patient to interpret. For instance, if her Glasgow Outcome Scale is 3, how much would she benefit from the new treatment? After all, no one is measured at 3.6 or 3.9. More seriously, for the same data, different effect sizes can be claimed if different people code the same data in different ways or different nonlinear monotone transformations are applied to the data. This can make the interpretation of treatment effect subjective and inconsistent among investigators. As a hypothetical example, suppose a study is testing whether a new treatment is helpful in reducing pain. One hundred patients are recruited with half of them randomized to receive the new treatment and the other half randomized to placebo. The following table gives responses from these 100 patients at the end of the study:

Group	Disabling	Severe	Moderate	Mild	None
Treatment	0	16	12	13	9
Placebo	6	10	17	15	2

Suppose two investigators analyzed these data separately. The first person coded the observations in linear scale as 0=disabling, 1=severe, 2=moderate, 3=mild, and 4=none. He obtained the estimated effect size of 0.326 and his two sample t-test gives a two-sided p value 0.103. He thus concluded that the treatment is not helpful in reducing pain. The second person did not think that the pain scale is linear. She thinks the differences between disabling and severe and between mild and none are greater than the differences between severe and moderate and between moderate and mild. She thus coded observations as 0=disabling, 4=severe, 5=moderate, 6=mild, and 10=none. She estimated an effect size of 0.522 and her two sample t-test gives a two-sided p value 0.008. Thus, she concluded that the treatment is helpful in reducing pain. Such inconsistent conclusions on treatment efficacy effect between the two investigators were due entirely to the different coding of the same data. This led to different estimates of a treatment's effect. Such illustrations highlight the difficulties in attempting to apply a continuous scale to ordered categorical data. Other approaches may be more robust as we shall see.

The limitation discussed above is mainly a consequence of the effect size's lack of invariance and lack of robustness to the measurement scales. Several authors [9, 10] proposed to use a scale-free measure, the probability of improvement, as a unified measure of treatment difference. This measure, denoted as p, is the same parameter used in the traditional Mann-Whitney-Wilcoxon test. For example, a treatment's effect is described using statement like "a patient's outcome will improve by 70% of the time if he/she switches from treatment A to treatment B". The advantage of using such measure has been outlined in Wolfe and Hogg [10] and Acion *et al.* [9]. For example, for data in preceding table, no matter how investigators code the data, there is a p=46% chance that the treatment is better than control, a q=31% chance the control is better than the treatment, and a s=23% chance that two groups yield the same results. Obviously, we must have p+q+s =100%. Further-more, p=46% alone is not sufficient to quantify a treatment beneficial effect: if the probability to yield tied observations were zero (s=0), then we would have had q=1-p=54%, implying that control group is better than the treatment group. If the probability to yield tied observations was s=50%, then q=1-46%-50%=4%, implying that treatment is much better than the control. Because of this potential for tied observations, Huang, Woolson, and O'Brien [11] suggested use the difference θ = (p-q) as a measure of treatment benefit. When there are multiple outcomes, compute such θ for each outcome and then take an average $\overline{\theta}$ of these θ values. This $\overline{\theta}$ value, called the *global treatment effect* (GTE) in Huang, Woolson, and O'Brien [11], provides a single measure of a treatment's global effect on multiple outcomes when all outcomes are considered equally important. If it is commonly accepted that some outcomes are more important than others, then the GTE can be defined as a weighted average of those θs. To simplify our discussion, we focus on the case when all outcomes are equally weighted, but the reader should keep the weighted generalization in mind.

There are a number of advantages in using GTE to measure a treatment's benefit rather than the use of the mean treatment difference or the effect size. First, treatment effect can be reported more objectively. This avoids inconsistent conclusions of treatment benefit as shown in the above ordered categorical data example. Second, the scientific conclusion is more robust or repeatable since one does not need to make unnecessary mathematical assumptions. Furthermore, the estimation of treatment effect is less affected by outliers compared to other scale-dependent measures such as outcome means. Third, the GTE makes it easy to combine treatment effects across different types of outcomes. This is a crucial advantage since different scales used by different outcomes can make it difficult

to summarize a treatment's global effect even when all outcomes are standardized. For example, consider the case when we are testing whether a treatment is preferred over a control therapy to treat acute ischemic stroke based on two outcomes: one is a binary indicator of the occurrence of Glasgow Outcome Scale of I (good recovery), and the other one is a continuous Modified Barthel Index score. If the treatment improves the binary indicator of Glasgow Outcome Scale I occurrence by an odds ratio of 1.5 and worsens the Modified Barthel Index score by 1.5 standard deviation (effect size), one would find it difficult to summarize the preference of this treatment because it is difficult to interpret a combination of odds ratio and an effect size. In contrast, GTE uses θ = (p-q), the difference between the probability that the treatment is better than the control and the probability that the control is better than the treatment, to quantify a treatment's global effect on both outcomes. Because θs for each outcome have the same interpretation, i.e., the probability of better outcome, we can easily combine them and still provide a sound scientific interpretation to this combination. In addition, it is easier to explain treatment effect using GTE to patients: the GTE tells a patient the probability that his clinical outcomes will be improved if he switches from the control to the treatment. If instead, both the effect size and odds ratio are used to interpret a treatment's effect, patients may find it confusing. GTE provides a direct and more relevant appraisal of treatment benefit to a patient.

Another major strength in the use of GTE is that it is easier for investigators to explicate specific hypotheses for sample size computation. The magnitude of treatment effect specified by the alternative hypothesis is used to control the statistical power. It is crucial to determine what will be an appropriate value for the alternative hypothesis when designing a future study. If this value is too close to the null hypothesized value, it can result in unnecessarily large sample size, as well as trial cost, and yet the trivial difference claimed by the study may not be clinically significant. If this value is too far away from the null hypothesized value, the trial may end up with low power to detect smaller, but important changes. Investigators often use information from literature or pilot studies as reference when determining this alternative hypothesis value. There are danders in this. The strong mathematical assumptions made regarding the association between past data and future data can easily be violated. For example, the effect size approach often assumes that the treatment effect sizes and variances of outcomes in the pilot study and the future study are essentially the same. This may not be true due to fundamental differences in how the pilot and full studies are conducted, to the improvement of the medical care system, or to alternations in clinical practice. The GTE approach does not require such restrictive assumptions, thus making the information transition from the pilot study to the actual study more robust and reproducible than the traditional effect size approach. In the next section, we briefly describe how to use this GTE approach to help investigators to determine an appropriate value $\bar{\theta} = \bar{\theta}_a$ for the alternative hypothesis.

Determination of the alternative hypothesis global treatment effect $\bar{\theta}_a$ for power and sample size development

A GTE $\bar{\theta}$ takes value between -1 and 1 with $\bar{\theta} = 0$ implying no global treatment benefit, $\bar{\theta} = 1$ implying the treatment is preferred, and $\bar{\theta} = -1$ implying the control is preferred. Larger positive $\bar{\theta}$ value corresponds to higher treatment preference. The alternative hypothesis generally specifies a clinically meaningful value $\bar{\theta}_a$ of $\bar{\theta}$ where the statistical power is to be controlled. In general, $\bar{\theta}_a$ should be chosen based on a series of different considerations including scientific rationale, budget and time constraints, as well as information from pilot data and other related studies. Here we describe how to compute $\bar{\theta}$ from pilot data (if they are available) or summary statistics from the literature (if no pilot data are available) using formulas previously published by Huang, Woolson, and O'Brien [11]. A $\bar{\theta}_a$ value can be derived by incorporating information from this $\bar{\theta}$ value.

Since $\bar{\theta}$ is the average of θ values from individual outcomes, one only need also present the method of computing the θ value for a single outcome. When there are pilot data, the steps to compute the observed θ are as follows:

1. Code all endpoints so that larger observation values are preferred clinical conditions.

2. Similar to usual rank tests, combine all observations from both groups and rank within each outcome. Give the largest rank to the largest observation.

3. Compute each patient's total rank across all outcomes.

4. Sum the total ranks from all patients in the treatment group. Denote this sum as R.

5. Compute θ using formula:
   $$\theta = \frac{2R - m_2(m_1 + m_2 + 1)}{m_1 m_2}, \text{ where } m_1 \text{ is the}$$
   number of patients in the control group and m_2 is the number of patients in the treatment group.

When there are no pilot data, investigators often estimate the treatment effect based on information from the literature. In most cases, such information is presented in terms of mean and standard deviation using normal approximation, or presented using summary statistics of other parametric distributions. In some studies, nonlinear monotone transformations (e.g., log transformation, square root transformation, etc.) were applied to the data to obtain a better parametric approximation, and only summary statistics of the transformed data were reported. In this case, it is generally impossible to derive the treatment's effect size under the original (untransformed) measurement scale since the effect size is not invariant to nonlinear transformation. However, this will not be a problem when the GTE is used to measure a treatment's effect: no matter what monotone transformation (linear or nonlinear) is applied to the data, the GTE is unchanged since the GTE is computed only from the observation ranks. Because of this, we can compute θ using the parametric distribution approximation for the transformed data. For example, if μ_1 and σ_1 are the mean and standard deviation from the control group, μ_2 and σ_2 are the mean and standard deviation from the treatment group respectively, and the transformed data are approximately normally distributed, then

$$\theta = 2\Phi\left(\frac{\mu_1 - \mu_2}{\sqrt{\sigma_1^2 + \sigma_2^2}}\right) - 1 \tag{1}$$

where Φ is the cumulative distribution function of the standard normal distribution. For other distributions, Huang, Woolson, and O'Brien [11] have presented a list of computational formulas of θ and a table of θ values under various other parametric settings: symmetric and nonsymmetric, continuous and discrete distributions, skewed to the left and skewed to the right, as well as bell shaped and U-shaped distributions.

USE OF GLOBAL STATISTICAL TESTING IN DATA ANALYSIS: TECHNICAL SET-UP

O'Brien's rank-sum-type GST is a simple useful method to compare a treatment's global effect on multiple outcomes. Once an appropriate $\bar{\theta}_a$ value for the target magnitude of treatment effect is determined, one is ready to set up the hypotheses, compute the sample size needed, and test the treatment's global effect using O'Brien's GST after the data are collected. The null hypothesis is H_0: $\bar{\theta} = 0$. The sample size computation is presented in the next session. Here we provide the necessary framework. We use the notation T to denote the new treatment group, and notation C to denote the control (or placebo) group. Suppose we are testing whether T is better than C based on the global effect of T on K outcomes V_1, V_2, ..., V_K. Using O'Brien's GST, one needs to code all K outcomes V_1, V_2, ..., V_K in the same direction. That is, larger outcomes are the preferred clinical conditions for each of the K outcomes. If there are n_1 patients in C and n_2 patients in T, the data collected at the end of the study have the form displayed in Table 1. For each column under V_1, V_2, ..., V_K, we first rank all $N = (n_1 + n_2)$ observations without regarding to group membership. Then replace the outcomes by their corresponding ranks. Thus the largest observation is given rank $n_1 + n_2$ and the smallest observation is given rank 1. Next, for each subject, we compute the rank sum across all K outcomes. The worksheet is displayed in Table **2**. To apply O'Brien's GST, one simply applies the t-test to the two samples of ranks: R_{11}, R_{12}, ..., R_{1n_1} and R_{21}, R_{22}, ..., R_{2n_2}. If group T and group C have quite different shapes in distribution, one can use an adjustment to the O'Brien's GST as described by Huang, Tilley, Woolson, and Lipsitz [12]. This is operationalized with the Splus function GST.parameter and the Splus code given in Appendix C.1 of Huang, Woolson, and O'Brien [11] to compute the GST statistic Z:

```
x<- GST.parameter(data, n₁)

Z<- sum(x$theta)*sqrt(N)/2/sum(x$Sigma)

Z
```

Here, the Splus data frame data has K columns with the first n_1 rows being observations from all patients in group C and the rest n_2 rows being observations from all patients in group T. The p-value of the GST is obtained by comparing the value of Z to the critical values from the normal distribution. For example, Z=1.645 corresponds to p=0.05 for the one-sided test and p=0.10 for the two-sided test; Z=1.960 corresponds to p=0.025 for the one-sided test and p=0.05 for the two-sided test.

Table 1.   Data Collected at the End of the Study. The K Outcomes are Denoted by V_1, V_2, ..., and V_K. The Entries are Observations from Patients

Group	Patient	V_1	V_2	...	V_K
C	1	X_{111}	X_{112}	...	X_{11K}
	2	X_{121}	X_{122}	...	X_{12K}
	...	...	...	...	...
	n_1	$X_{1n_1 1}$	$X_{1n_1 2}$	...	$X_{1n_1 K}$
T	1	X_{211}	X_{212}	...	X_{21K}
	2	X_{221}	X_{222}	...	X_{22K}
	...	...	...	...	...
	n_2	$X_{2n_2 1}$	$X_{2n_2 2}$	...	$X_{2n_2 K}$

SAMPLE SIZE COMPUTATION: BACKGROUND AND CALCULATIONS

Sample size generally depends on the target treatment effect size, the significance level α, the desired power $(1-\beta)$ for a specified alternative treatment effect size, the correlation among multiple outcomes, and finally, the randomization ratio $r = n_2/n_1$. For GST, the treatment effect size is replaced by the GTE parameter $\bar{\theta}$. Thus, our one-sided hypotheses are H_0: $\bar{\theta} \leq 0$ and H_1: $\bar{\theta} > 0$ and the two-sided hypotheses are H_0: $\bar{\theta} = 0$ and H_1: $\bar{\theta} \neq 0$. We use symbol α to denoted the significance level α and $(1-\beta)$ to denote the desired power at $\bar{\theta} = \theta_a > 0$.

When there are no pilot, or appropriate historical, data and following Huang, Woolson and O'Brien [11], the total required sample size N=(n_1 + n_2) for testing the one-sided hypothesis problem is

$$N = \frac{1 - \min(\theta_{1a}^2, \theta_{2a}^2, \cdots, \theta_{Ka}^2)}{\bar{\theta}_a^2} \left\{ \rho + \frac{1-\rho}{K} \right\} \frac{(1+r)^2}{r} (z_\alpha + z_\beta)^2 \quad (2)$$

Here $\theta_{1a}, \theta_{2a}, \cdots, \theta_{Ka}$ are the hypothesized θ values of the K outcomes respectively where the power is controlled at, $\bar{\theta}_a = (\theta_{1a} + \theta_{2a} + \cdots + \theta_{Ka})/K$; $\min(\theta_{1a}^2, \theta_{2a}^2, \cdots, \theta_{Ka}^2)$ is the smallest value among $\theta_{1a}^2, \theta_{2a}^2, \cdots, \theta_{Ka}^2$; ρ is the maximum correlation among the K outcomes, z_α and z_β are (1-α)x100 and (1-β)x100 percentiles of normal distribution. For example, if the significance level is set at α=0.05 and the power is (1-β)=0.90, then z_α=1.645 and z_β=1.28. For two-sided hypothesis test, the z_α in the formula is replaced by $z_{\alpha/2}$. When α=0.05, we have $z_{\alpha/2}$=1.960. When no individual $\theta_{1a}, \theta_{2a}, \cdots, \theta_{Ka}$ values are available and data have continuous distributions, the sample size can be computed using

$$N = \frac{1}{3\bar{\theta}_a^2} \left\{ \rho + \frac{1-\rho}{K} \right\} \frac{(1+r)^2}{r} (z_\alpha + z_\beta)^2 \quad (3)$$

When there are some pilot data, one can estimate the GTE from the pilot data and use this information to select a θ_a value for sample size calculation. A major advantage of using GTE in sample size computation is that it does not require outcome means or variances between the pilot data and the future data to be the same. The only requirement for GTE is that the rank correlation structures between pilot data and the future data be similar. This makes the GTE more user-friendly since change of medical care conditions and change of clinical practice over time can alter the values of mean difference and standard deviation and thus change the value of effect size – the most commonly used quantity for sample size computation. Conventional statistical methods often assume this effect size (or at least, the standard deviation) remains the same between the pilot data and the future data. If this assumption is violated, the statistical power based on effect size will be poorly, if not inaccurately, assessed. The relaxation of these unrealistic assumptions in GTE makes it possible to use pilot data from trials with similar treatment agents in new trial design (see example at the end of this section).

As described in Section 3, one needs to code all K outcomes in the same direction so that larger outcomes corresponding better clinical conditions. If an outcome variable is not in the correct order with preferred clinical conditions, then oft times, we can simply multiply by negative one (-1) for this outcome. Additionally, we can use the Splus function GST.parameter in Huang, Woolson, and O'Brien [11] and Splus command:

```
x<- GST.parameter(pilot.data, m₁)

x$delta
```

to obtain an estimate of GTE from the pilot data. Here, as before, the Splus data frame `pilot.data`, contains pilot data with K columns. Its first m_1 rows contain observations from all patients in group C and the rest m_2 rows contain observations from all patients in group T. Based on this GTE, one can determine an appropriate $\bar{\theta}_a$ value for the sample size computation. Save this $\bar{\theta}_a$ value to Splus variable `theta.bar`. The required total sample size N can be computed using the following Splus code:

```
z.alpha<- qnorm(1-alpha)

z.beta<- qnorm(1-beta)

x<- GST.parameter(pilot.data, m1)

d1.m1m2<- r0*(m1-1)*(m2-1)

d2<- (z.alpha+z.beta)^2/k^2/theta.bar^2

gamma1.m1m2<-(4*m1+4*m1^2*r0)*

    sum(x$S1.n1n2)+(4*m2^2 +
    4*m2*r0)*sum(x$S2.n1n2) - (m1*m2^2 +

    m1^2*m2*r0)*sum(x$S3.n1n2)

gamma2.m1m2<- 4*m1^2*sum(x$S1.n1n2) +

    4*m2^2*sum(x$S2.n1n2) -
    m1^2*m2^2*sum(x$S3.n1n2)

N<-ceiling((1+r0)*d2*gamma1.m1m2/2

    /d1.m1m2* (1+sqrt(1-4*d1.m1m2

    *gamma2.m1m2/d2/gamma1.m1m2^2)))

N
```

We close this section using the following example to illustrate how to compute sample size when there are multiple primary outcomes. NIH/NINDS has sponsored a series of neuroprotective exploratory clinical trials in Parkinson's disease (NET-PD) to identify the most promising compounds that can slow, stop, or even reverse the progression in Parkinson's disease (http://www.ninds.nih.gov/parkinsonsweb/matrix_2003_all.htm). Data from two NET-PD phase II futility trials [13, 14] and several past PD clinical trials were used for the design of a phase III NET-PD trial. This is a multicenter, double-blind, parallel group, placebo controlled study of creatine in subjects with treated Parkinson's disease. The primary objective of the study is to determine if there is a slowing of clinical decline in creatine treated PD patients defined by a combination of cognitive, physical, and quality of life measures. Active treatment will be compared to placebo control against a background of dopaminergic therapy and usual medical care. There are multiple primary outcomes in this phase III NET-PD trial: the changes from baseline visit to the end of 5-year follow-up in the measures of modified Rankin, symbol digit modalities (verbal), Schwab and England ADL scale (SEADL), Parkinson disease quality of life (PDQ-39), and ambulatory capacity. The GST is specified as the primary statistical analysis method.

There were no pilot creatine 5-year data to give effect size estimates for the five primary outcomes. If the conventional sample size computation method with Bonferroni adjustment for multiple primary outcomes is used, it is evident that the conservativeness of this approach would yield unreasonably large sample sizes. This is true since all 5 outcomes are likely to be positively correlated. However with GTE, one can pull information from pilot data with similar treatments when determining the alternative hypothesis for power analysis, and calculate more appropriate sample sizes. For example, the mean treatment differences and standard deviations of PDQ-39 score, modified Rankin, SEADL, ambulatory capacity, and symbol digit modalities were reported separately by Olanow *et al.* [15], NET-PD investigators [16], Parkinson Study Group [17, 18], and Kieburtz *et al.* [19] respectively in similar studies. These give target mean treatment differences of 3±9, 0.2±1, 2±11, 0.33±2.11, and 1.5±8.0 for each of the scales described above. The corresponding θ values, based on formula (1), are 0.1863, 0.1125, 0.1023, 0.0881, and 0.1055 respectively. Their weighted mean value is (0.1863 + 0.1125 + 0.1023 + 0.0881 + 0.1055)/5 = 0.1189. This value was used as the target treatment effect $\bar{\theta}_a$ = 0.1189 (alternative hypothesis value) in NET-PD phase III trial in sample size/power analysis. If we set significance level

Table 2.   Worksheet for Rank Sum Computation

Group	Patient	V_1	V_2	...	V_K	Rank Sum
	1	R_{111}	R_{112}	...	R_{11K}	$R_{11} = R_{111} + R_{112} + ... + R_{11K}$
C	2	R_{121}	R_{122}	...	R_{12K}	$R_{12} = R_{121} + R_{122} + ... + R_{12K}$
	...	...	...	...	...	... ...
	n_1	R_{1n_11}	R_{1n_12}	...	R_{1n_1K}	$R_{1n_1} = R_{1n_11} + R_{1n_12} + \cdots + R_{1n_1K}$
	1	R_{211}	R_{212}	...	R_{21K}	$R_{21} = R_{211} + R_{212} + ... + R_{21K}$
T	2	R_{221}	R_{222}	...	R_{22K}	$R_{22} = R_{221} + R_{222} + ... + R_{22K}$
	...	...	...	...	...	... ...
	n_2	R_{2n_21}	R_{2n_22}	...	R_{2n_2K}	$R_{2n_2} = R_{2n_21} + R_{2n_22} + \cdots + R_{2n_2K}$

α=0.05 (two-sided) and control power (1-β)=85% at the alternative hypothesis value $\bar{\theta}_a$ =0.1189, the estimate of the total sample size, based on formula (3), ρ=0.5 and r=1 (equal randomization allocation to both groups), is N=509 patients.

COMPARISONS OF GST WITH OTHER MULTIVARIATE TECHNIQUES–TWO ILLUSTRATIVE TRIAL EXAMPLES

A major feature of GST is that it generally has higher statistical power when treatment shows the same direction of change in all outcomes, but it reduces power when treatment shows both beneficial and detrimental effects in different outcomes. In this section, we demonstrate these properties in assessing a treatment's global effect using two clinical trial data sets.

1. Example 1 –Treatment has the same direction of effects across multiple outcomes

The primary objective of the Multi-center Effects of Coenzyme Q_{10} (CQ_{10}) study [20] was to determine whether CQ_{10} was safe and well tolerated and if it could slow the functional decline in Parkinson's disease. Eighty early Parkinson disease patients were selected to receive either one of the active treatments (doses of 300 mg, 600 mg, and 1200 mg) or placebo with sample sizes of 21, 20, 23, and 16 respectively. Patients were evaluated at screening, baseline, and 1-, 4-, 8-, 12-, and 16-months visits or until the subject had developed disability requiring intervention with levodopa therapy. The primary outcome was the change in the total Unified Parkinson's Disease Rating Scale (UPDRS) from baseline to the last visit at 16 months or the visit before starting levodopa therapy. Secondary outcomes included UPDRS sub-

Table 3.   Comparison Between 1200mg CoQ_{10} Group and Placebo Group Using QE2 Trial Data. All Tests are Two-Sided

	Outcome[‡]	GTE ($\bar{\theta}$)	P value[‡]
	Motor	0.207	0.28
Univariate	Mentation	0.242	0.18
Wilcoxon	ADL	0.457	0.02
Test	SEADL	0.397	0.03
Hotelling T^2	All*		0.11
Bonferroni	All*		0.08
GST	All*	0.370	0.02

*Outcomes included in Hotelling's T^2 test, Bonferroni, and GST were: Motor, Mentation, ALD, SEADL, BDI, and MMSE.
[‡]Motor, mentation and ADL are reverse coded by multiplying (-1).

scales in mentation, motor, and the activities of daily living (ADL), and the Schwab & England activities of daily living scale (SEADL). One of the secondary analyses was to compare each active treatment group with the placebo group in the mean change of the total UPDRS. We obtained the data from the QE2 trial investigators with permission for re-analyses using GST. Table 3 compares 1200mg CoQ_{10} group and the placebo group using both univariate (Wilcoxon) test for each of the four outcomes and multivariate tests (the Hotelling's T^2 test, Bonferroni adjustment, and GST) for all four outcomes together. The CoQ_{10} group yielded better clinical measures in all four outcomes. However, none of the measures was considered significant at the significance level of 0.05 using Bonferroni adjustment. Hotelling's T^2 did not identify significant improvement in the CoQ_{10} group either. Since all GTE values were positive, it is clear that the GST combined the treatment's beneficial effects across all outcomes. We concluded that CoQ_{10} had a globally beneficial effect.

2. Example 2 –Treatment has different directions of effects across multiple outcomes

This setting is more complex in general, but there are cases, like the following, where a GST can still help in data analysis and interpretation. This next example, taken from the Multicenter Randomized Controlled Trial of Remacemide Hydrochloride as a Monotherapy for PD (RAMP), has the primary objective to assess the short-term tolerability and safety of remacemide treatment [21]. Two hundred patients were randomized to receive either the active treatments or placebo. Patients were followed for five weeks. Treatment comparison was made using changes from baseline to week 5. Outcomes of interest included the UPDRS subscales in mental, motor, and ADL, the Schwab & England activities of daily living scale (SEADL), Beck Depression Inventory (BDI), and Mini-mental State Exam (MMSE). We obtained the data from the Parkinson

Study Group with permission for re-analyses using GST. There were 12 patients who either had no baseline measures or no week-5 measures. Hence, we consider only the remaining 188 patients (49 in placebo and 139 in remacemide).

Since GST requires that larger values correspond to better observations for all outcomes, we coded mental, motor, ADL, and the BDI in reverse by multiplying (-1) so that larger observations are preferred for all outcome variables. Table 4 gives the analyses of the RAMP trial data using both the univariate (Wilcoxon) test for each of the six outcomes and multivariate tests (Hotelling's T^2 test, Bonferroni adjustment, and GST) for all six outcomes together. The different signs of GTE values for the six outcomes imply that remacemide exhibited different directions of treatment effect on these outcomes. The GST lowers its statistical power under this setting and does not claim global treatment difference (p=0.22) in drug tolerability. However, the single p-value from the mentation outcome was sufficient for the Bonferroni adjustment to conclude that remacemide was significantly worse than placebo when considering all six outcomes together. Hotelling's T^2 test does not find significant treatment difference. It is worth noting that, after a thorough analysis of the trial data, the RAMP investigators concluded that remacemide hydrochloride was generally well tolerated and safe in this 5-week trial.

Table 4. **Analysis of RAMP Trial Data Using Both Univariate and Multivariate Tests. All Tests are Two-Sided**

	Outcome[‡]	GTE $\bar{\theta}$	P value[‡]
	Motor	-0.0163	0.86
Univariate	Mentation	-0.2355	0.004
Wilcoxon	ADL	0.0019	0.99
Test	SEADL	-0.0980	0.18
	BDI	-0.0552	0.18
	MMSE	0.0421	0.64
Hotelling T^2	All*	-	0.52
Bonferroni	All*	-	0.02
GST	All*	-0.0602	0.22

*
Outcomes included in Hotelling's T^2 test, Bonferroni, and GST were: Motor, Mentation, ALD, SEADL, BDI, and MMSE.
[‡]Motor, mentation, ADL, and the BDI are reverse coded by multiplying (-1).

DISCUSSION

In medical applications, several strategies have been used to compare treatments when multiple outcomes are evaluated jointly. One strategy is to choose a single outcome as the primary outcome. Sample size is computed based on this primary outcome while other outcomes are analyzed as secondary outcomes. This strategy may be lacking in many neurological settings since a treatment effective for several secondary outcomes might be dismissed prematurely, simply because the primary outcome measure fails to yield significant evidence of efficacy. This strategy also does not generate a *global* assessment of the treatment's benefits. A second strategy is to construct a composite outcome which compiles information from each of several outcomes and fold them into a single variable. This strategy has the advantage in controlling type I error easily and attaining higher statistical power; however, the global treatment benefit derived from the composite outcome could be difficult to interpret when outcomes are of different types (e.g., discrete, continuous, event time, and non-event time). A third approach is to perform multiple tests with adjustment to the overall type I error. While this strategy is appropriate to test whether a treatment has any type of effect, it comes at the expense of lower

statistical power when treatment shows improvement in majority of outcomes. This is demonstrated in the Coenzyme Q_{10} study (Section 6.1). On the other hand, when treatment shows different directions of change, any omnibus conclusion could be driven by observations from a single outcome, and often misses the larger picture of whether the tested treatment should be adopted. This is demonstrated in RAMP data analysis (Section 6.2) where the single negative treatment effect on mentation was sufficient to reject the use of remacemide hydrochloride. The trial investigators, however, recommended the use of remacemide hydrochloride after reviewing its effects on other outcomes. Many multivariate tests (e.g. Hotelling's T^2 test, Wald-type tests, and χ^2-type tests) share the same limitations as the Bonferroni adjustment. When both positive and negative treatment effects are observed from different outcomes, these tests do not indicate whether the treatment is preferred. A fourth strategy is to use latent models or Bayes models. These models often assume that all outcomes are associated through a common latent parameter or hyperparameter so that treatment benefit is measured by the improvement of this latent parameter. This strategy is very flexible mathematically in analyzing different types of multiple outcomes. However, it can be difficult to verify whether the mathematical assumptions required by these models hold. A final approach, the global statistical test (GST) is a useful nonparametric method to test whether one treatment has overall benefit over the other treatment when multiple outcomes are studied together. It does not require restrictive mathematical assumptions. The characteristics of GTE and the corresponding GST discussed in this article make them flexible in summarizing a treatment's global effect when outcomes are measured in different scales.

The GST approaches have been used in clinical research in neurologic diseases, HIV, cancer, health services research, psychiatric diseases, and autoimmune diseases [22-27]. In an NIH/NINDS sponsored randomized, double-blind, placebo-controlled trial of recombinant tissue plasminogen activator (rt-PA) for patients with acute ischemic stroke [22], since no single measure of disability is sufficient to characterize all dimensions of recovery for stroke patients at 3 months after stroke, five outcomes are specified as the primary outcomes: Barthel Index, Modified Rankin Scale, Glasgow Outcome Scale, and National Institutes of Health Stroke Scale. NINDS held a workshop on statistical methods for this trial data analysis. The workshop led to a consensus that GST would be used to test the trial's primary hypothesis that tPA could improve clinical outcomes at three months. The workshop also recommended familiarizing the clinical/scientific community with the global statistical test approach [23]. We believe that GST's will play a significant role in medical research and future scientific findings. While these approaches may have considerable merit, it is important to remember that GST approaches are likely to be most beneficial when most outcome variables are going in the same direction for a treatment. Situations with mixed directions may still benefit from the GST approach, but the interpretation of the data is inherently more complex.

ACKNOWLEDGE

The authors acknowledge the research support of National Institutes of Health Grants AG023630 from NIA, NS43127 from NINDS, RR01070 from NCRR, HL072377 from NHLBI, CA06973, CA109282, CA091409 from NCI, and DE016631. We thank RAMP and QE2 trial investigators in providing the data for re-analysis.

REFERENCES

[1]   Adams HP, Woolson RF, Clarke W, *et al.* Design of Org 10172 in acute ischemic stroke treatment (TOAST): implications for other trials of treatments of persons with acute ischemic stroke. Controlled Clinical Trials 1997; 18: 358-77.

[2]   Publications Committee for the Trial of Org 10172 in Acute Stroke Treatment (TOAST) Investigators. Results of a randomized, placebo-controlled trial of the low molecular weight heparinoid, Org 10172, in improving outcome after acute ischemic stroke. J Am Med Assoc 1998; 279: 1265-72.

[3]   Tilley BC, Alarcon GS, Heyse SP, *et al.* Minocycline in rheumatoid arthritis: A 48-week double-blind, placebo controlled trial. Ann Intern Med 1995; 122: 81-9.

[4]   O'Brien P, Geller N. Interpreting tests for efficacy in clinical trials with multiple endpoints. Control Clin Trials 1997; 18: 222-7.

[5]   O'Brien P. Procedures for comparing samples with multiple endpoints. Biometrics 1984; 40:1079-87.

[6]   Tang D, Gnecco C, Geller NL. Design of group sequential clinical trials with multiple endpoints. J Am Stat Assoc 1989; 84(407): 776-9.

[7]   Tilley BC, Marler J, Geller NL, *et al.* Use of a Global test for multiple outcomes in stroke trials with application to the National Institute of Neurological Disorders and Stroke T-PA stroke trial. Stroke 1996; 27(11): 2136-42.

[8]   Lefkopoulou M, Moore D, Ryan L. The analysis of multiple correlated binary outcomes: application to rodent teratology experiments. J Am Stat Assoc 1989; 84(407):810-5.

[9]   Acion L, Peterson JJ, Temple S, Arndt S. Probabilistic index: an intuitive non-parametric approach to measuring the size of treatment effects. Stat Med 2006, 25: 591-602.

[10]   Wolfe, DA, Hogg, RV. On constructing statistics and reporting data. Am Stat 1971; 25: 27-30.

[11]   Huang P, Woolson RF, O'Brien PC. A rank-based sample size method for multiple outcomes in clinical trials. Stat Med 2008; 27: 3084-104.

[12]   Huang P, Tilley BC, Woolson RF, Lipsitz SR. Adjusting O'Brien's test to control type I error for the generalized nonparametric Behrens-Fisher problem. Biometrics 2005; 61: 532-9.

[13]   The NINDS NET-PD Investigators. A randomized, double blinded, futility clinical trial of creatine and minocycline in early Parkinson's disease. Neurology 2006; 66: 664-71.

[14]   The NINDS NET-PD Investigators. A randomized clinical trial of Coenzyme Q_{10} and GPI-1485 in early Parkinson's disease. Neurology 2007; 68: 20-8.

[15]   Olanow CW, Kieburtz K, Stern M, *et al.* Double-blind, placebo-controlled study of entacapone in levodopa-treated patients with stable Parkinson disease. Arch Neurol 2004; 61: 1563-8.

[16]   The NINDS NET-PD Investigators. A randomized, double blinded, futility clinical trial of creatine and minocycline in early Parkinson's disease. Neurology 2006; 66: 664-71.

[17]   Parkinson Study Group. Impact of deprenyl and tocopherol treatment on Parkinson's disease in DATATOP patients requiring levodopa. Ann Neurol 1996; 39: 37-45.

[18]   Parkinson Study Group. Pramipexole vs levodopa as initial treatment for Parkinson disease: a 4-year randomized controlled trial. Arch Neurol 2004; 61: 1044-53.

[19]   Kieburtz KK, McDermott M, Como P, *et al.* The effect of deprenyl and tocopherol on cognitive performance in early untreated Parkinson's disease. Neurology 1994; 44: 1756-9.

[20]   Shults CW, Oakes D, Karl KM, *et al.* Effects of Coenzyme Q10 in Early PD: Evidence of Slowing of the Functional Decline. Arch Neurol 2002; 59: 1541-50.

[21]   Parkinson Study Group. A multicenter randomized controlled trial of remacemide hydrochloride as monotherapy for PD. Neurology 2000; 54(8): 1583-8.

[22]   The National Institute of Neurological Disorders and Stroke rt-PA Stroke Study Group. Tissue Plasminogen Activator for Acute Ischemic Stroke. N Engl J Med 1995; 333: 1581-7.

[23]   Tilley BC, Marler J, Geller NL, *et al.* Use of a global test for multiple outcomes in stroke trials with application to the National Institute of Neurological Disorders and Stroke t-PA stroke trial. Stroke 1996; 27: 2136-42.

[24]   Kaufman KD, Olsen EA, Whiting D, Savin R, De Villez R, Bergfeld W. Finasteride in the treatment of men with androgentic alopecia. J Am Acad Dermatol 1998; 39: 578-89.

[25]   Li DK, Zhao GJ, Paty DW. Randomized controlled trial of interferon-beta-1a in secondary progressive MS: MRI results. Neurology 2001; 56(11): 1505-13.

[26]   Shames RS, Heilbron DC, Janson SL, Kishiyama JL, Au, DS, Adelman DC. Clinical differences among women with and without self-reported perimenstrual asthma. Ann Aller Asth Immunol 1998; 81: 65-72.

[27]   Tilley BC, Pillemer SR, Heyse SP, *et al.* Global test for comparing multiple outcomes in rheumatoid arthritis trials, Arthritis Rheum 2000; 42(9): 1879-88.

Index

A

Acid-sensing ion channels   **11, 14, 16, 19, 20**

Aging **9, 94, 99, 114**

Akt   **21, 22, 24-28, 31, 32, 39, 77, 103**

Alzheimer's disease   **94**

AMPA **1, 95**

Ang-2 **31, 32, 34, 37, 78**

Angiogenesis   **30- 43, 49, 52, 71, 75-82, 87, 88, 91, 92, 98, 100-103, 105**

Angiopoietin 1   **98**

Antagonists   **11-13, 16-18, 26, 59, 95, 96, 99**

Apoptosome   **3**

Apoptotic pathways   **7, 22, 27**

ASIC **14, 15, 18, 19, 20**

ATP   **2, 5, 11-13, 18, 60, 110**

B

Bak   **2, 6**

Basal lamina   **31, 44-46, 49-51, 53, 57, 64**

Bax   **2, 4-10**

BBB   **30-39, 44-46, 47, 53-57, 64, 75, 101, 107-112**

Bcl-2   **2, 4-9, 25, 28, 81, 82**

Bcl-XL   **2, 4-9**

BDNF **32, 36-38, 40, 43, 72, 78, 79, 82, 87, 88, 92**

Blood brain barrier   **30, 44, 45, 53, 64, 75, 101, 107**

BMCs **33, 34, 38**

BMSCs   **72, 75, 76, 79**

BrdU   **49, 77, 84-91, 96, 102**

C

CA1 region   **84, 89, 95, 104**

Calcium   **1, 2, 4, 7-19, 59, 60**

Calpain   **1-10, 22, 27, 112**

CBF   **24, 25, 27, 63, 75, 108, 109, 110**

CCA   **22-25**

CECs **53, 55**

Cell death   **1-14, 17, 22-28, 44-47, 51, 53, 57, 60-97**

CEPO **101, 102, 103**

Cerebral blood flow   **25, 30, 34, 42, 53-59, 63, 75, 83, 105, 107**

Cerebral endothelial cells   **53, 103**

Cleavage   **2, 5, 9, 17**

CNS   **11, 14, 17, 30-33, 38, 44, 48-56, 72, 76-104**

CT   **35, 92, 93, 105, 107, 112**

CXCR4   **33, 38, 40, 88, 93, 98**

Cytochrome *c* **2, 3, 4, 5, 6, 7, 11, 16, 22, 25, 27**

www.ingramcontent.com/pod-product-compliance
Lightning Source LLC
Chambersburg PA
CBHW041718210326
41598CB00007B/700